MW01155938

Introduction to Clinical Medicine

A Student-to-Student Manual

Third Edition

Roger M. Macklis, M.D.
Chairman and Director of Radiation
Oncology, and Senior Staff Physician,
Department of Radiation Oncology, The
Cleveland Clinic Foundation, Cleveland

Michael E. Mendelsohn, M.D.
Associate Professor of Medicine, Tufts
University School of Medicine; Director of
Molecular Cardiology Research Center, New
England Medical Center, Boston

Gilbert H. Mudge, Jr., M.D.
Associate Professor of Medicine, Harvard
Medical School; Director of Clinical
Cardiology Service, Brigham and Women's
Hospital, Boston

Student Editors
Rushika Fernandopulle
Bradley Marino
Harvard Medical School, 1994

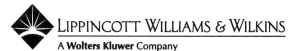
LIPPINCOTT WILLIAMS & WILKINS
A **Wolters Kluwer** Company
Philadelphia · Baltimore · New York · London
Buenos Aires · Hong Kong · Sydney · Tokyo

Library of Congress Cataloging-in-Publication Data

Macklis, Roger M.
  Introduction to clinical medicine : a student-to-student manual / Roger Macklis, Michael Mendelsohn, Gilbert Mudge ; student editors, Bradley Marino, Rushika Fernandopulle. — 3rd ed.
      p.   cm.
  Includes bibliographical references and index.
  ISBN 0-316-54243-1 : 26.50
  1. Clinical medicine—Handbooks, manuals, etc.   2. Diagnosis—Handbooks, manuals, etc.   I. Mendelsohn, Michael E.   II. Mudge, Gilbert H.   III. Title.
  [DNLM: 1. Internal Medicine—handbooks.   2. Clinical Medicine—handbooks.   WB 39 M158m 1994]
  RC55.M24   1994
  616—dc20
  DNLM/DLC
  for Library of Congress   94-14222
                                                                              CIP

10 9 8 7 6 5 4 3

Printed in the United States of America

Editorial: Evan R. Schnittman, Kristin Odmark
Production Editor: Karen Feeney
Copyeditor: Julie Hagen
Indexer: Nancy Weaver
Production Supervisor: Louis C. Bruno, Jr.
Cover Designer: Hannus Design Associates

An air of excitement and some measure of anxiety mark the transition from the preclinical to clinical years. The anxiety may be openly expressed or hidden by a white coat of cultivated sophistication. It may range from passive bewilderment to uncomfortable levels of assertiveness. You are leaving the tidy world of the library, the seminar, and the laboratory to face the infinite variations of illness and the human condition. You are a student and something more; you are a doctor and something less. You are no longer merely a spectator; as an observer you become part of another person's life, for good or ill. You will find that Hippocrates had something in that old aphorism, "The art is long, decision difficult." You will make mistakes that others will forgive but you will remember.

You have weathered many years of academic competition; now for these last all too brief years of medical school, enjoy what you have earned. If you feel too put upon, take some time for yourself. Remember Kipling's words about a doctor's work: "It seems to be required of you that you must save others. It is nowhere laid down that you need save yourselves."

J. Gordon Scannell, M.D.

Contents

Preface

The practice of medicine in the 1990s is undergoing a series of profound changes. As managed health care systems and the framework for a universal health network are implemented, medicine is being transformed. A new focus on primary and preventive care is emerging, and the roles of tertiary care specialists and high-tech medical strategies are being redefined. Yet, the fundamental principles of the doctor-patient relationship remain unchanged. Despite all the technologic and philosophic advances, the process of meeting the patient, listening intently and respectfully to his or her history, focusing the diagnostic work-up, and instituting a therapeutic plan is still the cornerstone of each doctor-patient relationship. One central challenge of the 1990s is to continue to provide this level of individual service and communication while recognizing that health care expenses must be controlled and interventions must be justified.

The role of the medical student on the ward is becoming ever more complex. In the eighteenth century, the student was primarily a clerk, transcribing the attending physician's instructions and following the patient's progress. Later, the student became an apprentice, exerting only a minimal level of autonomy in patient care decisions. More recently, medical students have become integral parts of the treatment team, often more knowledgeable about their patients' lives and histories than either the resident or the attending physician.

For this third edition, *Introduction to Clinical Medicine* has been revised and extensively rewritten to update both the information and the tone of the book. Philosophically, it remains a student-to-student manual, and for that reason we felt it important to obtain the assistance of two superb medical students, Bradley Marino and Rushika Fernandopulle, in organizing the revision. They carefully and creatively dissected the previous editions, augmenting and editing the material to more closely reflect the realities of medical clerkship in the 1990s. New sections on the pediatric exam, drug classes, and AIDS serve as examples of the many topics that have been extensively revised and updated. We hope that the clinical clerk will be able to function more effectively on the wards with this manual as a roadmap to the teaching hospital, a guide made all the more important by the accelerated pace of medicine in the 1990s.

As authors, we are indebted to our families and friends for offering the sort of supportive environment that allowed us to undertake this project. As academic physicians, we are indebted to our colleagues and our mentors for teaching us the intellectual and medical skills that we use daily in our professional lives. We are indebted as well to Kristin Odmark and her colleagues at Little, Brown and Company for helping us to push this project to completion. And we are indebted to our patients, who continue to teach us that it is a privilege to be entrusted with their care.

R.M.M.
M.E.M.
G.H.M.

Acknowledgments

We would like to thank Drs. Macklis, Mendelsohn, and Mudge for giving us the opportunity to revise this book, as well as Kristin Odmark, Robert Stuart, and Karen Feeney at Little, Brown for being so patient in helping us through the publishing process for the first time. We are indebted to our professors and colleagues at Harvard Medical School for imparting to us the love of clinical medicine and to our friends for helping us survive our years as medical students. Finally, we would like to thank our families, without whose support none of this would be possible.

R.F.
B.M.

The Hospital Environment

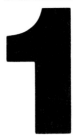

The Hospital Environment

The transition from the classroom to the clinical setting is one of the most important and dramatic steps in the long road to becoming a physician. Though in many ways it is an incredibly exciting period, it can be a very difficult transition as well, with unclear expectations, long hours and little sleep, and sometimes unpleasant encounters both with patients and with other health care providers. This section will discuss your roles and responsibilities, and those of the other members of your team on the wards, as well as a crucial topic for your own safety—universal precautions.

I. Roles and responsibilities

A. Your role. One of the biggest changes in going from learning in the classroom to learning on the wards is that on the wards you have a much larger responsibility to others—to your patients and to members of your team. Your particular responsibilities will change from service to service and year to year, as you gain experience. Always ask, early on, what is expected of you.

1. As a **second-year student,** in most programs your role, through your Introduction to Clinical Medicine (ICM) course, is to learn to interview and examine patients. Frequently you will be given the name of an inpatient and asked to take a history and do a physical exam. You may be asked to write an admission note or perhaps to give an oral presentation on your findings.

2. As a **third-year student** doing a rotation, you are more integrated into the team that is taking care of patients. You will do admission histories and physicals, follow your patients' progress and perhaps write orders for tests and interventions, present your patients on rounds, and be expected to read about their problems.

B. The **other members of the team** will most certainly include:

1. The **intern,** who is in his or her first year of post–medical school training (sometimes called PGY-1, or postgraduate year 1), is responsible for most of the day-to-day work of taking care of patients on the service. Though usually very overworked, interns are great sources from whom to learn the details of patient management. Remember, they were in your shoes not very long ago.

2. The **resident,** who is in the second year or higher of post–medical school training, is responsible for supervising the interns. It is usually the resident's responsibility to teach the medical students as well, and he or she will be able to answer broader questions about your patients.

3. **Fellows** have completed their residency and are undergoing further specialty training. Though they usually do not have direct teaching responsibility, many are happy to answer any questions, especially in their field, about your patients.

4. The **attending physician** is an experienced doctor who is responsible for all the patients on the service, and most major decisions on management are discussed with him or her before they are made. The attending is also the person responsible for teaching and evaluating the medical students, the interns, and the residents.

5. **Nurses** can be your best allies on the wards. Though you will no doubt hear stories of nurses taking out their frustrations concerning doctors on medical students, if you treat them like professionals they will no doubt treat you similarly. As a second-year, always check with a patient's nurse before going in for an interview—this can alleviate many interruptions later. As a third-year, learn the names of the nurses caring for your patients, and remember that they have a lot to teach you as well.

6. **Others.** Respiratory therapists, physical therapists, nutritionists, pharmacists, and others are also part of the patient care team. They, too, can be a huge resource for you on particular aspects of patient care. As a second-year, your interviews will frequently be interrupted by therapists and others. Ask them politely if they can return later, but remember that, like you, they are very busy and that they play an important role in getting your patient out of the hospital.

II. Universal precautions

A. **Your own safety** is one of the most important things to keep in mind when you are on the wards. While a medical student, you will almost inevitably come into contact with many patients who have transmissible diseases, including HIV and hepatitis. You are at risk for contracting these diseases through contact with bodily fluids. You should make sure that you have been immunized against hepatitis B before you enter the wards, but remember that even the full series of immunizations is not 100 percent effective. Because of this, and because of the increasing presence of HIV, for which there is still no vaccine, you need to observe certain precautions while on the wards.

B. Since it is impossible to tell at all times who is infected and who is not, you should practice **universal precautions**—that is, you should act as if every patient you encounter is potentially infectious. Specifically, you should wear protective clothing and use devices to prevent contamination of your skin and mucous membranes whenever you handle certain bodily fluids. It is crucial for you to understand how the HIV virus can be transmitted and how it cannot. Blood, semen, vaginal secretions, and lab preparations of HIV, cerebrospinal, amniotic, synovial, pleural, peritoneal, and pericardial fluids have all been implicated in the transmission of HIV. Currently it is thought that feces, nasal secretions, breast milk, sweat, tears, urine, and vomitus carry a very low risk of transmitting the HIV virus [9]. Hepatitis B, while formerly thought to be transmitted only parentally and through sexual contact, now is thought to be infectious through the oral route as well, though much more rarely.

C. **Specific measures you should take** while on the wards include:

1. **Gloves** should be worn whenever handling any blood or body fluid. After each use, gloves should be discarded carefully, without touching the outside of the gloves with your bare hands. Most hospitals have gloves available in each patient room; if not, carry some with you.

2. **Wash your hands,** with soap, before and after each patient contact. Patients especially like to see their doctor washing his or her hands before examining them. Get into the habit of doing this early; it's good both for you and your patients.

3. Be extremely careful with **sharp instruments** like needles and scalpels. They should be disposed of immediately after use, in a puncture-resistant container. **Do not recap needles under any circumstances.** Be especially careful during codes, when chaos reigns and inadvertent needle sticks are more likely. Always check for sharp objects before handling used materials after a procedure. If you use any sharp object, it is your responsibility to dispose of it.

4. Wear **protective eyewear and a mask** if there is potential for blood or body fluid to splash into your eyes, nose, or mouth.

5. To avoid contamination during **mouth-to-mouth resuscitation,** use a barrier device or a resuscitation bag; these should be available.

6. If you do get splashed, wash the area immediately. If you think you have been exposed, for example through a needle stick, you should **act on it immediately.** Data indicate that the chance of getting HIV from a single contaminated needle stick is about 1 in 250. Make sure you know the procedures at your institution for reporting exposures. There is some evidence that AZT given within a few hours after an exposure might reduce the risk of infection. Treat this incident as a crisis and seek assistance immediately.

D. All of this is meant not to scare you but to stress the importance of protecting yourself. Some providers trained in the pre-AIDS era may not follow these safety guidelines, and you may feel pressure to follow their example. Do not. These recommendations could save your life, so get into good habits early and practice universal precautions.

III. **Some words of advice**

A. Your role as a second-year student on the wards doing ICM is a particularly hard one, as you may frequently feel your presence is simply a burden, and at times patients may even refuse to talk to you. Remember that they are not feeling well; think back to the last time you were sick and remember how miserable you felt. Though at times you may not think so, **your presence is really valuable.** Learning to do interviews and perform physicals on actual patients is an important part of your training. Patients will also benefit from your work; it is rare that anyone in a busy hospital takes the time to talk with them and hear their story.

B. You need to **take control of your own education.** Never be afraid to ask questions, whether about your patients, your responsibilities, or medicine in general. There is a lot you need to learn and experience before you graduate, so take advantage of every opportunity. To do well on the wards, try to be enthusiastic, dependable, an advocate for your patients, well prepared, and, especially, a team player.

C. Finally, in the midst of taking care of all the patients, remember to **take care of yourself.** Work on the wards can expand to take up your whole life if you allow it to. Try to eat and sleep well, exercise, and keep up with at least one aspect of your life outside the hospital. The road ahead is a long one, and this is a good time to learn how to balance your life inside and outside of medicine.

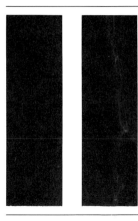

The Medical Work-up

The *medical work-up* is a term used to refer to the sequence of diagnostic inquiries and laboratory tests that are implemented during the evaluation of any specific medical problem. The primary job of the medical student starting clinical work is to become familiar with the work-up process and to learn to conduct a patient work-up thoroughly and efficiently.

Although the specific details of the work-ups for various problems may be quite different, the **sequence of data acquisition and analysis** is always the same: first a **history** is taken, then a **physical examination** is performed, then **diagnostic tests** are conducted and analyzed, and finally an **assessment and a therapeutic plan** are formulated. This sequence of history, physical examination, diagnostic tests, assessment, plan is at the heart of every work-up.

Part II of this book is organized in a sequence roughly parallel to that of the work-up. Chap. 2 outlines the content and technique of the medical interview, while Chap. 3 presents a brief outline of the general physical examination. Chap. 4 contains a detailed description of the physical exam, arranged by organ system. Finally, Chap. 5 describes how to alter your basic exam when seeing children of different ages.

Turning from the bedside work-up to the clinical laboratory, the next seven chapters present, first, a general discussion of when to order lab tests, and then brief overviews of the principles and interpretation of the six most common diagnostic tests: the hematologic screen, the serum chemistry battery, the urinalysis, the electrocardiograph, the chest x-ray, and the arterial blood gas determination. In each of these chapters, an attempt has been made to simplify the interpretation of the lab results and to concentrate only on the more common and significant findings. These chapters do not, of course, take the place of the more rigorous treatments found elsewhere.

Chap. 13 is a discussion of the medical case write-up and includes a sample student write-up as well as specific advice on how to construct a good write-up. The medical case presentation is described in Chap. 14, which contains specific advice on how to present medical cases on hospital rounds and in formal didactic sessions.

Because the information in many of these chapters is of two types, objective and subjective, some chapters are divided into two parts: Part A, which contains generally objective information and will be useful as a memory aid and pocket reference; and Part B, which contains subjective advice and the kind of pragmatic information that traditionally has been passed informally from student to student. The purpose of Part B in these chapters is to help students "learn the ropes" of clinical work early in their careers, to give them more time to concentrate on the factual information that must be mastered. As much as possible, Parts A and B of each chapter parallel each other and should be read together.

This book contains no specific therapeutic information; for this the student is referred to the *Washington Manual of Medical Therapeutics* (also published by Little, Brown and Company). For the novice clinician this latter book is indispensable.

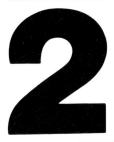

Taking a History

> *"Listen to the patient. He will tell you the diagnosis."* This well-known
> admonition of Dr. Hermann Blumgart to generations of medical students
> underscores the importance of an empathetic and sensitive history, but the
> patient will teach the receptive physician more than the simple identity
> of his illness. Given a prepared and responsive listener, the patient will
> also reveal for his examiner the most intimate workings of his disease
> process. A sick patient is an experiment of nature. The sapient clinician
> must reserve one corner of his mind for clues the patient will provide to
> unresolved questions about his disorder. The patient who manifests an
> unusual feature of his illness, no matter how humdrum the diagnosis, or
> the patient who presents with an uncommon diagnosis, or the patient with
> a mystifying illness and no clear diagnosis—any of these may provide
> the acute observer with new understanding of a previously stubborn and
> frustrating question. The patient is prepared to teach professor and student
> alike; they must be prepared to be his pupils.
>
> **Edwin W. Salzman, M.D.**

The patient interview, usually referred to as the **history,** is the first step in
the diagnostic work-up. Taking a good history is probably the single most
important task in the work-up, both because of its importance in diagnosis
and because the history is the portion of the work-up in which the physician-
patient relationship is first established. The job of the medical student is not
only to learn how to conduct a thorough interview but also to develop a professional manner that will put the patient at ease. Whether the patient will
regard the student as an unnecessary third party or as a vital member of the
medical team often depends on the tenor and style of the initial interview.

Part A of this chapter is a point-by-point review of the subjects and style of
each part of the formal medical interview. Part B contains a collection of
practical advice intended to help the student conduct and interpret the interview.

The parts of the medical interview that should be memorized early in the
clinical career are outlined in Table 2-1. Chap. 13 presents information and
formats useful in subsequently writing up the case for the medical record.

A	The History and Review of Systems

I. **Introductory information.** Begin by collecting the identifying data about a
patient from both the existing medical record and the patient, especially including the patient's name, age, sex, race, occupation, and, if the patient has
been referred from elsewhere, the source of and reason for the referral.

Table 2-1. Outline of the patient interview

I. Introductory information
II. Chief complaint
III. History of present illness
IV. Past medical history
   A. Other medical problems
   B. Injuries, hospitalizations, operations
   C. Medications
   D. Habits
   E. Allergies
   F. Major childhood illnesses
   G. Immunizations
V. Family history
VI. Social history
   A. Lifestyle
   B. Home life
   C. Occupational life
   D. Sexual history
VII. Review of systems
VIII. Conclusion

II. Chief complaint and its duration. The chief complaint is traditionally defined as that problem or set of problems that makes the patient decide to seek medical attention. Questions concerning the chief complaint follow the physician's greeting of the patient (see **Part B.I.E**) and the brief questions about introductory information. The chief complaint is elicited by asking an open-ended question, such as "What made you decide to come to the hospital?" "What brings you here today?" or "What seems to be the trouble?" The **duration** of the chief complaint provides an important temporal framework for the physician and should be inquired about at this time.

III. History of the present illness. The logical continuation and expansion of the chief complaint is the history of the present illness (HPI). The HPI is recounted by the patient to the interviewer, who is predominantly a listener at this point in the interview, and, when appropriate, interjecting questions or phrases that may facilitate the flow of information.

   A. Symptoms. The crux of the HPI is a detailed exploration of the symptoms that constitute the chief complaint. Each symptom should be investigated thoroughly, first by listening to the patient's unfolding story and then by asking specific questions to discover any dimensions of the symptoms that may have been omitted. The dimensions to be explored are detailed in Table 2-2.

   B. Review of pertinent systems. The chief complaint and HPI usually suggest the involvement of one or more organ systems in the patient's illness. It is useful to inquire about other symptoms that relate to the organ systems involved while discussing the present illness. This implies that inferences about the disease process must be made during the history-taking procedure (probable organ systems involved must be identified). It is also therefore necessary to be familiar with the topics and symptoms related to the various organ systems, in order to review the pertinent systems during the HPI (see Table 2-3). The purpose of reviewing the pertinent organ systems at this point is to accumulate further support for or evidence against diagnoses being considered by the interviewer. For example, if a patient enters with a chief complaint of "spitting blood," the interviewer

Table 2-2. Symptom analysis

Dimension	Typical question	Synonyms and related ideas
1. Location	Where is the pain located?	Main site, region, radiation
2. Quality	What is it like?	Character
3. Quantity	How intense is it?	Severity, frequency, periodicity, degree of functional impairment
4. Chronology	When did it begin and what course has it followed?	Onset, duration, frequency, periodicity, temporal characteristics
5. Setting	Under what circumstances does the pain take place?	Relation to physiologic functions
6. Aggravating-alleviating factors	What, if anything, makes the pain worse or better?	Provocative-palliative factors
7. Associated manifestations	What other symptoms or phenomena are associated with this pain?	Effects of disease, related concerns

will inquire about each topic in the respiratory systems review. It then becomes diagnostically useful to note a recent history of tuberculosis (TB) exposure (a pertinent positive) or to discover that the patient does not smoke (a pertinent negative).

C. **Concluding the HPI.** To close this part of the interview, you should summarize your understanding of the patient's story and ask him or her if this is accurate. You should end with a question that gives the patient a further chance to air concerns, such as, "Is there anything else about these recent pains that you would like to bring up?"

IV. **Past medical history.** The past medical history (PMH) is devoted to defining and describing medical problems that may be related to the present illness, problems that are active but unrelated to it, and problems that existed at one time but are inactive at present. Although some patients may remember and provide much of the information during this part of the interview, portions of the past medical history are often discovered in and elaborated by the existing medical record.

A. **Other medical problems** are sought by the interviewer, with a particular effort toward discovering any existing medical problems that may relate to the present illness. For instance, a 10-year history of hypertension may be of particular interest in a patient who enters complaining of chest pain. This is the point to get the patient to elaborate on any other medical problems that may have been identified during the review of pertinent systems.

The interview for other problems should include questions concerning date of onset, diagnostic procedures, and major therapy for the problem in question. For each medical problem discovered, it is also important to gain an understanding of the current status of the problem. For the patient with hypertension, for example, it would be important to inquire about how well the hypertension has been controlled since its diagnosis and treatment 10 years before and to ask for the most recent blood pressure measurement.

B. **Injuries, hospitalizations, and operations** are also sought in this portion of the interview. Included is any history of auto or other accidents, broken

Table 2-3. Review of systems

System	Master list	Clinical points
Constitutional	Weight change	Recent change important.
	Anorexia	Acute or chronic?
	Fatigue	
	Weakness	
	Fever	Pattern (intermittent, remittent, sustained, or relapsing)? How documented?
	Sweats	Night? Drenching or mild? Frequency?
	Chills	Goose bumps vs. shaking (rigors)?
	Insomnia	Acute or chronic? When during night?
	Irritability	
Integument	Rashes	Local or generalized? Characterize.
	Itching	Diffuse?
	H/O skin trouble	Occupational? Allergic?
	Sores that do not heal	Squamous cell carcinoma? Poor diet? Drugs (e.g., steroids)?
	Bruising	Recent change?
	Bleeding disorders?	FHx?
Head	Headaches	
	Loss of consciousness	Cardiovascular vs. neurologic? Hx crucial.
	Seizures	Focal vs. general? Motor vs. absence?
	H/O trauma	When? Sequelae?
Eyes	Vision	Recent change? Glasses?
	Date last eye exam	
	FHx of glaucoma	Glaucoma often asymptomatic; hereditary with high penetration.
	Photophobia	Meningeal irritation?
	Pain	
	Redness	
	Irritation	
	Excessive tearing	
	Diplopia	
	Scotomata	
Ears	Hearing	Recent change?
	Discharge or pain	H/O otitis? Trauma?
	Vertigo	Sensation of movement (vertigo) vs. dizziness.
	Tinnitus	Drug-related (aspirin)?
Respiratory Upper	Frequent colds	
	Sinus trouble	
	Postnasal drip	
	Nosebleeds (epistaxis)	Trauma? Other bleeding problems?
	Obstruction	Snoring history?

Table 2-3 (continued).

System	Master list	Clinical points
Lower	Cough	Chronic? A.M.? Productive? Recent change? Smoking history?
	Sore throat	
	Sputum	Amount? Color? Character? Recent change?
	Shortness of breath	Dyspnea? Rest or exertional? Accompanying chest discomfort?
	Wheezing	Seasonal? Episodic? Known allergens?
	Hemoptysis	Oral (e.g., dental) vs. pulmonary (e.g., bronchitis) vs. cardiac (e.g., mitral stenosis)). Frank blood vs. tinged sputum vs. pink sputum?
	H/O chest illness	TB exposure? Bronchitis? Emphysema? Asthma? Pneumonia(s)?
	H/O smoking	Quantitate no. of pack-years. If "no," quit recently?
Lymphoreticular	Increased node size	Tender vs. painless? Location? Reactive (infections? systemic disease? drug?) vs. infiltrative? How first noticed? Any AIDS risk factors?
Breasts	Swelling	Unilateral or bilateral? Associated changes? Tender?
	Lumps	Recent change? Transient or persistent? Menstrually related?
	Pain	Unilateral or bilateral? Trauma?
	Discharge	Milk (galactorrhea) vs. serous vs. blood? Unilateral or bilateral?
	Do you do self-exam?	Be able to teach during PE.
Cardiovascular	Chest pain or discomfort	Major DDx: cardiovascular vs. gastrointestinal vs. musculoskeletal.
	Palpitations	If ⊕, ask patient to tap out rate and rhythm. Syncope history? Any particular time when increased?
	Blood pressure	Usual range? H/O ↑ or ↓ ? FHx? Medications?

Table 2-3 (continued).

System	Master list	Clinical points
	Shortness of breath	Paroxysmal nocturnal dyspnea? Exercise tolerance? Exertion induced?
	Orthopnea	No. of pillows? If ⊕, what happens when patient reclines without pillows?
	Edema	Generalized (e.g., CHF, liver disease, nephrotic syndrome) or localized?
	Leg pain, cramps	Relieved by rest (intermittent claudication) vs. unremitting or night time (muscular)?
	Other cardiac Hx	H/O murmur(s), thrombophlebitis, "blood clots," varicose veins, "large" heart. Other cardiac medications? Rheumatic fever?
	Risk factors	Smoking, hypertension, hypercholesterolemia, DM, gout, obesity, FHx?
	Nocturia	Quantitate.
Gastrointestinal	Dentures, problems with teeth, oral lesions	Bleeding gums, ulcers, sores.
	Dysphagia	Where? (Have patient point and describe.) Invariably heralds organic disease.
	Heartburn (pyrosis)	How does patient find relief?
	Other symptoms of indigestion	Bloating, belching, flatulence; food-related Hx critical.
	Nausea	Relation to food. H/O GI disease and surgery, associated symptoms and signs.
	Vomiting	All medication, H/O weight loss, psychosocial factors.
	Hematemesis	Color? H/O ulcer disease? H/O gastritis? (Lesion usually proximal to ligament of Treitz.)
	Abdominal pain, discomfort	Hx critical. Acute vs. chronic? GI vs. reproductive?
	Food intolerance	Milk products? Gluten-containing fried or fatty foods? H/O gallbladder disease?

Table 2-3 (continued).

System	Master list	Clinical points
	H/O GI disease	Hepatitis, ulcer disease, gallbladder disease, pancreatitis, diverticulitis, hemorrhoids?
	Hematochezia	Often suggests distal lesion; hemorrhoids most common, but R/O neoplastic.
	Jaundice	FHx? Viral-drug exposure? Associated Sx and/or signs?
	Change in stool	Color, consistency, unusual odor, oiliness, mucus? Caliber?
	Diarrhea	Acute vs. chronic? Infectious, drug or laxative? Dietary, inflammatory?
	Constipation	Mechanical vs. systemic illness vs. drug-induced vs. neurologic?
Genitourinary		
Urinary	Polyuria	Recent change? (Common causes: DM, renal disease, iatrogenic.)
	Dysuria	UTI "triad" (dysuria, frequency, urgency), but R/O genital disease.
	Hematuria	Painless (primary renal disease) vs. painful (e.g., UTI, stones, renal infarct)?
	Nocturia	How often? Recent change?
	Hesitancy	In older men, along with ↓ stream, dripping, incontinence, consistent with prostatic hypertrophy. Medications?
	Other renal Hx	UTIs? Stones or gravel in urine? Flank pain?
	Testicular swelling	Painful vs. painless?
Menstrual	Menarche	Cycle length, regularity, duration and amount of bleeding.
	Amenorrhea	Primary vs. secondary?
	Menorrhagia (profuse)	
	Metrorrhagia (intermenstrual)	
	Date last period	
	Date last Pap smear	
	Pregnancies	Gravida ___ Para ___ Abortions ___ Miscarriages ___
	Vaginal discharge	H/O vaginal infections? Itching?

Table 2-3 (continued).

System	Master list	Clinical points
Venereal disease	H/O VD	If ⊕, what Rx did patient receive?
	H/O penile discharge	
	H/O chancre	
Sexual history		Must be tailored to patient (see **Part B.VI.C**). AIDS risk?
Musculoskeletal Joints	Pain	Location? Acute vs. chronic? H/O trauma? H/O previous infection? Present medication? FHx? H/O gout? Morning vs. evening stiffness?
General	Weakness	
	Cramping	
	H/O back difficulties	Low back strain, osteoarthritis, and disc disease are common causes.
	H/O trauma, fracture	
	H/O endrocine disease	
	Diabetic symptoms	Weight change, polyuria, polyphagia, polydipsia.
	Thyroid symptoms	Goiter, heat-cold intolerance, change in metabolic rate.
	Change in head, glove, shoe size	Acromegaly; change in head size only may be consistent with Paget's disease.
Nervous system	Neuro. difficulties in past	H/O stroke, seizures, childhood illness.
Motor	Atrophy	Location, time course, change in normal function.
	Weakness	Location, asymmetries? (Quantitate.)
	Involuntary movements	Tremor, fasciculations, seizure Hx.
Sensory	Anesthesia	Recent burns?
	Parasthesia	
	Hyperesthesia	
Mental status	Cortical function change	Memory change? Reading, writing change?

Note: *At the end of the ROS, it is useful to ask two questions:* (1) "Is there anything else bothering you?" (2) "Is there anything you would like to bring up or ask about before I do a physical exam?"

bones, trauma, or surgery. Information about previous hospital admissions should be sought, and the reason for the admission, the date and year, and the hospital involved should be systematically explored.

C. Medications. The name, dosage, and regimen of each drug the patient is using should be discussed. Any drugs that have been recently discontinued or used intermittently should be inquired about as well. Patients frequently need to be reminded about their use of birth contol pills, over-the-counter analgesics (aspirin, acetaminophen), laxatives, sleeping medication, and diet pills.

D. Habits. Tobacco smoking should be quantitated, as should ethanol intake. Also ask about the use of recreational drugs as well as habits that may be relevant physiologically, such as coffee and tea usage. See **Part B.IV** for some hints on how best to approach this subject.

E. Allergies should be documented carefully, and the patient should be specifically questioned about drug reactions and reactions to prior blood transfusions or hospital procedures. When a patient notes an allergy, it is extremely important to obtain a description of the specific allergic reaction. Is a penicillin allergy manifested with a rash on the upper trunk or with spasm of the larynx and difficulty breathing?

F. Major childhood illnesses such as tuberculosis, rheumatic or scarlet fever, polio, chicken pox, mumps, measles, rubella, and whooping cough should be investigated.

G. Immunizations for polio, measles, mumps, diphtheria, pertussis, tetanus, and so on are inquired about in the PMH portion of the patient interview, especially with pediatric patients.

V. Family history. The history turns to questions about the family after the patient's medical problems have been explored. This part of the interview has two goals: to find out about the health of immediate family members, and to discover certain common diseases with a familial pattern.

A. The age and health of the patient's parents, siblings, spouse, and children are first discussed. If a family member is deceased, the cause of death is noted.

B. The occurrence of any disease like that described in the patient's HPI is sought in other family members. Important diseases with a strong hereditary component or a tendency for family clustering are also sought, including coronary artery disease, heart disease, diabetes mellitus, high blood pressure, stroke, asthma, allergies, arthritis, anemia, cancer, kidney disease, and mental illness.

VI. Social history. Although some of the information sought in this portion of the interview emerges from simply speaking with the patient while taking the history, several goals exist for the social history. Specifically, insights into the patient's lifestyle, home life, occupational life, and attitude toward the disease and the hospitalization are sought. This is also the portion of the interview in which many physicians choose to take the sexual history (see **D**).

A. Lifestyle. An attempt should be made to understand what constitutes a typical day for the patient, what recreation the patient engages in, and what religious beliefs he or she holds. The patient's school and military experience may be discussed at this point.

B. Home life. Housing, the emotional atmosphere at home, marriage and family, and significant others should be briefly explored. An attempt should be made to identify factors that have influenced the relationship between the patient's disease and home life. Such questions may range from concerns about the physical layout of the home to the impact of the disease on the family.

C. **Occupational life.** Two goals exist here. First the nature of the patient's occupation is explored, and second, when relevant, the likelihood of a toxic exposure related to the patient's job is investigated.

   1. **Nature of the occupation** is evaluated through questions about what the patient does for work and by attempting to gain insight into the relative satisfactions and dissatisfactions associated with the work and the workplace.

   2. **Toxic exposures** may be especially relevant in patients with respiratory or dermatologic disease without obvious etiology (e.g., silicosis in a cement plant worker or contact dermatitis on a surgeon's face or hands). Occupational exposures may occasionally be associated with disease of the liver (e.g., hepatitis in a hospital worker), central nervous system (e.g., polyneuropathy in an insecticide worker), and other organ systems. Exposures may also play a role in oncologic illness (mesothelioma in a shipyard worker with brief asbestos exposure, or hematologic malignancy in a worker exposed to radiation).

D. **Sexual history.** The sexual history is one of the hardest parts of the patient interview for most medical students, but is also one of the most important. It may be taken during the psychosocial history, the genitourinary part of the review of systems, or the past medical history. The goal is to find out about the patient's sexual preferences and habits, sexual history, and any physiologic or psychological concerns he or she might have. The sexual history is particularly important in cases with possible venereal, gynecologic, or psychological problems, but it should be addressed with all your patients.

   1. **Questions to ask:** Is the patient sexually active? Does he or she relate sexually to men, women, or both? Is there any history of sexual difficulties or sexually transmitted diseases? Does he or she engage in any high-risk sexual behavior? What type of birth control, if any, does the patient use? Does the patient have any concerns about his or her sexual functioning? Ask especially about the effect of any chronic diseases (like diabetes) or medications (e.g., antihypertensives) on the patient's sex life. Part B contains further discussion of how to conduct this important and difficult part of the patient interview.

VII. **Review of systems.** In this portion of the history interview, all organ systems not already discussed during the HPI are systematically reviewed. The review of systems (ROS) is the last portion of the interview, and it serves three purposes: (1) to provide a thorough search for further, as yet undiscovered disease processes, (2) to remind the patient of possible, as yet unmentioned symptoms or difficulties he or she may be experiencing, and (3) to remind the physician in a logical manner of points of inquiry that may have been inadvertently omitted. The ROS purposely contains some redundancy in the interest of thoroughness, and it is a final methodic inquiry prior to the physical examination. Table 2-3 contains a master list of the topics in the ROS, as well as selected clinical points of emphasis. Performance of the ROS and usage of the ROS table are discussed further in Part B.

VIII. **Conclusion of the history.** After the ROS, the physician concludes the history by offering the patient an opportunity to question or comment further, by asking a question such as, "Is there anything else you would like to discuss before I examine you?"

B   **Practical Points Concerning
                                              the Patient Interview**

> *The complaint I hear most often about doctors is that they will not talk to
> their patients adequately.* A friendly and sincere interest in a patient's
> problem breaks the ice. Keep your appearance such that a patient will
> trust you. ("If he doesn't button up his shirt, how will he sew up my head?")
> Explain every move of the physical examination before it is done. Be cour-
> teous, respectful, and confidential. Show continued interest while in contact
> with the patient. Reappear frequently and at predictable times. Be
> reachable.
>
> **John Shillito, Jr., M.D.**

I. Introduction: Before the interview

A. Patient's chart. The patient's medical record is still known as the *chart* in
many institutions, a holdover from the days when all information was
recorded on a chart kept at the foot of the bed. Often you will be assigned
a patient who has accumulated a substantial chart from previous admissions that includes recent notes concerning the present admission. Should
you read the chart before seeing the patient, and if so, how much of it
should you read?

   1. In general, it is not a good idea to read the information concerning the
present admission, especially when first learning how to interview
and take a history.

   2. There is nothing wrong with having knowledge of **previous admissions** or problems, provided that the HPI is respected and faithfully
taken. The present admission may be for new disease processes; it may
also concern new nuances of previous problems. Being forearmed with
some knowledge of the patient's prior problems may be an advantage
and can prompt further insightful questions during your interview.

   3. The chart that has accumulated during the present admission may be
especially useful after you have finished your HPI and physical exam.
Use it to compare your understanding of the patient's story, as well as
your physical findings, with those of more experienced physicians.

   4. Despite **(1)** above, as you become more comfortable with interviewing
and begin to do admissions, you will realize that the chart can be very
useful for gaining a rapid introduction to a patient's case. Do not assume that something has been "unfairly provided"—the work-up is
not an exam. Similarly, realize that your responsibilities as an interviewer and as a caregiver are not lessened by the chart and by other
persons' input into the patient's care. Always confirm with the patient
any information you read in the chart before assuming it is true.

B. Approaching the patient. Although the patient in a teaching hospital generally knows that he or she may be seen by a medical student, you are still
obligated to explain your status. This is usually done by introducing yourself and saying, for instance, "Hello, Mr. Jones. I'm Wendy Mogan, the
medical student who will be working with Dr. Thomas on your case." Remember, however, that the hospitalized patient is undergoing a threatening and uncomfortable experience and that your visit may be seen as an
irrelevant intrusion. If you sense hostility, it may be prudent to have the
patient's main doctor introduce you as a member of the team. Adamant

refusal to see a medical student is uncommon, and if you encounter it often, it may be time to reevaluate your approach.

C. When first learning to interview, you will occasionally be sent to interview a patient who is **clearly too ill** to be subjected to yet another history and physical exam. At such times it becomes necessary to take the initiative and, after a brief visit with the patient, return to your preceptor, explain the situation, and find a new patient to interview.

D. **Do not introduce yourself as a doctor.** If the patient wishes, he or she may call you "doctor" after you have explained your medical student status, but it is misleading and legally unwise to introduce yourself as a physician. Patients will respect you for being a medical student; the discomfort students feel when explaining this is a part of the natural insecurity involved with learning to be on the wards. It will not be uncommon for other physicians to introduce you as a doctor; in general, that moment is not the time to redefine your position. However, you may explain to the patient at a later time that you are, in fact, a medical student.

E. **Greeting the patient.** When you first enter the room and greet the patient, begin with an introduction of yourself, followed by a brief conversation that is not medical but is rather an exchange of pleasantries, an attempt to find out how the patient is feeling in general without yet pursuing the specific. The point here is to help both you and the patient feel a bit more at ease before you begin with the introductory information and your questions about the chief complaint.

F. Always call a patient by the proper title and his or her last name (e.g., Mr. Jones or Ms. Smith), unless they tell you to do otherwise.

G. It is your responsibility to ensure a good setting for the interview. Though this is difficult in a crowded, busy hospital, try to find a quiet, private place in which to talk to your patient. (This may require asking visitors to leave, or moving to a location other than the patient's room, if that is possible. Always sit down when interviewing a patient, and make sure that you are both comfortable.

H. In the course of your clerkships you will inevitably have to interview some patients who do not speak English. The best solution to this problem is to get an official translator, who will translate everything that is being said. It is better not to depend on fragmentary conversations and broken English, and one should be careful about having family members translate, as they may change the meaning of what the patient said.

I. It is a good idea to take a **clipboard** and scratch paper into the interview so that you can jot down brief notes during the HPI, record information that will be difficult to remember, and note points to which you wish to return. You will find such notes especially useful when inquiring about the past medical history, the family history, medications and habits, and the review of systems. In the beginning, you will find yourself writing down much of what is said, but try to devote yourself more to the patient than to the notes. When discussing particularly sensitive or emotional topics, it is best to put your clipboard down and simply listen.

II. Chief complaint and its duration

A. Many clinicians recommend using the **patient's own words** to describe the chief complaint (CC) in the write-up. This is the time to record just what is said in response to your questions about why the patient has come to the hospital.

B. **The chief complaint may not be immediately obvious,** since patients will not uncommonly complain of several things. Listen for a minute and try to pinpoint or determine the main problem that caused the patient to seek medical attention. **Taking a stance** is central to developing clinical skill.

Therefore, choose a chief complaint and record other complaints to be placed after the HPI in your write-up (see Chap. 13). Drawing conclusions that prove to be erroneous and emphasizing inappropriate data are expected consequences of learning to organize a case, and thoughtful mistakes will be respected.

C. Realize that the chief complaint may be very different from what you subsequently consider to be the patient's **most serious problem.** When a patient with a history of leukemia enters with a mouth ulcer, you may be more concerned about a possible relapse, while the chief complaint remains "my mouth is very sore."

III. History of the present illness

A. As a student, your primary goal in taking the HPI should be to get the patient to relate for you a clear **sequence of the events** that led the patient to seek medical attention. This information should be both **specific** and **quantitative** ("I felt the pain all across my chest and down my left arm"; "I can only walk half a block before I get tired"). To obtain this sort of HPI, you will have to use a combination of careful listening and skillful, goal-oriented questioning.

B. At first, when the interviewing process seems overwhelming, and later, when time is precious, it is easy to be too tired or harried to **listen well.** We cannot overemphasize that respect for and attention to the patient's story are central to any thoughtful work-up. Failure to listen to the patient's story and then to react with refining questions is perhaps the most common difficulty for the beginning clinician. Do not allow the history to drown in the flood of concerns about further diagnostic steps (physical exam, lab work) that it rightfully sets in motion.

Let the patient do as much explaining as possible without interrupting. Interject to clarify and prompt, but avoid leading questions. Give your patient several uninterrupted minutes before you delve into a dissection of the symptoms or attempt to order the events.

Also, be wary of patient's use of **medical jargon;** ask about symptoms, not about diagnostic phrases that may be offered by the patient.

C. There are specific **techniques in interviewing** that will help you encourage and maintain the flow of information. Basically, the interviewer can follow the patient's own lead by using these techniques, which include facilitation, reflection, clarification, responding with empathy, interpretation, and, occasionally, confrontation. We recommend the discussion in Bates [4].

D. In your mind, try to **organize the evolving story around calendar dates and clock times.** Realize that your first clue in this regard is the duration of the chief complaint. The history (and its subsequent write-up) are built on a chronological foundation. If you are clear about the course of the patient's problems, two things result. First, the case will be logically organized for yourself and later for your readers. Second, you will have further insight into the tempo of the disease, one of the cornerstones of diagnosis.

E. Symptom analysis is explained in detail in Part A of this chapter. The scheme for symptom analysis in Table 2-2 is thorough and worth learning, but a mnemonic device to use when considering a symptom can be useful. Such a mnemonic (created for the attributes of the symptom "pain") is presented in DeGowin and DeGowin (see **Appendix D**). The mnemonic is **PQRST:**

Provocative-palliative factors
Quality of the pain
Region of the pain
Severity of the pain
Temporal characteristics

F. Do not be afraid to **requestion** the patient about points that are unclear or that seem crucial to your understanding of the case. People forget to mention things and may be reminded of them the second time, or they may have dismissed what seemed unimportant to them. Generally, the first time you ask a question you will take an open-ended stance ("Did you have any blood in your urine?"). The second time you can be more direct ("And you have seen blood in your urine only once?").

G. It is useful to stop and **summarize** your understanding of the details the patient has recounted at select points during the interview and especially as you conclude the HPI and get ready to begin the past medical history. Say something such as, "Let me see if I have this straight now," then pause and summarize aloud the patient's HPI, as you understand it. This will encourage you to construct the story in a concise, uncluttered form, and it allows the patient to edit out errors and supplement areas of omission. Once you become good at the summarizing process, the write-up of the HPI will be a lot easier.

H. At some point during the interview you should ask directly **what the patient thinks is wrong** and what features of the symptoms are causing the most worry. If the patient's fears are not addressed, the patient will undoubtedly leave the interview with some measure of anxiety. In addition, you may gain a new insight into the nature of the problem.

IV. Past medical history

A. The best way to **begin the past medical history** (PMH) is to ask a question such as, "Now, have you had any other medical problems or illnesses besides what we just discussed?" Often patients, especially older ones, will have trouble recalling their earlier medical history and will forget to mention illnesses that are chronic and treated, such as diabetes. It may help to prompt them with questions about prior admissions, but it will often be necessary to refer to the old chart. Turn to the PMH section of the typed discharge summary from the previous admission, which provides a good place to begin constructing a list of other medical problems.

B. Although other medical problems may have been brought up during the discussion of the present illness, **specific discussion of each problem** identified takes place at this point. Make a quick note of various diagnoses or problems poorly remembered by the patient, and consult the chart later for further details.

C. Patients commonly deny any **allergies,** but there are instances when more specific questions are important. For instance, if you think antibiotics may be important in a patient's management, you might ask, "Have you ever taken penicillin before?" Because penicillin or penicillin derivatives are extremely useful and allergic reactions are their biggest disadvantage, a specific inquiry is merited. Similarly, patients admitted for cardiac catheterization should be asked about past allergic reactions to shellfish. It is also important to distinguish between drug allergies and allergies to environmental factors. You need to make it clear that you are asking about drugs or asthma, as the case may be.

D. **Childhood illnesses** may be revealed with a general question such as, "Were you ever seriouslly ill as a child?" If the patient gives a positive response, it is important to determine how the diagnosis was made, how long the problem lasted, and whether there were any sequelae. Patients who claim to have had rheumatic fever, for instance, should be asked whether they have had a rash (erythema marginatum), painful joints, uncontrolled movements especially of their hands (Sydenham's chorea, or St. Vitus' dance), or any evidence of heart difficulties since that time.

E. In gathering information about previous hospitalizations, a question that seeks a specific history of **prior surgery** often will jog the patient's memory.

F. As the patient lists **medication** out loud, jot down each entry on a note pad in three columns. For example:

Drug name	Dose	Regimen
propranolol	40 mg	bid

   1. If a patient cannot remember the name of a medicine, ask for a description of the medicine and the reason for its use; you can later describe it to a more experienced clinician, who will probably be able to identify the drug. Also, you can ask patients if they have brought along their pill bottles, on which you will find the information you seek. **Appendix B** contains a list of common drugs and their actions, which may be helpful in this part of the interview, and the **inside covers** of this book list some common abbreviations found on medication labels.

G. While it is important to quantitate your patient's **alcohol intake,** realize that many patients may underestimate this number. A more sensitive set of screening questions for problems with alcohol is called the CAGE questions:

"Have you ever felt the need to **C**ut down on your drinking?"
"Have you ever felt **A**nnoyed by criticism of your drinking?"
"Have you ever had **G**uilty feelings about drinking?"
"Have you ever taken a morning **E**ye-opener?"

One positive answer to these questions should lead to further inquiry about problem drinking, and two should be considered good evidence for a diagnosis of alcoholism (*American Journal of Psychiatry* 1974;131:1121).

H. Quantitate **smoking** in pack-years (1 pack-year equals 1 pack per day for 1 year). For example, a patient who smoked 2 packs per day for 3 years but cut back to 1 pack every other day for the past 2 years has a 7 pack-year history.

V. Family history

A. Record the information given about the patient's family by constructing a quick, simple **pedigree diagram.** Males are represented with squares, females with circles. Living relatives' ages are recorded within the circles or squares, and deceased relatives' circles or squares have slashes drawn through them. Specific diseases are noted next to the appropriate symbol for the relative with the history of that disease. The patient is included on the diagram and identified with an arrow. For examples, see the FHx portion of the sample write-up in Chap. 13.

VI. Social history

A. The social history is perhaps the most variable portion of the medical history. It is the section of the interview that focuses on the patient's lifestyle, home life, work, and anxieties, in an effort to develop a more complete idea of the patient as a person. Because you may have gained some of the information in a less formal manner during the course of your conversation, the time required for the psychosocial history varies. **The key insights are those that relate to the ways in which the patient's daily life may interact with his or her disease and treatment, both physiologically and psychologically.** A sedentary 70-year-old man with occasional back pain when bending will have very different therapeutic needs from those of an active 40-year-old with similar pain.

B. As in other portions of the history, asking **general, open-ended questions** is a good way to initiate a discussion. For example, "How do you spend a typical day?" or "Tell me about your life at home" may be a useful starting point. In asking about occupation, both general questions ("What sort of work have you done in your life") and directed ones ("Have you ever worked in a place where you were exposed to fumes or chemicals?") may be appropriate.

C. In beginning the **sexual history,** the ease with which the patient is able to discuss his or her private life will be related to your own ease in discussing and asking about sexual matters. It is important to not make any assumptions in asking questions. Do not assume people are attracted to others of the opposite gender, or that they have a traditional family structure. Questions like "Who are the important people in your life?" are better opening questions than "Tell me about your wife." Also do not assume that just because someone is elderly he or she is no longer sexually active.

In asking about people's sexual lives, it is crucial to pay attention to both verbal and nonverbal responses. Generally you will be able to sense whether or not people have more to say on the subject; if they do, you can facilitate the discussion by being receptive and understanding. On the other hand, a patient who is comfortable with his or her sexual life will usually make that fact clear. It is well worth reading a more thorough discussion concerning the sexual history, such as that found in Bates [4] or Billings and Stoeckle [5].

VII. Review of systems

A. Conduct this portion of the history **quickly and efficiently.** Explain to patients that you must ask a long series of questions, but that they may simply answer "no" after each question that does not apply to them. Some people like to conduct this review of systems as they are doing each part of the physical exam.

B. Avoid unnecessary repetition. Although some redundancy will occur, as explained earlier, it is not necessary to review the organ system(s) you covered during the HPI interview unless there is a particular point you want to clarify.

C. Recent changes are the most important points to glean from the ROS. Has the patient's exercise tolerance decreased recently, or has climbing stairs fatigued her for several years? Did the patient begin to have night sweats this year, or has he always had them in the summertime? Patients may bring up several issues in one or more organ systems. It takes experience to know which complaints are more significant, but those that have not appeared or changed recently will usually assume a lower place on your list of priorities as you organize the case.

D. If a patient points to a lesion during the ROS, state that you will return to it while doing the physical exam, and continue your questioning.

VIII. Concluding the history. The patient is offered a chance to ask questions at the end of the history. Realize that you can always return to history questions later, during the physical exam or on a subsequent visit. The sequence explained in this chapter is designed to help retrieve most of the important data necessary for working up a patient's case and to begin constructing a logical framework for considering the case. The next step in that framework is the physical examination.

The Physical Exam: An Overview

The best physical exams are quick, thorough, and follow a logical sequence that maximizes both efficiency and the patient's comfort. A minimum number of position changes during the physical exam, especially when examining sick individuals, is highly desirable. The purpose of this chapter is to lay out the physical exam in broad strokes so that a formalized structure can be developed and used in the future. The hope is that by internalizing this broad schematic of the physical exam, through repetition your physical exam will begin to flow smoothly.

Before the specific details concerning the examination of a particular organ system are learned, it is an absolute imperative that the examiner know when each organ system is examined over the course of the physical exam and what the appropriate patient position for examining that organ system. A useful analogy here would be to think of the physical exam as a tree. The trunk and largest branches are the information in this chapter. In Chapter 4, a detailed account of the physical exam, we will add the leaves that cover the tree. Remember: **Make your tree, then add the leaves.**

I. **Exam sequence: head to toe**

  A. **Patient position 1.** Patient is sitting on the edge of the examining table, stretcher, or bed, and you stand in front of the patient, moving to either side as needed. **Exam segments:**

    1. **General inspection**

    2. **Vital signs**

    3. **Skin**

    4. **HEENT** (head, eyes, ears, nose, and throat) and **neck,** including cervical nodes and cranial nerves.

    5. **Breast exam** (inspection with patient's hands on hips and over head), with examination of axillary and epitrochlear nodes.

  B. **Patient position 2.** Move behind the sitting patient. **Exam segments:**

    1. **Thyroid gland**

    2. **Posterior thorax** and **posterior lung fields**

    3. **Back**

  C. **Patient position 3.** Patient is supine; you should stand on the patient's right side. **Exam segments:**

    1. Continue **breast exam** (palpation)

    2. **Anterior thorax** and **anterior lung fields**

    3. **Cardiovascular system** (jugular venous pressure [JVP], heart, radial and brachial pulses)

      4. **Abdomen,** and palpate inguinal nodes and femoral pulse

      5. **Musculoskeletal system,** and palpate dorsalis pedis, posterior tibial, and popliteal pulses

  D. Patient position 4. Patient is standing; you should sit on a chair or stool. **Exam segments:**

      1. Continue **musculoskeletal system** exam; examine alignment of back, legs, knees, and feet

      2. **Rectal** exam for men

      3. **Genital exam** for men

      4. Screening **neurological exam** (gait, Romberg)

  E. Patient position 5. Patient is sitting. **Exam segments:**

      1. Continue **neurological exam** (sensory, motor, cerebellar, and deep tendon reflex [DTR] exams)

  F. Patient position 6. Lithotomy position. **Exam segments:**

      1. **Pelvic** and **rectal exams** for women

II. Summary

Patient positions 1 and 2: **sitting**
Patient position 3: **supine**
Patient position 4: **standing**
Patient position 5: **sitting**
Patient position 6: **lithotomy**

Remember: head to toe

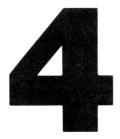

Annotated
Physical Exam

The physical examination follows and complements the history in the sequence of the patient work-up. Chap. 3 described the general **head-to-toe** flow of the exam and discussed how to conduct the exam with the minimum of inconvenience. In this chapter we will more fully discuss each part of the exam, what to look for, and how to address some common problems faced by students new to the wards.

Part A is an outline of the physical examination arranged by organ system, presented telegraphically for bedside use. It parallels the order in which the exam is usually presented in both written and oral form, and it contains comments on exam procedure and on positive and normal findings. Its goal is not to explain how to do the exam, which is carefully detailed in the recommended physical diagnosis textbooks (see **Appendix D**), but rather to answer some questions and address some concerns that frequently emerge during the specific exam sequence. Part B of this chapter contains some practical advice concerning the physical exam for the student who is inexperienced in physical diagnosis. It gives hints both on the general conducting of the exam, as well as on particularly difficult sections of it.

A   **Annotated Outline of the
Physical Examination**

I. General exam

A. Appearance

1. State of **health and nourishment**

2. Obvious **distress or affect problems**

3. Apparent **age and vigor**

4. **Grooming and expression**

5. **Hair distribution**

6. **State of consciousness**

7. Note speech patterns, lethargy, stupor, coma, intoxication, or anything else that will affect interpretation of the rest of the physical examination.

B. Vital signs and measurements

1. **Height and weight.** Weight is useful for following nutritional status and fluid balance.

2. **Oral or rectal temperature.** Fever means infection until proved otherwise. Normal oral temperature fluctuates diurnally between 35.8°C (96.4°F) and 37.3°C (99.1°F).

3. **Pulse strength, rate, and rhythm.** Taking the radial pulse is an un-threatening way to initiate physical contact. Note if irregularities are regularly irregular or irregularly irregular. Do beats drop occasionally? Sporadically? Note if the pulse is strong or weak. Compare to apical pulse during the cardiac exam.

4. **Blood pressure.** Hypertension is defined as >90 mm Hg diastolic and/or >140 mm Hg systolic. In patients with possible or known asthma, pericardial effusion or tamponade, or emphysema, check for pulsus paradoxus (an inspiratory fall in systolic arterial pressure that exceeds 10 mm Hg). In patients with suspected hypotension, check pressure sitting or lying down as well as standing. If initial reading is elevated, check pressure in other arm, and recheck at some later point in the exam.

5. **Respiratory rate and character.** Note any respiratory patterns while taking the pulse. Do not announce your intention to "count breaths," which may increase the patient's anxiety and alter the normal breathing pattern.

C. **Hands.** Note temperature, color, appearance, nails, clubbing, nodes, contractures, degenerative changes.

1. Compare general **palm color** to your own, especially if considering anemia. Try to describe any **degenerative changes** seen. Note which **interphalangeal joints** are involved and which are spared. Note location of any **nodules, swelling, or contractures;** presence or absence of **tenderness;** and **degree of motion** remaining in the affected digits or limbs.

2. Examine and describe for yourself changes in the **nails,** especially clubbing, deformities, or discolorations. **Clubbed nails** are consistent with (c/w) numerous pulmonary, cardiovascular, and other diseases. **Spoon nails** (koilonychia) are c/w iron deficiency or hypochromic anemias. **Mees's lines** are c/w renal insufficiency, MI, infectious fevers, and poisonings, among other conditions.

D. **Integument.** Note skin color, temperature, turgor, moisture, and lesions.

1. **Skin color.** If suspicious of cyanosis, check for blue especially around mouth, nails, lips. Look for the yellow of jaundice especially in the sclera. Decreased skin turgor is c/w dehydration and old age.

2. **Skin lesions.** Note type (see Fig. 4-1), shape (round, irregular), arrangement with respect to each other (discrete, clusters), and distribution on body (legs, trunk, face). Note especially lesions with irregular borders, heterogeneity of colors, and inflammatory regions. The majority of skin malignancies do not cause pruritis or pain. If a suspicious lesion is found, ask the patient: How long has it been present? Has it changed? Does it seem not to heal? (See also Colorplates E–I.)

The skin exam may be continued throughout the physical exam. Draw quick diagrams on your clipboard and quantitate when possible.

II. **HEENT.** Many parts of this exam overlap with the neurologic exam. This is a convenient time and place to check cranial nerves.

A. **Head**

1. Skull shape, scalp, hair distribution, lesions

2. Characteristic facies, including the edematous, myxedematous, cushingoid, acromegalic, and parkinsonian

B. **Ears**

1. External ear exam; check for any discharge, pain on movement

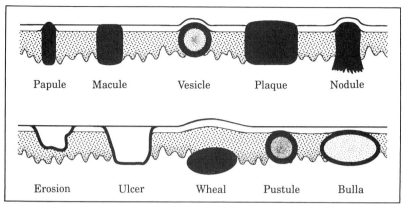

Fig. 4-1. The most common structural changes in the skin. (Modified from R. D. Judge, G. D. Zuidema, and F. T. Fitzgerald [17], p. 95.)

2. Otoscopic look at auditory canal, tympanic membranes; check for a light reflex and for fluid behind the eardrum

3. Hearing (can use whispered numbers or tuning fork). **Weber** (tuning fork held at midline) and **Rinne** (air versus bone conduction) **tests,** if indicated.

C. Eyes

1. **Eyelids, conjunctivae, and sclera.** Look for xanthelasma (suggests hypercholesterolemia), unequal palpebral fissures (clue to ptosis), scleral yellowing (implies jaundice), redness of eyes, discharge, congestion of lacrimal glands.

2. **Visual acuity.** Measure with and without glasses. Can use pocket Snellen's chart.

3. **Pupils.** Check size, symmetry, direct and consensual pupillary reaction to light, and accommodation. **Anticholinergics** cause dilated pupils. **Opiate intoxication** causes pinpoint pupils. **Argyll-Robertson** pupil (reacts to accommodation but not to light) is c/w syphilis, diabetes, central nervous system (CNS) disease.

4. **Extraocular movements.** See Figure 4-2 for muscles and nerves associated with each direction. Check for **nystagmus;** remember, a few beats of nystagmus on horizontal gaze is within normal limits.

5. **Visual fields.** Use confrontation technique with tip of a pen, looking for gross field deficits.

6. **Ophthalmoscopic exam of fundi.** Note opacities of the lens and funduscopic abnormalities (arteriovenous nicking, hemorrhages, exudates, arteriolar narrowing); check for papilledema. The funduscopic exam is especially important in diseases with microvascular sequelae, such as hypertension and diabetes mellitus (DM). See hints on this exam in **Part B.II.A.**

D. Nose

1. Note **septal position, nasal discharge, sinus tenderness, turbinate exam, airway patency**

2. **Sinusitis** may be brought out by having patient flex neck and lower head or by tapping over ethmoid, maxillary, and frontal sinuses. If it

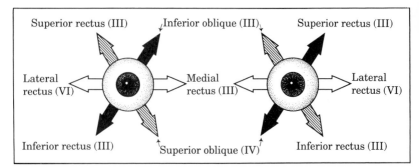

Fig. 4-2. Extraocular movements and their controlling nerves. Cranial nerves noted in parentheses. (Modified from R. D. Judge, G. D. Zuidema, and F. T. Fitzgerald [17], p. 133.)

is suspected, ask the patient whether sinus difficulties have been a problem.

3. The most common cause of **epistaxis** is nose picking.

E. Mouth and throat

1. **Lip conditions, cheilosis, gum and mucous membrane condition.** Check for **mucosal lesions** (petechiae, apthous ulcers, areas of induration). **Gingival hypertrophy** is c/w puberty, pregnancy, dilantin therapy, leukemia, gingivitis. Note any **bleeding of gums.**

2. **Tongue color and condition.** An abnormally smooth, red tongue is c/w vitamin B_{12} or iron deficiency (atrophic glossitis).

3. **Dentition.** Note the state of the teeth and whether any are missing.

4. **Oropharynx.** Note especially any unusual breath odor, hoarseness, lesions and excessive salivation (ptyalism) or redness (injection).

III. Neck and axilla

A. Lymphadenopathy. Characterize cervical and axillary adenopathy: note number, location, tenderness or lack of tenderness, texture (rubbery versus soft), and mobility. Recall that some "shotty" adenopathy is common, especially in inguinal area and in children. Remember to check supraclavicular nodes (Virchow's node can indicate thoracic malignancy).

B. Trachea position. Tracheal deviation may suggest a mass effect, pneumothorax, loss of lung volume, or fibrotic change.

C. Thyroid. Note thyroid size, mobility, and symmetry. It is often easier to see and feel the thyroid when the patient swallows (provide a cup of water). The thyroid may be palpated either from in front of or when standing behind the patient.

D. Carotids. Listen for bruits, palpate pulses. Be careful when palpating older patients, and only check one carotid artery at a time.

IV. Back

A. Spinal column curvature and tenderness. Forward flexion of trunk may make scoliosis and kyphosis more obvious.

B. Costovertebral angle (CVA) tenderness. Extreme CVA tenderness is c/w acute kidney disease. Minor CVA tenderness is c/w low back pain of any etiology.

V. Respiratory exam

A. Inspection

1. **Symmetry and shape of chest** (note how it moves with inspiration)

2. **Respiratory pattern.** Note rate, rhythm, regularity, and depth. Normal rate is 12–18 cycles/min for adults; it may be 35–40 in infants. Resting shallow tachypnea is c/w restrictive lung disease. Hyperpnea is commonly c/w anxiety or exertion. Rapid, deep Kussmaul breathing is seen in metabolic acidosis. Decreased respiratory rate is c/w a CNS respiratory depression. Cheyne-Stokes breathing (alternating hypernea and apnea) is c/w normal sleep, heart failure, uremia, and CNS dysfunction.

B. Palpation of thoracic wall.
Note by inspection and palpation the presence or absence of symmetry and excursion of the thoracic wall. In trauma patients check for pneumothorax, tension pneumothorax, hemothorax, flail chest (paradoxical inward buckling of chest during inspiration).

C. Percussion

1. **Diaphragmatic descent.** Normal descent is approximately 3–6 cm with full inspiration. Compare both sides and note any gross asymmetries in movement.

2. **Resonance.** Compare percussion notes of right and left lung fields. Dullness is often caused by pleural thickening or consolidation. Palpate for tactile fremitus if consolidation is suspected.

D. Auscultation

1. **Posterior chest.** Compare the corresponding sites in right and left fields. Check for presence of breath sounds at both bases and for adventitious sounds (crackles, wheezes, or rubs). Listen for egophony, whispered pectoriloquy, when appropriate.

   Airway deflation and pulmonary consolidation often lead to egophony, crackles, and/or increased fremitus. Bronchitis and asthma often cause crackles, wheezes, and an increased expiratory-inspiratory ratio.

2. **Anterior chest.** Always check apices of lungs; some diseases have primarily apical findings (e.g., TB).

VI. Breast exam

A. Inspection.
Have patient perform several maneuvers: arms at side, over head, pressed against hips. Dimpling, contour asymmetry, venous prominence, redness, and nipple retraction or discharge may all be c/w breast cancer.

B. Palpation.
Use a systematic manner of palpating. Note tenderness, nodularity, nipple discharge. Nodules may be c/w fibrocystic breast disease, benign fibroadenomas, or carcinoma. Malignant lesions are typically firm, irregular, and neither well encapsulated nor mobile. Superficial signs of breast tissue retraction may be present. Draw diagrams indicating findings and specifying position with respect to the nipple.

VII. Cardiovascular exam

A. Inspection

1. **Jugular venous pulsation level.** Often best performed when patient's upper body is elevated with pillows to a 30-degree angle (see Fig. 4-3). The normal JVP meniscus, measured at this angle, can be seen one-third to one-half of the way up the neck. Increased JVP is c/w elevated right-side pressures (consider elevated pulmonary pressures, right ven-

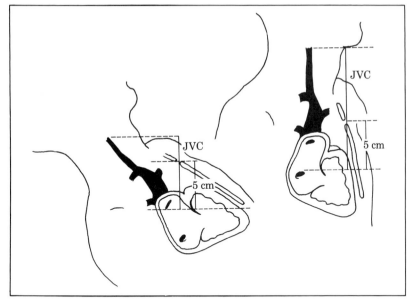

Fig. 4-3. The jugular venous pulse can be used as a manometer to measure right atrial pressure. Since the distance from the right atrium to the sternal angle is 5 cm, regardless of the patient's position (see above), right atrial pressure can be estimated by measuring the distance in centimeters from the sternal angle to the top of the jugular venous column (JVC). Then, right atrial pressure = 5 cm + JVC (cm). (Modified from R. Judge and G. Zuidema, *Methods of Clinical Examination: A Physiologic Approach,* 3rd ed. Boston: Little, Brown, 1974.)

tricular failure, pericardial tamponade or constriction, or tricuspid valve disease).

   2. Point of maximal impulse (PMI), or apex beat. Search for the apex beat visually before palpating.

B. **Palpation**

   1. Apex beat (PMI). Note the position and character of the apex beat. An enlarged, prolonged, or displaced apex beat may indicate right or left ventricular hypertrophy or dilatation. Note any other impulses or thrills, and whether they occur in systole or diastole.

C. **Auscultation**

   1. Heart sounds

      a. **First sound (S₁)** created by closure of mitral, tricuspid valves.

      b. **Second sound (S₂)** created by closure of aortic, pulmonic valves. Note splitting of sound, best heard at high left sternal border (third interspace).

      Normally, S₂ splits during inspiration, as increased venous return slows closing of pulmonic valve. **Fixed splitting** occurs with any condition that delays closure of the pulmonic valve, like pulmonary stenosis, atrial septal defect (ASD), right bundle branch block (RBBB). **Paradoxical splitting** (split disappears on inspiration) oc-

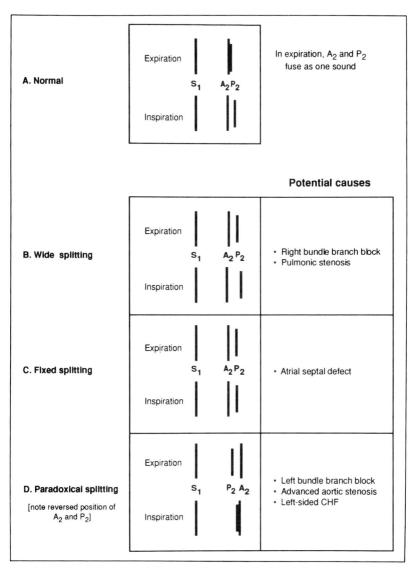

Fig. 4-4. Splitting patterns of the second heart sound (S_2). S_1 = first heart sound; A_2 = aortic component of S_2; P_2 = pulmonic component of S_2. (Reproduced with permission from L. S. Lilly [19], p. 21.)

curs with delayed closure of aortic valve, as with aortic stenosis (AS), left ventricle (LV) myopathy, and left bundle branch block (LBBB). See Fig. 4-4.

   c. Third sound (S_3) a low-pitched sound in early to mid diastole, heard best at the apex using the bell of the stethoscope, with the patient in the left lateral decubitus position. S_3 is generated by the sudden termination of excessively rapid filling of the left ventricle, usually in the dilated heart. While S_3 may be heard in children and adolescents with normal hearts, in mature patients it is considered pathologic and can indicate ventricular failure, MI, or valvular heart disease. When S_1, S_2, and S_3 are heard in sequence, the sound has a cadence like the syllables of the word "Ken-tuc-ky," in which the final "ky" represents S_3. A pathologic S_3 is frequently called a ventricular gallop.

   d. **Fourth sound (S_4)** a low-pitched sound in late diastole, also heard best with the bell at the apex, with the patient in the left lateral decubitus position. S_4 is generated by decreased ventricular compliance and the atrial systole, which ejects an atrial jet of blood against the stiff ventricle and thus generates a sound. An S_4 implies myocardial disease. When S_4, S_1, and S_2 are heard in sequence, the sound has a cadence like the syllables of "Ten-nes-see," with S_4 represented by the initial "Ten." A pathologic S_4 heard in the setting of tachycardia is commonly called an atrial gallop.

   e. **Rubs** usually indicate pericardial inflammation. They sound like squeaky leather, heard both in systole and diastole. Heard best with diaphragm over sternum, with patient sitting up, leaning forward, and holding breath after exhaling.

   f. Other sounds to listen for include: **opening snap** (rheumatic involvement of mitral or tricuspid valves; heard in diastole), **pericardial knock** (constrictive pericarditis), **tumor "plop"** (especially with left atrial myxomas), and **ejection clicks** (heard in systole; represents most common valvular disease). See Fig. 4-5 for a diagram of the relationship of some of these sounds to the cardiac cycle.

2. **Murmurs.** Describe timing, location and radiation, loudness, pitch, duration, quality (crescendo/decrescendo, musical, etc.). Table 4-1 shows how to grade murmurs by loudness.

   a. **Systolic murmurs** (see Fig. 4-6)

      (1) **Midsystolic.** Usually ejection murmurs, caused by valve stenosis (aortic or pulmonic), increased stroke volume (SV) dilation of vessel just distal to valve.

      (2) **Holosystolic.** Regurgitant murmurs; commonly mitral regurgitation/tricuspid regurgitation (MR/TR) or ventricular septal defect (VSD).

      (3) **Late systolic.** Heard in mitral valve prolapse, usually preceded by a click.

   b. **Diastolic murmurs** (see figure 4-7)

      (1) **Early diastolic.** Aortic regurgitation (AR) or pulmonic regurgitation (PR). AR is high-pitched, heard best with diaphragm at left sternal border while patient is sitting up and holding breath after exhalation. PR of similar quality, heard better at pulmonic area.

      (2) **Mid to late diastolic.** Mitral stenosis (MS) or tricuspid stenosis (TS). MS gives a low-pitched rumble heard best at apex with bell, patient on left side; falls then rises in intensity during diastole. TS has similar quality, heard best at tricuspid area; louder on inspiration.

   c. **Continuous and to-and-fro murmurs.** (See figure 4-8.) Continuous murmurs begin in systole, and continue without interruption into diastole; seen in patent ductus arteriosus, other arteriovenous (AV)

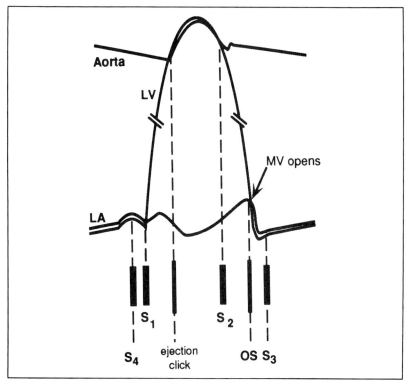

Fig. 4-5. Timing of extrasystolic and diastolic heart sounds. S_4 is produced by atrial contraction in the case of a "stiff" left ventricle (LV). An ejection click follows the opening of the aortic or pulmonic valve in cases of valve stenosis or dilation of the corresponding great artery. An S_3 occurs during the period of rapid ventricular filling; it is normal in young individuals, but its presence in adults implies LV contractile dysfunction. The timing of an opening snap (OS) is shown for comparison, but it is not likely that all of these sounds would appear in the same individual. LA = left atrium; MV = mitral valve. (Reproduced with permission from L. S. Lilly [19], p. 23.)

Table 4-1. Grading of heart murmurs

Grade	Description
I/VI	Heard only after special maneuvers and "tuning in"
II/VI	Faint, but readily heard
III/VI	Loud, but without a thrill
IV/VI	Associated with a thrill, but stethoscope must be fully on chest to be heard
V/VI	Heard with stethoscope partly off the chest; palpable thrill
VI/VI	Heard with stethoscope entirely off the chest; palpable thrill

Reproduced with permission from R. D. Judge, G. D. Zuidema, and F. T. Fitzgerald [17], p. 291.

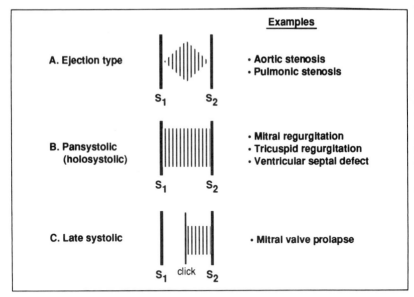

Fig. 4-6. Classification of systolic murmurs. Ejection murmurs are crescendo-decrescendo (or "diamond-shaped") in configuration, whereas pansystolic murmurs are homogenous throughout systole. A late systolic murmur often follows a midsystolic click, and suggests mitral-valve (or tricuspid-valve) prolapse. (Reproduced with permission from L. S. Lilly [19], p. 25.)

fistulas. To-and-fro murmurs do not extend through S_2 and have discrete systolic and diastolic components.

    d. Maneuvers. Various maneuvers that can alter hemodynamics to help differentiate murmurs and heart sounds are described in Part B of this chapter.

VIII. Abdominal exam

  A. Inspection. Draw a brief diagram on your clipboard on which to note data from the abdominal exam (see Chap. 14, sec. III). Note any distention, scars, superficial lesions, or venous prominence. Venous prominence is seen with portal hypertension.

  B. Auscultation.

    1. Note: Auscultation precedes palpation and percussion in the abdominal exam, so that you can listen to the bowels while they are undisturbed.

    2. Listen for **bruits** (especially over liver, spleen, abdominal aorta) and **bowel sounds;** absence of bowel sounds for up to 1 minute may be normal.

  C. Palpation. Palpate first lightly, then more deeply. Start away from any painful areas. Note any rigidity, guarding, tenderness, rebound tenderness, organomegaly, masses; watch the patient's face for change in expression as you palpate, to help quantify degree of tenderness. Note any kidney tenderness or enlargement. Palpate the liver edge for texture, contour, and tenderness. Remember that the spleen is usually not palpable in the adult.

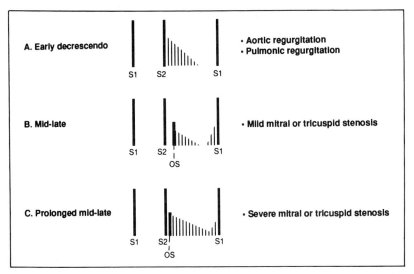

Fig. 4-7. Classification of the diastolic murmurs. A. An early diastolic decrescendo murmur is typical of aortic or pulmonic valve regurgitation. B. Mid or late low-frequency "rumbling" murmurs are usually due to mitral or tricuspid valve stenosis, which follows a sharp opening snap. Presystolic accentuation occurs in patients in normal sinus rhythm, because of forceful propulsion of blood across the stenotic valve by atrial contraction. C. In more severe mitral or tricuspid valve stenosis, the opening snap and diastolic murmur occur earlier, and the murmur is prolonged. (Reproduced with permission from L. S. Lilly [19], p. 28.)

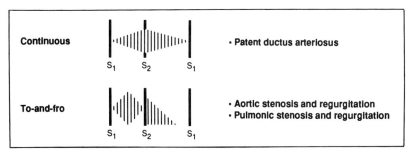

Fig. 4-8. A continuous murmur peaks at and extends through the second heart sound (S_2). A to-and-fro murmur is not continuous; rather there is a systolic component and a distinct diastolic component, separated by S_2. (Reproduced with permission from L. S. Lilly [19], p. 29.)

D. Percussion

1. **Percussion note.** Note character of percussion note (gas percusses with a hollow, tympanitic sound; fat, fluid, and underlying tissue percuss with dull sounds).

2. **Liver and spleen.** Percuss for size of liver and spleen, and define the extent to which they extend below the costal margin. Liver size can also be determined by scratch test.

3. Shifting dullness. In cases with possible ascites, check for dullness that shifts as patient changes position. Look also for a fluid wave.

IX. Peripheral vascular pulses

A. Note carotid, brachial, radial, femoral, popliteal, dorsalis pedis, and posterior tibial pulses.

1. Weak pulses **(pulsus parvus)** are c/w shock, heart failure, aortic stenosis. Increased pulse pressure is c/w aortic regurgitation and high-output states like thyrotoxicosis, fever, anemia. Delayed carotid upstroke is c/w significant aortic stenosis **(pulsus tardus)**. Alternating strong and weak pulses **(pulsus alternans)** are c/w LV failure. Right-left asymmetries in pulses suggest vascular diseases or shunts.

B. Bruits. Listen for bruits, which may be heard with atherosclerosis or aneurysms. Check the carotid and femoral arteries, and listen in the abdomen for aorta and renal artery bruits.

X. Hematopoietic system.
Check for **adenopathy** in cervical, axillary, epitrochlear, inguinal nodes. Note location, size (use a ruler), degree of tenderness, fixation to underlying tissue, and texture (hard, soft). Usually each set of nodes is examined when examining its region of the body (e.g., cervical nodes checked during neck exam).

XI. Musculoskeletal exam.
This exam is one in which it is particularly important to **focus on the symptomatic or suspicious areas** pinpointed by the general screening questions and exam. For example, complete, quantitative range-of-motion testing is warranted only by specific history or findings consistent with musculoskeletal disease.

Ask again about joint or bone pain, and have patient point to the specific area involved. Listen throughout this exam for crepitations; inspect for joint swelling or deformities; and evaluate strength and range of motion.

A. Head and neck. If neck pain is present, especially with headache, suspect meningitis and check Kernig's, Brudzinski's signs.

B. Shoulders. Pain may be generated from or referred to local structures (e.g., processes involving the diaphragm may be referred to the shoulder).

C. Elbows. Warm, tender joints with subcutaneous nodules around the olecranon process suggest rheumatoid arthritis.

D. Hands and wrists. Palpable enlargement of bones in the hands and Heberden's nodes on the distal interphalangeal (DIP) joints are seen most commonly in degenerative joint disease (osteoarthritis). Bilateral wrist swelling and proximal interphalangeal (PIP) involvement is seen usually in rheumatoid arthritis.

E. Spine. Always inspect contour carefully and test range of motion.

F. Hips. Pain and limitation of motion are common arthritic sequelae.

G. Knees. Note presence of *genu varum* (bowlegs) or *genu valgum* (knock knees).

H. Feet and ankles. Gout commonly affects the metatarsophalangeal joint of the first (big) toe.

XII. Neurologic exam

A. Mental status. Use the mnemonic looks-speaks-feels-thinks to remember the four main parts of the exam.

1. Looks—general appearance and behavior. Check level of consciousness, posture, dress and grooming, facial expressions, and manner; orientation to person, place, and time.

2. **Speaks**—speech and language. Note quantity, rate, volume, fluency, and modulation of speech. Note especially circumlocutions, neologisms, dysarthria, pressured speech, perseveration, clanging, echolalia.

3. **Feels**—mood and affect. Ask about mood; note patient's affect throughout interview: is it flat, euphoric, depressed, inappropriate, labile? If you suspect depression, you must assess risk of suicide. Ask directly if the patient has thought of killing him or herself. Does he or she have a plan?

4. **Thinks**

   a. Thought process and content. Check thought content (hallucinations, delusions, obsessions), thought process (loose associations, tangentiality, flight of ideas, confabulation).

   b. **Cognitive functions**

      (1) **Attention.** Check with serial sevens or threes, or digit span.

      (2) **Memory.** Test **recall:** give patient three items to remember and explain you will ask for them again in 5 minutes, and then do so; **recent memory:** ask about occurrences in the past 24 hours; **remote memory:** ask about date of marriage, childhood events, name of high school principal.

      (3) **Construction ability.** Ask patient to draw a cube or a house. Ask him or her to copy a figure you draw.

      (4) **Higher functions.** Test **judgment** ("What would you do if you found a stamped addressed envelope on the sidewalk?"); **proverbs** (ask patient the meaning of common proverbs, like "A stitch in time saves nine"); **calculations; fund of knowledge.**

B. **Cranial nerves.** The cranial nerves that have not yet been tested are examined at this point (all may have been tested earlier in the exam, while examining the head and neck).

   1. **I, olfactory.** Smell; not routinely tested. Use nonirritating scents. Most significant in unilateral loss.

   2. **II, optic.** Vision; test acuity, visual fields, pupils.

   3. **III, oculomotor.** Most extraocular muscles; pupillary constriction.

   4. **IV, trochlear.** Movement of eye down and in (superior oblique muscle).

   5. **V, trigeminal.** Sensory to face; motor to temporal and masseter. Palpate masseters on forced closure of jaw; touch cornea for corneal reflex; test all three divisions for sensation on face.

   6. **VI, abducens.** Lateral movement of eye (lateral rectus muscle).

   7. **VII, facial.** Motor to most of facial muscles; anterior tongue taste. Check smile, strength of eye closure, symmetry of forehead wrinkling and nasolabial folds.

   8. **VIII, vestibulocochlear.** Hearing and balance. Use 256-cps or 512-cps tuning fork for low frequency, ticking watch for high frequency, whispered voice for medium frequency.

   9. **IX, glossopharyngeal.** Pharynx, sensory and motor; posterior tongue taste.

   10. **X, vagus.** Motor to palate, pharynx, larynx; sensory to pharynx and larynx. For nerves IX and X, test swallowing, phonation ("me," "la," "ga"); check gag reflex, midline uvula.

11. **XI, spinal accessory.** Sternocleidomastoid and trapezius motor. Test shrug, turning of head, head flexion.

12. **XII, hypoglossal.** Motor to tongue. Check symmetry of tongue protrusion, look for tongue fasciculations, strength in pushing tongue against cheeks.

C. **Sensory exam.** Check symmetric areas in both right and left limbs; symmetric loss is c/w peripheral neuropathy. With pinprick and vibration, if sense is intact in the distal part of extremity you need not proceed proximally.

1. **Pinprick.** Use only broken tongue depressor, *not* reusable pins.

2. **Vibration.** Use 128- or 256-cps tuning fork on joints. Be sure patient is really sensing vibration (check this with a "sham" vibration caused by pressing the extremity with a nonvibrating tuning fork).

3. **Position sense.** Grasp sides of toe or finger and move it up or down, asking patient which way you moved it.

4. **Light touch.** Use cotton wisp.

5. **Temperature.** Differentiate between tuning fork (cold) and rubber of reflex hammer (warm). Usually corresponds to pinprick sensation.

6. **Cortical discrimination.** Examples of tests include graphesthesia (blindly identify letter or number "written" on palm), stereognosis (blindly identify object, like coin or key, placed in hand).

D. **Motor Exam**

1. **Muscle strength.** Strength is usually graded on scale of 1 to 5 (see Table 4-2).

2. **Tone.** Test resistance to passive motion. For Parkinson's disease, look for "cogwheel" rigidity.

3. **Bulk.** Compare one side of body to the other, but remember to allow for handedness, occupation-induced differences. Look for fasciculations, tenderness, wasting.

E. **Reflexes.** Note any right-left asymmetries. Record the findings on a clipboard by drawing a stick figure (see the sample write-up in Chap. 13).

1. **Biceps** (C5, 6), **triceps** (C6, 7, 8), **brachioradialis** (C5, 6), **patella** (L2, 3, 4), **Achilles tendon** reflexes (S1, 2). Upper motor neuron lesions cause spasticity; lower motor neuron lesions cause flaccidity. Leg reflexes can be reinforced by isometric, opposed arm pulls. Graded 1 +

Table 4-2. Testing for muscle strength

100%	5	N (normal)	Complete range of motion against gravity with full resistance
75	4	G (good)	Complete range of motion against gravity with some resistance
50	3	F (fair)	Complete range of motion against gravity
25	2	P (poor)	Complete range of motion with gravity eliminated
10	1	T (trace)	Evidence of slight contractility; no joint motion
0	0	0 (zero)	No evidence of contractility

Reproduced with permission from R. D. Judge, G. D. Zuidema, and F. T. Fitzgerald [17], p. 419.

to 4+ (1+ = present but difficult to elicit; 2+ = average; 3+ = hyperactive but not necessarily pathological; 4+ = very hyperactive, with clonus).

2. **Babinski reflex.** Positive Babinski reflex is c/w upper motor neuron disease.

3. Other reflexes not routinely tested include: **upper abdominal** (T7, 8, 9), **lower abdominal** (T11, 12), **cremasteric** (T12, L1), **jaw,** and **anal wink.** Presence of grasp, suck, or rooting reflexes usually indicate frontal lobe disease.

F. **Cerebellar.** Test finger-nose, heel-shin coordination.

G. **Gait.** Include heel-to-toe walking, Romberg's sign.

XVIII. Genital and rectal exam

A. Male

1. **Penis.** Note the presence of any penile lesions or discharge.

2. **Scrotum.** Check for scrotal lesions, varicosities; palpate spermatic cord.

3. **Testes.** Check testes bilaterally, and evaluate shape and firmness.

4. **Hernia.** Inspect for hernia; this is best done with patient standing. Ask patient to cough, and feel for weakness of wall.

5. **Rectum.** Anal lesions, sphincter tone, stool color, prostate size. Prostate exam is especially important in men more than 50 years old. Always check for occult blood with a guaiac test.

B. Female

1. **External exam.** Labia, urethral orifice, introitus, perineum. Careful inspection conducted here for irritation, discharge, lesions.

2. **Speculum exam.** Cervix and os specimens (endocervical swab, cervical scrape, and vaginal pool), vaginal canal exam. The Pap smear and gonococcal cultures are taken here. The vaginal canal may be inspected as the speculum is removed.

3. **Bimanual exam.** Cervix, fornix, uterus, ovaries.

4. **Rectal exam.** The rectal exam is often done with simultaneous placement of a finger in the vagina to palpate the interposed tissue. Change gloves before doing this exam, to decrease the likelihood of spreading infection.

B	Practical Points For the Physical Examination

I. General Advice

A. Many patients have negative expectations about physical exams, and it is important that you **make patients comfortable** throughout the process. Patients should be completely disrobed, except for underwear, to allow for proper exposure, but parts of the body not being examined should be kept covered for modesty's sake. Get into the habit of washing your hands before and after each exam; patients are reassured if you do this in their presence. Make sure your hands and stethoscope are warm before allowing them to touch the patient. Always let the patient know what you are about to do, and why.

B. The physical examination is an art that is learned only by constant repetition. You will learn a great deal through careful study of one of the many available physical examination manuals, but the only way to get comfortable with the techniques of the exam is to practice. The best way to learn physical diagnosis is through **repeated proctoring** of your methods. An experienced clinician can show you how to hold your hands just so; it is always easier to demonstrate than to explain.

C. Although there are many individual styles and methods of conducting the general screening exam, a good physician will choose one examination sequence and stick to it. Most people prefer to work in a head-to-foot order, with exceptions made as necessary for convenience and completeness. Most physicians stand at the patient's right side. As each part of the body is examined, it is usually best to follow an orderly sequence of **inspection, palpation, percussion, and auscultation.** This routine will help ensure thoroughness, and also will aid in putting the patient at ease by minimizing the unexpected.

D. The physical examination should always be conducted and assessed in the context of the patient's clinical history. The range of what is normal varies from patient to patient, and physical findings cannot be gathered and interpreted in a vacuum. Think in advance about **what you expect to find** in any given part of the exam. What kind of peripheral neurologic exam might you expect of a long-term diabetic? Are there other physical exam findings that might help you gauge the progress of the disease?

E. Do not be alarmed if, during the first few weeks, the complete exam takes you much longer than expected; first concentrate on learning each subsection, then work on stringing all the parts together smoothly. Do not be afraid to **repeat** parts of the exam if the findings are equivocal. Realize, however, that the diagnostic success of your exam depends on the cooperation of the patient, and that it is tedious and uncomfortable to be poked and maneuvered for hours at a time. It is often useful to repeat parts of the physical exam after looking at the results of the physical diagnostic tests; a patient whose chest x-ray shows some lobar consolidation provides a good opportunity to fine tune your auscultatory abilities.

F. Practice your exam techniques when you are away from the bedside. Take the time to familiarize yourself with your equipment, so that you will not, for example, fumble around with an inside-out blood pressure cuff. Practice on other medical students to get a good idea of the normal range.

G. Realize that the physical exam provides a perfect opportunity to **question** the patient concerning ROS topics you may have forgotten or you may be unclear about. It is often quite natural to introduce your next step with a general question concerning the organ system being examined (e.g., begin the otoscopic exam with, "So you've had no difficulties with earaches or infections?").

H. Each exam you do is **tailored to the patient** involved and directed by his or her problems. You will learn to run rapidly through the organ systems that you do not suspect to be involved and quickly decide whether findings are within normal limits. This takes practice, but it is certainly possible to do a brief, general screening physical in 10 minutes, once you are familiar with and can conduct easily the various parts of the exam.

I. A knowledge of **surface anatomy** is important in performing the physical examination. Note the relation of the internal organs in Figs. 4-9 and 4-10 to the spinal column landmarks on Fig. 4-11.

II. Specific points concerning the physical examination
There are six traditionally difficult or **problematic sections** of the physical examination: the funduscopic exam, the cardiac exam, the neurologic exam,

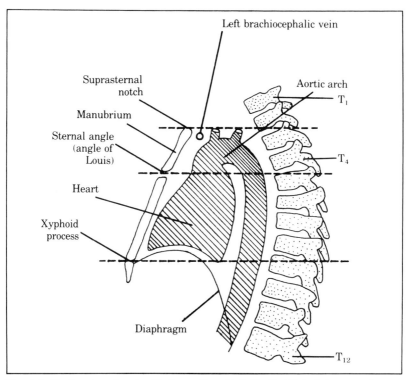

Fig. 4-9. The heart and aorta. (Redrawn from R. S. Snell, *Clinical Anatomy for Medical Students,* 2nd ed. Boston: Little, Brown, 1981.)

the rectal exam, the pelvic exam, and the breast exam. Each of these is discussed specifically below.

A. The **funduscopic exam** is very difficult to master. Work first on getting the "**red reflex.**" If you have a cat at your house, practice by looking into its eyes, since the cat's pupil remains relatively dilated. If you are around when a patient's eyes are pharmacologically dilated for some reason, ask to be permitted to examine his or her eyes as well.

Once you can elicit the red reflex easily, concentrate on **visualizing the disc** and then tracing its perimeter. Dial up and down 1 or 2 diopters in each direction on the funduscope after you have visualized an edge of the disc, and try to get a sense of how the disc relates to the retinal surface. Remember, the beautiful textbook pictures of fundi are generated with a special ophthalmoscope that allows visualization of much more of the fundus than your handheld model.

Finally, begin to follow the course of the **vessels** from the fundus outward into the four quadrants. Do not subject your patient to too long an exam; divide it into two parts if necessary. Note where veins and arteries cross; look for nicking and other abnormalities. The funduscopic exam takes months to learn and years to master. In some patients it is impossible to visualize the fundi without dilating their pupils. (The ophthalmologist usually insists on dilating a patient before performing an exam.)

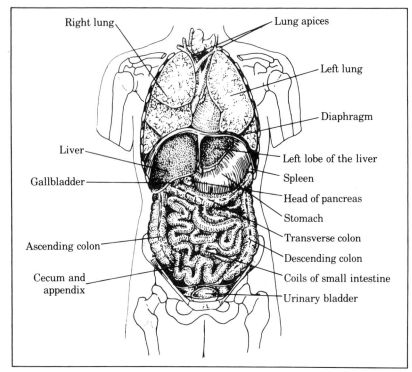

Fig. 4-10. The thorax and abdomen. (Redrawn from R. S. Snell, *Clinical Anatomy for Medical Students,* 2nd ed. Boston: Little, Brown, 1981.)

   B. The **cardiac exam** is made up of several parts. Of these, auscultation of the heart usually takes the longest time to master.

   1. The first goal of auscultation of the heart is **distinguishing systole from diastole.** This aim may sound simplistic, but it is not. Here are a few hints to make the distinction easier.

   a. Begin auscultating with the stethoscope held on the apex with one hand while your other hand gently feels the carotid pulse; the first heart sound, corresponding to closure of the atrioventricular valves and onset of systole, just precedes the carotid pulsation. This often can help you to distinguish S_1 (and therefore systole).

   b. In the absence of valvular pathology, the **intensity** of S_1 is greater than that of S_2 at the apex of the heart, while the intensity of S_2 is greater than that of S_1 at the base. (Listen at the aortic and pulmonic areas for the two components of S_2 and at the mitral area or PMI for S_1.)

   c. Although more subtle, the **pitch** of S_1 is discernibly lower than that of S_2 in most patients. Remember, high-frequency sounds are best heard with the diaphragm of your stethoscope, while low-frequency sounds are better appreciated with the bell.

   d. Remember that the PMI correlates with systole. This means that S_1 just precedes the onset of the apical impulse, which you may both see and feel with your hand and your stethoscope.

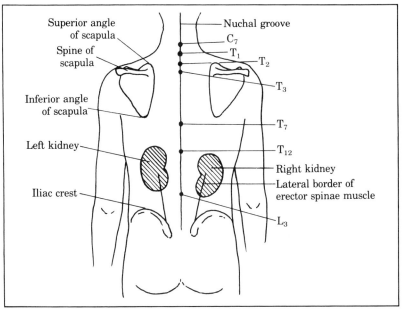

Fig. 4-11. The back. (Redrawn from R. S. Snell, *Clinical Anatomy for Medical Students,* 2nd ed. Boston: Little, Brown, 1981.)

2. **"Inching."** Once you are oriented to systole and diastole, you can begin a systematic exam. It is helpful to base this assessment on an initial, routine path of movement of the stethoscope from the aortic to the pulmonic area and down the left sternal border (tricuspid area) to the mitral area (see Fig. 4-12).

   a. Develop a specific sequence at each step in this path, in which the components of the cardiac cycle are systematically sought. Thus, at each stop along the inching "path," **listen selectively** to: S_1, S_2, other heart sounds, murmurs. It is crucial to learn to listen selectively to each of these components. Concentrate on *each* item individually in the above list, starting with S_1, at *each* step of the way. Inching will be lengthy, even tedious at first, but it will soon become routine, and it is the best way to "hear" heart sounds effectively.

3. **Maneuvering and murmur analysis.** Although a thorough description of murmur analysis is beyond the scope of this section, there are several basic points to remember from the start. Examine the patient first in the **supine position,** then the **left lateral decubitus position,** and then the **sitting position.** The murmur of aortic insufficiency is often appreciated only with the patient sitting up and leaning slightly forward. Murmurs at the apex are best heard with the patient in the left lateral decubitus position, which brings the heart closer to your stethoscope.

   It is possible to alter the character of murmurs heard by **maneuvering** your patient in certain ways. Maneuvering is the physiologic alteration of venous return, peripheral arterial resistance, or cardiac output. For instance, the hand grip increases peripheral arterial resistance, which in turn decreases the gradient across the aortic valve in systole or

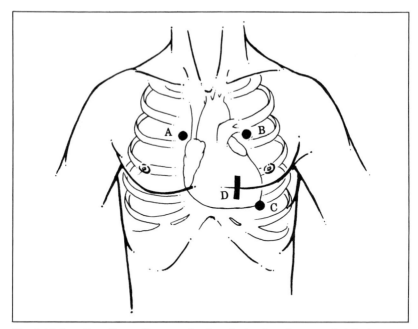

Fig. 4-12. Locations for cardiac auscultation. A. Aortic valve; second right interspace. B. Pulmonic valve; second left interspace. C. Mitral valve; apex. D. Tricuspid valve; lower left sternal border. (Modified from R. D. Judge, G. D. Zuidema, and F. T. Fitzgerald [17], p. 274.)

increases the degree of mitral regurgitation. Therefore, an aortic systolic ejection murmur can sometimes be heard to decrease in intensity with the patient doing the hand grip maneuver, while that of mitral regurgitation may increase. See Table 4-3 for a list of common maneuvers, their physiologic effects, and how they affect common murmurs.

C. The **neurologic exam** has five main parts: the mental status, motor, sensory, cranial nerve, and reflex exams. Because a thorough neurologic exam has so many specific parts, confusion often results, largely because the neurologic exam is approached in a shotgun manner during a typical physical exam sequence.

Most patients will only require a screening neurologic exam. When it is warranted, however, consider performing on appropriate patients a more complete neurologic exam, separate from and in addition to the usual screening physical exam. With the neurologic examination as your specific (and only) task, it is much easier to organize your thoughts and your work-up.

D. The **rectal exam** is sometimes difficult simply because it is unpleasant for both patient and physician; it is not hard to learn or to execute, however. (It does take practice to learn how to palpate the prostate and judge its size and firmness, but this becomes much easier over time.)

Relax yourself and your patient, be firm and gentle, and be sure to guaiac the small bit of stool that is invariably on your glove after the exam. In men, especially older men, practice defining the lobes of the prostate, assess its texture, and search for focal areas of induration. The normal prostate

Table 4-3. Effect of some physical maneuvers on cardiovascular dynamics and heart sounds

Maneuver	Peripheral resistance (afterload)	Left ventricular volume (preload)	Murmur of aortic stenosis	Murmur of hypertrophic obstructive cardiomyopathy	Murmur of mitral regurgitation	Click murmur of mitral valve prolapse	Murmur of mitral stenosis	Murmur of aortic insufficiency and Austin Flint
Supine with passive leg raising	— or ↑	↑	↑	→	—	↑	↑	—
Sitting or standing	↑	→	—	←	—	↓	—	↑ or —
Prompt squatting	↑	↑	— (early) → (late)	→	←	↑	→	←
Isometric exercise (e.g., handgrip)	↑	↑	→	→	←	↑	→	←
Valsalva maneuver	↑	→	→	↑ or → or —	→	↓	→	→
Exercise	→	→	←	←	—	↓	←	→
Amyl nitrite	→	→	←	←	→	↓	←	→

↑ = increased; ↓ = decreased; — = no change; → = later in systole; ← = earlier in systole.
Reproduced with permission from R. D. Judge, G. D. Zuidema, and F. T. Fitzgerald [17], p. 304.

should have the consistency of the tip of your nose; a harder nodule may be pathologic. In women the rectal exam is part of the pelvic exam in many cases, and it is especially important when defining the extent of gynecologic tumor and for the stool guaiac.

Do not be tentative about doing a rectal exam; it is a brief exam but a very important one. On the other hand, when first learning, you will often examine patients who have already had several rectals. It is prudent to check the chart ahead of time to see how many rectals have been done, and to defer if one has already been performed that day.

E. The **pelvic exam** is often considered separately for two reasons: it requires a special setup, and it is an examination that is extremely sensitive and personal.

  1. A male should never perform a pelvic examination without a **female chaperone** (nurse or physician) present.

  2. The exam is best learned by spending a concentrated period of time doing **several pelvic examinations each day,** for example through going on an obstetrics-gynecology rotation or by arranging to work for several consecutive days in an outpatient gynecology clinic.

  3. Traditionally, the most difficult part of the exam is the **speculum insertion.** The speculum exam should be observed several times and then practiced, paying special attention to warming and moistening the speculum before insertion, the angle at which the speculum is introduced, and opening the speculum after it is fully inserted.

F. The **breast exam.** Like the blood pressure measurement, the breast examination is one of the few parts of the physical exam that will frequently yield crucial information prompting major medical interventions in the entirely asymptomatic patient. Nearly one of nine American women will develop breast cancer, and every medical student should be familiar with its signs.

  1. **Inspection.** The patient should be disrobed to the waist and both breasts should be inspected concurrently to allow comparison. Pay particular attention to symmetry of the left and right breasts. Though it is quite common for one breast to be somewhat larger than the other, the asymmetry should not include major differences in the appearance or texture of the skin or the nipples, nor should there be lumpy irregularities in the normally smooth breast contours.

  Local areas of erythema and swelling may be due to tumor, inflammation, or merely to tight clothing, and should be carefully scrutinized. While breast cancer with lymphatic engorgement may produce only subtle changes (peau d'orange, best seen with a tangentially directed flashlight), direct skin invasion often produces an angry red cellulitic appearance that is unmistakable. Except in the nursing mother, any nipple discharge should be regarded as suspicious. Skin retraction is one of the most subtle findings in this part of the exam. It is often best appreciated in the arms-over-head and hands-against-hips maneuvers. A small, innocuous-looking bulge in the upper outer quadrant that moves up into the axilla when the arms are raised is a classic early finding in breast carcinoma.

  2. **Palpation.** Though many different sequences of breast palpation are used, all are thorough, systematic, and bimanual. One good technique for the novice involves starting at the nipple and following a clockwise spiral pattern around the breast and into the axilla. The fingertips are used alternately to compress and push the breast tissue toward the other hand. The palms of the hand are less sensitive and do not play

a major role in this technique. If a suspicious area is felt, it is localized under the examiner's fingertips with the patient's arms down. The arms are then slowly raised over the head to allow an assessment of mobility of the lesion.

In addition to a careful breast exam, it is critical to investigate thoroughly the possibility of associated lymphadenopathy in the axillary and supraclavicular regions in all patients.

The **axilla** must be deeply palpated with the patient's arm draped across the chest to accomplish maximal relaxation of the pectoral muscles. Once again, asymmetry between the left and the right breast may be the only clue to an abnormal finding.

3. **Recording the exam.** Accurate recording of the breast exam is absolutely crucial and may spare the patient unnecessary surgery at some point in the future. It is usually best to accompany a verbal description with diagrams and precise polar coordinates (e.g., "a 2-cm by 3-cm freely mobile mass located in the 3 o'clock position, 2.5 cm from the areolar edge"). For premenopausal patients, the exact position in the menstrual cycle at the time of the exam should also be noted.

4. **Benign processes,** including chronic cystic mastitis and fibroadenomas, are common in the breast, and the vast majority of breast masses are not malignant. However, serial breast exams with mammographic correlation provide the best means of detecting this very common malignancy in its early stages.

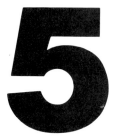

Pediatric History and Physical Exam

There are three issues which must be understood and addressed in *the care of adolescent–young adult patients*. First, the history must be given by the patient alone. Parents may, of course, make their contribution, but not initially. Second, the physical examination is not complete unless the sexual maturation stage is noted and recorded. Third, the patient must be informed at the close of the evaluation what the diagnostic possibilities are, what tests and studies are necessary and why, and what treatment is planned, giving the responsibility to the patient, not the parents, for carrying out the therapy. Following these simple guidelines will open up the opportunity for you to talk about and counsel in the more sensitive areas of behavior, sexuality, education, career decisions, drugs, and alcohol. Care for your adolescent patients—don't delegate and triage!

Robert P. Masland, Jr., M.D.

The toughest pediatric patients to examine are young toddlers aged 9 months to 2½ years. Even the most experienced and skilled physicians will usually be met by a screaming child who continues to scream even if the child is repeatedly examined by the same person.

In this age group I have always found it helpful to begin the examination with the child in a parent's lap, on a chair rather than on the examining table. A brief period might be spent trying to find ways to, at best, entertain the child and, at least, let them know you won't hurt them. The exam should begin with the heart since this may be the only opportunity to examine the child while he/she is not (yet) crying. After the cardiac exam, the physical assessment can be continued in any order as long as it remains systematic. As much of the exam as possible should be performed in the caretaker's lap, including abdominal and otoscopic examinations.

Michael Shannon, M.D., M.P.H.

In this chapter we will describe how to conduct those parts of the physical examination of infants and children that require a different approach or technique from those used in the physical examination of adults. When assessing an infant or a child, always consider where the patient is on the continuum of growth and development. In general it is helpful to think of the pediatric population as having **four developmental levels: infancy** (the first year), **early childhood** (age 1–4), **late childhood** (age 5–12), and **adolescence** (age 13–20).

| A | **Annotated Outline of Pediatric History and Physical Exam** |

I. The pediatric history

A. General approach

1. When conducting the history, establish a **rapport with both the patient and the parents.** All too often the examiner focuses on the parents and neglects the child, who should be the ultimate focus of the examiner's attention. Though the history is obtained from the child's primary caregiver, much valuable information can be elicited from the child. Inattention to the child during the history taking will make the physical examination much more difficult, from a comfort standpoint for the child and from an informational standpoint for the clinician.

2. When taking a history from an adolescent, be sure to **set some time aside to talk to the young adult alone,** to give the patient an opportunity to discuss problems or issues that he or she would not be comfortable discussing in front of a parent or guardian.

B. Past medical history. The amount of detail here depends on the nature of the problem and the age of the child. In general, the younger the child the more pertinent perinatal events become.

1. **Antenatal.** Health of mother during pregnancy (prenatal care, diet, weight gain, infections such as toxoplasmosis, syphilis, rubella, cytomegalovirus (CMV), hepatitis, AIDS, and toxemia), Rh typing and serology, other pregnancy outcomes. Medications taken, quantity taken. Drug, cigarette, or alcohol use.

2. **Natal.** Sedation and anesthesia used, labor description, type of delivery, Apgar scores, birth weight, gestational age.

3. **Neonatal.** Color, cry, cyanosis, excessive mucus, anemia, jaundice, twitching, paralysis, convulsions, fever, hemorrhage, congenital or acquired abnormalities, difficulty in sucking, rashes, excessive weight loss, feeding difficulties.

4. **Development.** Tailor assessment to the age and condition of child. For infants and toddlers, observe and evaluate development through the Denver Developmental Screening Test. For older children, compare development to that of siblings and peers, look at performance in school. With all children, inquire about any period of failure of growth or unusual growth (check percentile records if available).

5. **Nutrition.** This should be detailed for infants and toddlers.

   a. Breast milk or formula: type, duration, major formula changes, time of weaning, and difficulties.

   b. Vitamin supplements: type, when started, amount, duration.

   c. Solid foods: when introduced, how taken, types, how tolerated.

   d. Appetite: food likes and dislikes, allergies, reaction of child to eating, pica.

6. **Illness.** Contagious diseases: age; complications following measles, rubella, chicken pox, mumps, pertussis, scarlet fever.

7. **Immunizations.** Record routine and other immunizations, including age at time of administration and any adverse reactions. Record also tuberculin tests and responses.

8. **Operations.** Type, age, complications, reasons for operations, apparent response of child.

9. **Unintentional injuries.** Nature, permanent sequelae. **Note:** Many children present to physicians with "accidents." Most injuries are just accidents, but **be aware of the possibility of child abuse.** If you suspect child abuse, notify your preceptor or resident. You are legally bound to report suspected child abuse.

10. **Habits and behavior**

   a. Eating: appetite, food dislikes, how fed, attitudes of child and parents to eating.

   b. Sleeping: hours, disturbances, snoring.

   c. Exercise and play.

   d. Urinary and bowel: toilet training completion, accidents.

   e. Disturbances: excessive bed wetting, thumb sucking, nail biting, breath holding, temper tantrums, tics, nervousness, undue thirst; similar disturbances among other members of the family.

   f. Relations with other children: level of independence, ability to separate from parents, hobbies; negativistic, shy, submissive, easy or difficult to get along with.

   g. School progress: class, grades, nursery school, special aptitudes, reaction to school.

C. **Social history.** Who is child's primary caregiver? What adults live in the household with the child? If both parents do not live with the child, how much of a participant is the child's absent parent?

D. **Family history.** Critical in pediatric history, due to the abundance of inherited disorders.

II. **The pediatric physical exam.** Following is a step-by-step outline of the pediatric physical exam, highlighting what to look for in children that is different from adults.

A. **General appearance.** How the child is dressed; cleanliness; does the child look sick?

B. **Vital signs.** Temperature, pulse, respiratory rate, blood pressure, body length (to six years) or height, weight; head circumference in infants. Place height, weight, and head circumference in percentiles for age.

   1. **Temperature.** For infants and children younger than 5 years, rectal temperatures should be used almost exclusively because accurate oral temperature readings are difficult to obtain. Rectal temperatures may be one degree higher than oral temperatures. A rectal temperature up to 100° F may be considered normal in a child. Activity, apprehension, and fear may elevate the temperature.

   2. **Heart rate.** Obtain the heart rate in infants by observing the pulsations of the anterior fontanelle, by palpation of the carotid or femoral arteries, or by direct auscultation of the heart if the rate is very rapid. Palpate the radial artery in older children and in young children who are cooperative. The heart rate in infants and children is quite labile and more sensitive to the effects of illness, exercise, and emotion than that in adults.

   3. **Respiratory rate.** In infancy and early childhood, diaphragmatic breathing is predominant and thoracic excursion is minimal; therefore, you can more easily ascertain the respiratory rate by observing abdominal rather than chest excursion.

4. **Blood pressure.** With children, unlike adults, the point at which sounds first become muffled is recorded as the diastolic pressure. At times, especially in early infancy, the heart sounds are not audible, due to a narrow or deeply placed brachial artery; in such instances palpate the radial artery at the wrist to determine the blood pressure. The point at which the pulse is first felt is recorded as the systolic pressure. This is approximately 10 mm Hg lower than the systolic pressure determined by auscultation. The diastolic pressure cannot be determined by using the radial pulse method.

C. **Skin.** Color, texture, cyanosis, erythema, rash, edema, hemorrhagic manifestations, dilated vessels, hemangiomas and nevi, Mongolian blue spots, pigmentation, turgor and elasticity.

1. **Loss of turgor,** especially of the calf muscles and skin over the abdomen, is evidence of dehydration. Roll a fold of loosely adherent skin on the abdominal wall between your thumb and forefinger to determine its consistency, the amount of subcutaneous tissue, and the degree of hydration.

2. The soles and the palms are often bluish and cold in early infancy **(acrocyanosis);** this is of no significance.

3. The degree of **anemia** cannot be determined reliably by inspection, since pallor (even in the newborn) may be normal and not due to anemia.

4. To demonstrate **pitting edema** in a child, it may be necessary to exert prolonged pressure.

5. Use natural daylight rather than artificial light when evaluating for the presence of **jaundice** at any age. In borderline cases, press a glass slide against the infant's cheek. This will help you detect the presence of jaundice by producing a blanched background for contrast.

D. **HEENT**

1. **Head.** Size, shape, symmetry of face and skull, control, molding, hydrocephalus, craniotabes, cephalohematoma, fontanelles (size, tension, number, abnormally late or early closure, sutures).

   Examine the anterior fontanelle for tenseness and fullness while the baby is quietly sitting or being held in an upright position.

2. **Eyes.** Photophobia, visual acuity, muscular control, nystagmus, Mongolian slant, epicanthal folds, lacrimation, conjunctivae, pupillary size and reaction, fundi, fields by confrontation (older children and adolescents).

   a. The assessment of vision in **the newborn** is based on the presence of visual reflexes: direct and consensual pupillary constriction in response to light, blinking in response to bright light and to movement of an object quickly toward the eyes, and red reflex to rule out retinoblastoma.

   b. **Visual field assessment.** In infants and young children, this can be done with the child sitting on the parent's lap. Hold the head in midline while bringing a dangling object or a toy into the child's field of vision from several points behind, above, and below. Deviation of the eyes in the object's direction indicates that the child has seen the object.

3. **Ears.** Pinna, canals, tympanic membranes (landmarks, perforation, inflammation, discharge), hearing acuity. Note position of ears in relation to eyes.

a. **Auditory acuity.** Elicit the acoustic blink reflex. This is positive when one observes a blinking of the eyes in response to a sudden sharp sound produced by snapping the fingers or clapping the hands at a distance of 12 inches from the ear.

b. **Allaying fear of the ear examination.** Before actually examining the ears, it is often helpful to place the otoscopic speculum gently into the external auditory canal, removing it instantly and repeating the procedure on the other canal. Then you can begin again, taking the necessary time in the actual examination, when the child's apprehensions have been allayed.

c. **Patient position.** Place the patient in a supine position and have parent or assistant hold the child's arms extended, close to the sides of the head, thus limiting movement from side to side. This position will be used for both the ear and the throat exam.

d. **Examination of the ear.** To examine the right ear, turn the child's head to the left and hold it firmly in this position with the lateral aspect of your right hand and wrist. Hold the otoscope in your right hand in an inverted position, and manipulate the auricle with your left hand, using the lateral aspect of your hand to help restrain movement of the child's head. In infancy and early childhood, the external auditory canal is directed upward and backward from the outside, and the pinna must be pulled upward, outward, and backward to afford the best visualization. The thumb and forefinger of your right hand, which holds the otoscope, should be buffered from sudden movements of the child's head by your restraining right hand and your forearm, which rests firmly on the examining table. The left ear is examined in a similar way.

e. **Pneumatic otoscopy.** This should be part of every otoscopic exam; it is accomplished by observing the tympanic membrane as the pressure in the external auditory canal is increased or decreased. You can do this by insufflating with a rubber squeeze bulb.

4. **Nose.** Exterior, mucosa, patency, discharge, bleeding, pressure over sinuses. Most infants are obligate nose breathers, so when checking patency of nares do not occlude both at the same time.

5. **Mouth.** Lips, teeth, mucosa, palate, tongue, mouth breathing.

6. **Throat.** Tonsils (size, inflammation, exudate, crypts, inflammation of the anterior pillars), mucosa, hypertrophic lymphoid tissue, postnasal drip, epiglottis, voice (hoarseness, stridor, grunting).

a. Before examining a child's throat, it is advisable to examine his mouth. Permit the child to handle the tongue blade and nasal speculum, to help him or her overcome a fear of the instruments. Then ask the child to stick out his tongue and say "ah," more and more loudly. In some cases this may allow an adequate examination. In others, if the child is cooperative enough, he or she may be asked to "pant like a puppy"; while the patient is doing this, the tongue blade is applied firmly to the rear of the tongue. Gagging need not be elicited to obtain a satisfactory examination. In still other cases, it may be expedient to examine one side of the tongue at a time, pushing the base of the tongue to one side and then the other. This may be less unpleasant for the child and is less apt to cause gagging.

b. Young children may have to be restrained to allow you to obtain an adequate examination of the throat. Eliciting a gag reflex may be necessary if the oropharynx is to be adequately seen. The small child's head may be satisfactorily restrained by having the parent place his or her hands at the level of the child's elbows, holding the child's arms firmly against the sides of the child's head. If the child can sit up, the parent is asked to hold the child erect in his or her lap, with the child's back against the parent's chest. The parent then holds the child's left hand in his or her left hand and the child's right hand in his or her right, and places them against the child's groin or lower thighs to prevent the child from slipping down in the parent's lap.

E. Neck. Thyroid, stiffness. To detect nuchal rigidity in early and late childhood, have the child sit with legs extended on the examining table. Normally children should be able to sit upright and voluntarily touch their chin to their chest.

F. Lymph nodes. Location, size, sensitivity, mobility, consistency. Enlargement of the lymph nodes occurs much more readily in the child than in the adult. Small inguinal lymph nodes are palpable in almost all healthy children.

G. Thorax. Shape and symmetry, retractions, paradoxical breathing.

H. Lungs. Type of breathing, expansion, flatness or dullness to percussion, fremitus, resonance, breath and voice sounds, rales, wheezing.

   1. Expiration is more prolonged in infants and children relative to adults.

   2. The stethoscope may be a very threatening instrument to a young child. Your success in placing it on the child's chest will be enhanced if you allow the child to manipulate it or listen through it first.

I. Heart. Carefully check peripheral pulses bilaterally to rule out murmurs, ventricular heave, evidence of right- or left-sided failure.

   1. Pediatric cardiac pathology often differs from that seen in an adult, and auscultation is much more difficult, since the heart rate is higher in the child. Nevertheless the examinations are the same.

J. Abdomen. Size and contour, visible peristalsis, respiratory movements, umbilicus, tenderness, rigidity, shifting dullness, hepatosplenomegaly.

   1. The abdomen may be examined while the child is lying in the prone position in the mother's lap or held over her shoulder, or seated on the examining table with his or her back to the physician. In the infant, the examination may be aided by having the child nurse at a bottle or a pacifier. These positions may be particularly helpful when tenderness or rigidity is present or a mass is suspected.

   2. Obtain abdominal relaxation by holding the infant's legs flexed at the knees and hips with one hand, and palpate with the other. You can avoid the spasm and rigidity encountered in palpating the abdomen of a crying infant by administering a bottle or a sugar nipple.

K. Genitalia

   1. Male. Hypospadias, phimosis, adherent foreskin, cryptorchidism, hydrocele, hernia, size of penis (midshaft diameter) and testes (length and width), testicular torsion, pubertal changes.

      a. Testicular retractibility can be overcome by having the child sit in a cross-legged squatting position on the examining table, as illustrated in Fig. 5-1. A diagnosis of undescended testicle should not be made until you have palpated the inguinal canal and scrotum with the patient in this position.

   2. Female. Vagina (imperforate, discharge, adhesions), clitoral hypertrophy, pubertal changes.

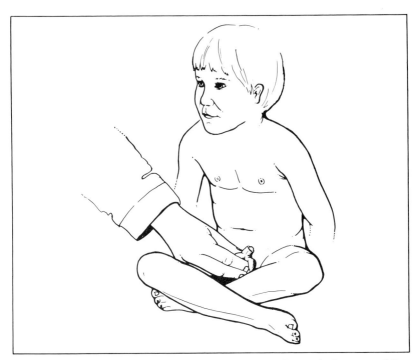

Fig. 5-1. Use the cross-legged squatting position to examine testicular retractibility. (Redrawn from B. A. Bates [4].)

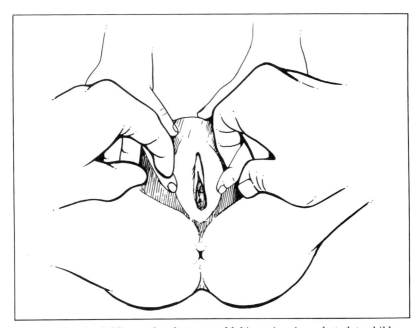

Fig. 5-2. Use the child's own hands to spread labia majora in early to late childhood, prior to puberty. (Redrawn from B. A. Bates [4].)

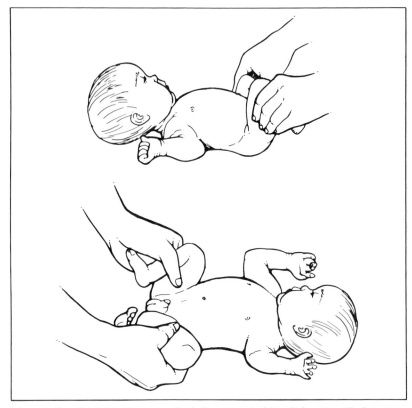

Fig. 5-3. Use the Ortolani test to check for congenital hip dislocation. (Redrawn from B. A. Bates [4].)

   a. Digital or speculum examination is rarely done until after puberty, but the vagina and cervix often can be visualized with infant in a knees-to-chest position.

   b. The examination of the genitalia in a child in early or late childhood can be made easier for you and more comfortable for the child by using the child's own hands to spread the labia majora, as shown in Fig. 5-2. This will both distract and reassure her.

L. Rectum. Imperforate anus, pinworms.

   1. In infants, **digital examination** is done only for a specific indication. Use little finger and insert slowly. Note muscle tone, character of stool masses. Examine stool on glove finger (gross, microscopic, culture, guaiac).

M. Extremities

   1. General. Deformities, hemiatrophy, bowleggedness, knock-knee, paralysis, muscle weakness.

   2. Joints. Swelling, erythema, pain, limitations, rheumatic nodules; hip dislocation or fracture and clavicular fractures may occur during the birth process.

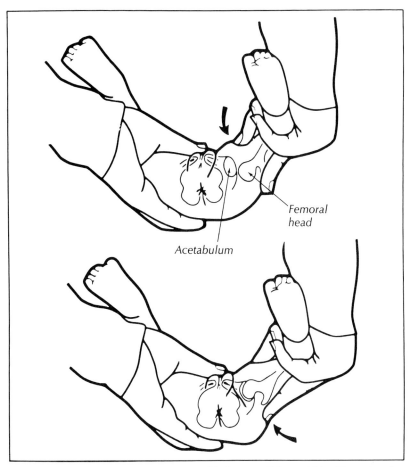

Fig. 5-4. Technique for detecting an unstable but not dislocated hip. (Reproduced with permission from J. W. Burnside, *Physical Diagnosis: An Introduction to Clinical Medicine,* 16th ed. Baltimore: Williams & Wilkins, 1981. P. 246.)

    a. To detect congenital dislocation of the hip in the infant, use the **Ortolani test** (Fig. 5-3). Place the baby in the supine position with the legs pointing toward you. Flex the legs to right angles at the hips and knees, placing your middle fingers over the greater trochanter of each femur and your thumbs over the lesser trochanter. Abduct (push in) and adduct (push out) each hip, one at a time, while stabilizing the other hip by putting the lateral aspect of the knee you wish to stabilize against the examining table. If there is congenital dislocation, you will hear a click and feel movement of the femoral head, as it lies in the posterior acetabulum.

    To detect an unstable (nondislocated but potentially dislocatable) hip, place your thumb medially over the lesser trochanter and use your index or middle finger laterally over the greater trochanter as shown in Fig. 5-4. Press your thumb backward and outward. Feel for movement of the head of the femur against some resistance, as it slips out onto the posterior lip of the acetabulum. Normally no movement is felt. Then, with your index or middle finger press the greater trochanter forward and inward. Feel for a sudden movement of the femoral head inward as it returns to the hip socket. Again, movement is not normally felt.

    3. **Hands and feet.** Extra digits, clubbing, simian crease, splinter hemorrhages, koilonychia.

N. Neurologic exam. Cranial nerves, reflexes, gait, ataxia, strabismus, nystagmus, muscle strength, sensation, developmental delay or reemergence of vanished responses.

The Babinski response and clonus are normal for the first year of life.

O. Spine and back. Posture, curvatures, rigidity, webbed neck, spina bifida, pilonidal dimple or cyst, Mongolian spot.

B   Practical Points for the Pediatric Physical Exam

I. **Approaching the child.** Time should be spent in becoming acquainted with the child and allowing the child to become acquainted with you. A friendly manner, quiet voice, and a slow and easy approach will help to facilitate the examination. If, however, you are not able to establish a friendly feeling between the child and yourself, and if you feel it is important that the examination be performed at that time, you should proceed with the physical examination in an orderly, systematic manner in the hope that the child will then accept the inevitable.

II. **Observation of the patient.** Although the very young child may not be able to speak, one may still gather a lot of information by observing the child. Much useful information can be gained by observing how the parent and child interact and how the patient relates to the examiner. The neurologic examination of a toddler may often consist mostly or even solely of watching the child play, run, jump, and so on. The need to observe the child cannot be overemphasized. Spend time watching the child and thinking about what you see.

III. **Developmental assessment.** It is best to perform the developmental assessment before subjecting the child to upsetting parts of the examination. It is important to observe what the child can and cannot do.

IV. **Holding the child for the examination**

    A. **Younger than 6 months:** examining table usually is well tolerated. **Never walk away and leave the child unattended.**

    B. **6 months to 3–4 years:** Often the examination may be carried out while the child is held in the caregiver's lap, over his or her shoulder, or with the caregiver standing at the head of the table while holding the child's hands.

V. **Removal of clothing.** Clothing should be removed gradually, in order that the child will not be chilled and to prevent the development of resistance in a shy child. To save time and to avoid creating unpleasant associations with the physician in the child's mind, undressing the child and taking his or her temperature are best performed by the parent or caregiver. The physician should respect the marked degree of modesty that may be exhibited by some children. Underpants may be left on during the examination and removed only when necessary.

VI. Sequence of examination. It is best to explain the purpose of the instruments and maybe even to permit the child to handle them before starting the various parts of the examination. In most cases it is best to begin the examination of the young child with an area that is least likely to be associated with pain or discomfort. **Heart and lungs should be examined first; ears, throat, and any other areas that will be sensitive or painful to the child should always be examined last.**

The Language of Labs

> Nothing is more important to the care of the patient than the personal attention of a competent and conscientious physician. There is no substitute for the information a physician can obtain from a careful history and physical examination. This information should guide all diagnostic and therapeutic efforts. Without it, laboratory tests cannot be used effectively, therapeutic plans lack direction, and serious errors in management are likely to occur. The greatest mistake in the practice of internal medicine these days is the tendency to let indiscriminate laboratory testing and diagnostic procedures replace the common sense of the doctor.
>
> **Arnold S. Relman, M.D.**

One of the most important skills that you need to learn as you begin on the wards is how to "work up" a patient. This involves interviewing and examining a new patient, and then determining what steps need to be taken to diagnose and treat the patient's illness. One of the primary tools for diagnosis, as well as for following the course of disease, is the laboratory test.

This chapter will discuss some of the things you need to keep in mind when deciding when to order tests and how to interpret their results. Some of this is quite complex, but the bottom line is simple: **Always know why you are ordering a test, and what you will do with each possible result, before you order it.** This will serve your patient, by reducing false-positive results and inconvenience, as well as society, by cutting down on wasteful medical spending.

I. Ordering tests

A. Routine tests. In the past, most admitted patients were given a battery of routine tests, and then, presented with this data, a clinician would make a diagnosis. Many studies have found little use for such "routine" tests. Durbridge and colleagues in Australia, for instance, randomly selected 1,500 patients to either receive a battery of 50 tests on admission, or to get only the needed ones. They found no difference in mortality, morbidity, length of stay, or any other clinical parameter between those who got the routine battery and those who did not, but they did see higher costs and lower patient satisfaction in the routine-test group [11].

B. Scientific method. Good clinicians use a variant of the scientific method in deciding when to order tests. As you take a history and examine the patient, you should be generating a list of hypotheses as to what is wrong. Further questions and physical signs may narrow this list of hypotheses, called the **differential diagnosis.** Next, you should order only those tests needed to either confirm or rule out these hypotheses; use their results to narrow your list further or to generate new hypotheses. The reiterative method will lead most efficiently to the proper diagnosis.

C. **Consequences.** In addition to thinking about the chances of getting a false positive or a false negative when ordering a test (see **II.B**), you should think about the consequences of each. The consequences of a false positive HIV test for an individual, for instance, could be huge, including loss of insurance and job, much anguish, and so on. In testing blood in a blood bank, on the other hand, the consequences of a false positive may be small (i.e., you throw away one unit of blood), while the consequences of a false negative may be huge (i.e., a recipient might get infected).

D. **Costs.** In an era of limited medical resources, you should keep in mind the cost of the lab tests you are ordering. Although most patients are insured and do not face the full cost of the work-ups you order, we all collectively pay for them through our insurance premiums and our taxes. Being able to conduct cost-effective work-ups will be a much valued skill for you in the future, and you should get into the habit of thinking about this aspect of medicine early in your career.

II. Interpreting tests

A. **Lab tests and probability.** Lab tests, like most things in life, are not perfect. The best they can do is affect what we think is the probability of some outcome. Before doing a test, we have some notion of how likely it is that a person has a given disease (called the pretest probability), and the test simply changes that likelihood (the post-test probability) either up or down.

For instance, suppose a 45-year-old man comes to you with chest pain. After taking a good history and physical, you conclude that there is a 64 percent chance that he is having a heart attack. To test this hypothesis, you check his serum creatine phosphokinase (CK), which is usually elevated with myocardial infarcts. If the test is positive (the patient has a serum CK above a certain cutoff), then you can raise the probability that he is having a heart attack to 93 percent, while if the CK is below the cutoff, you can drop the probability to 12 percent. The basic point is this: **A positive test does not guarantee the patient has the disease, and a negative test does not ensure absence of disease.**

B. **False and true results.** Let us go into this a little bit further, using the example of serum CK and myocardial infarction. Say we did a study in which we measured the CK of 360 men who had chest pain, and then also used another test to definitively diagnose whether they indeed had suffered a heart attack. (Such a definitive test is called a **gold standard,** as it is the basis of comparison for all other tests). The results of the test are summarized in the following table:

	MI	No MI	Total
Test positive (CK ≥ 80)	215 (a)	16 (b)	231 (a + b)
Test negative (CK < 80)	15 (c)	114 (d)	129 (c + d)
Total	230 (a + c)	130 (b + d)	360 (a + b + c + d)

1. **True positives** (a): those who tested positive and really had an MI.

2. **False positives** (b): those who tested positive but did not have an MI.

3. **True negatives** (d): those who tested negative and had no MI.

4. **False negatives** (c): those who tested negative but really did have an MI.

C. **Test characteristics.** How good a test is depends on its rates of false positives and false negatives. Ideally, one would like to have none of either, but in most cases there is a tradeoff between them. Thus, as you change the cutoff of the test, you change the ratio of false positives to false negatives. If we made the CK cutoff very high (e.g., called the test positive only if CK ≥ 200), we would have almost no false positives, but we would get many false negatives. If we made the cutoff low, on the other hand, we would get very few false negatives, but many false positives. We can quantify these characteristics of a test by two measures: the **sensitivity** and the **specificity.**

1. **Sensitivity** (a/[a + c]) tells how well the test does among those with disease; that is, of those who really had a heart attack, how many did we find with our test? In this case, the sensitivity is 215/(215 + 15) = 93 percent.

2. **Specificity** (d/[b + d]) tells how the test does in the world of the nondiseased; that is, of those without MI, how many tested negative? In this case, the specificity is 114/(114 + 16) = 88 percent.

D. **Predictive values.** These two statistics tell us about how good a test is, but in real life we do not know if a person really has the disease or not (if we did, we wouldn't have to do a test at all). What we really want to know is this: if a test result is positive or negative, what is the probability that the patient either has or does not have the disease?

1. **Positive predictive value** (a/[a + b]) tells us what proportion of those with positive test results really have the disease. Here, if you have a positive test, your probability of having an MI was 215/(215 + 16) = 93 percent.

2. **Negative predictive value** (d/[c + d]) tells us what proportion of those with negative test results really did not have an MI. In this case, if you had a negative CK test, your probability of not having an MI was 114/(114 + 15) = 88 percent.

E. **Back to probabilities.** Now we can go back to the statements we made earlier in the chapter. The pretest probability of MI in this situation is also called the:

1. **Prevalence** ([a + c]/[a + b + c + d]), which is the proportion of people in the test group (i.e., men with chest pain) who had an MI. Here, this is 230/360 = 64 percent.

   Now we see that a positive test makes the **post-test probability** 93 percent (the positive predictive value), while a negative test makes it 12 percent (1 minus the negative predictive value).

F. **Prevalence and probability.** Note that the positive and negative predictive values of a test are very dependent on the pretest probability or prevalence of disease. This is an especially important issue in **HIV testing.** The usual screening test used for HIV disease is called the ELISA (see Chap. 24), which has a sensitivity of 99.6 percent and a specificity of 99.2 percent.

Even with such good test characteristics, the positive predictive value of the ELISA test varies greatly with the pretest probability of disease. For instance, if we know that the prevalence of HIV in gay men in San Francisco is 50 percent, then the positive predictive value of the test in this group is 99.2 percent. (This calculation uses Bayes' theorem, which is beyond the scope of this book. You should review or learn it if you do not already know it; see the references at the end of this volume for help. The general idea involves creating grids like the one in **II.B.**) On the other hand, if the prevalence of HIV in male army recruits is only 0.16 percent, the positive predictive value of the test in members of that group is only 16.6 percent.

Thus, how you interpret a test, even one with extremely high specificity and sensitivity, depends greatly on what you think the pretest probability of the disease is. In gay men in San Francisco, a positive HIV test is more than 99 percent likely to indicate they are infected with the HIV virus, while in male army recruits, a positive test indicates a less than 17 percent probability of their having HIV, because there are many more false positives than true positives in this group.

G. In the next few chapters we will discuss several major categories of lab tests. For each category, we will look at the indications for ordering the tests, the basis for interpreting their results, and useful tips for a beginning student on the wards. While reading each section, and while in the hospital, you should keep in mind the concepts discussed in this chapter. Ordering the proper tests and interpreting them correctly is truly one of the hallmarks of an excellent clinician.

Hematologic Tests

Outline of Hematologic Tests

I. **Reasons for ordering general hematologic tests.** These tests provide useful information on four general categories of disease processes:

A. **Hematopoietic problems,** such as anemia and leukemia, both of which involve an alteration in the number and function of the blood cells.

B. **Systemic diseases,** especially renal and liver disease, which alter the hematologic environment, causing morphologic and functional changes in the blood cells.

C. **Infection,** which often results in increased total leukocyte count. Depending on whether this increase is predominantly toward early myeloid forms ("shift to the left") or toward lymphoid forms, one can draw a general conclusion about the nature of the insult.

D. **Hemostatic problems,** which often manifest themselves through a protracted clotting time on one or more of the clotting screens.

II. **Specific hematologic tests**

A. **Complete blood count (CBC) and red cell indices.** In most hospitals, the CBC is a mechanized spectrophotometric analysis of an anticoagulated specimen of the peripheral blood. It results in a reasonably accurate estimate of the number, size, and hemoglobin content of the erythrocytes. The reported results include the **hematocrit** (Hct), the **red blood cell count** (RBC) and **white blood cell count** (WBC), the **hemoglobin concentration** (Hgb), and the red cell morphologic indices **(mean corpuscular volume [MCV]**, **mean corpuscular hemoglobin [MCH]**, **mean corpuscular hemoglobin concentration** [MCHC])**. See Table 7-1 for normal values.

B. **Differential white cell count.** The differential (commonly called the "diff"), either done by machine or manually by a technician, is a quantitation of the proportions of different types of leukocytes in the smear of the patient's peripheral blood. It is reported as the percent of total leukocytes made up by each individual type of white cell.

C. **Blood smear analysis.** The smear analysis involves an inspection, under high magnification, of the size and appearance of the red and white cells.

D. **Platelet count and clotting indices.** The platelet count and the clotting indices are mechanized tests that screen for hemostatic problems. The usual battery of hemostatic tests includes, in addition to a platelet count, a **prothrombin time** (PT) and a **partial thromboplastin time** (PTT). Other clotting-factor tests may be ordered if the results of the initial screening battery are abnormal, or if a specific defect is suspected.

Table 7-1. Complete blood count: normal values and ranges

Hct: Men: 47 ± 7.0
Women: 42 ± 5.0

Hgb: Men: 14–18 gm/100 ml
Women: 12–16 gm/100 ml

MCV: 85–100 μm³; **MCH:** 28–31 μμg; **MCHC:** 30–35%

RBC: Diameter: 7.3–7.5 μ
Men: 4.2–5.4 × 10⁶ cells/mm³
Women: 3.6–5.0 × 10⁶ cells/mm³
Reticulocytes: 0.5–1.5%

WBC: Total: 4–11 × 10³ cells/mm³
Diff
PMN: 40–75%
Lymphocytes: 15–45%
Eosinophils: 1–6%
Basophils: 0–2%
Monocytes: 1–10%

Platelets: 145–375 × 10³/mm³

PT: Depends on lab; usually ~ 12–14 sec. Always given with control; should be within 2 secs of control.

PTT: Depends on lab; usually 25–45 sec. Always given with control; should be within 4 secs of control.

ESR: Wintrobe
Men: 0–5 mm/hr
Women: 0–15 mm/hr
Westergren
Men: 0–15 mm/hr
Women: 0–20 mm/hr

E. **Erythrocyte sedimentation rate.** The erythrocyte sedimentation rate (ESR) is a nonspecific test that is loosely correlated with the serum levels of fibrinogen and globulin. It is especially useful in screening for malignancy, connective tissue disorders, and infection, and in following the course of chronic inflammatory disease states.

III. **Analyzing and interpreting results of hematologic tests**

A. **Complete blood count and indices**

1. The **hematocrit** and the **red blood cell count** are reflections of the concentration of erythrocytes in the blood. Although the hematocrit will usually indicate whether or not the patient has some degree of anemia, you must analyze it together with the hemoglobin concentration and the red cell indices to determine the class of anemia (e.g., hypochromic microcytic versus normochromic normocytic) and thereby to gain insight into the etiology of the anemia.

2. The **red cell indices** represent average values for the size and hemoglobin content of the red cells. They are calculated as follows:

$$MCV = \frac{Hct\,(\%) \times 10}{RBC\,(millions/mm^3)}$$

Normal range is 85–100 μm³.

$$MCH = \frac{Hgb\,(gm/100\,ml) \times 10}{RBC\,(millions/mm^3)}$$

Normal range is 28–31 μμg.

$$\text{MCHC} = \frac{\text{Hgb (gm/100 ml)}}{\text{Hct (\%)}}$$

Normal range is 30–35%.

Fig. 7-1 represents an approach to the differential diagnosis of anemia based on the red cell indices and the reticulocyte count.

3. The **total white blood cell count** is useful both as a diagnostic tool and in following the course of diseases. Shown below are the most common types of processes associated with decreased and increased WBC values.

  a. Processes consistent with **WBC decrease:**

  (1) Infections, especially overwhelming bacterial infection, septicemia, and so on.

  (2) Viral infections: infectious mono, hepatitis, influenza.

  (3) Drugs, for example, sulfonamides, antibiotics.

  (4) Radiation and cytotoxic chemotherapy.

  (5) Hematologic diseases: pernicious and aplastic anemia.

  b. Processes consistent with **WBC increase:**

  (1) Acute infections: pneumonia, meningitis, rheumatic fever, septicemia.

  (2) Intoxications: uremia, acidosis, eclampsia, chemical poison, drugs (e.g., prednisone).

  (3) Leukemia.

B. **Differential white blood cell count.** This reflects the response of the bone marrow hematopoietic feedback systems to physiologic and pathologic processes. Although the differential is usually too nonspecific to suggest an exact diagnosis, it is a fairly convenient way of following the course of many types of diseases, especially infections and neoplastic processes. For these two types of disease, it is also useful to analyze the maturity of the various leukocyte types. In general, high numbers of immature cells in the peripheral blood reflect either a "push on the marrow" to produce these cells in large quantities (e.g., a common manifestation of a bacterial pneumonia is a "shift to the left," with high numbers of immature granulocytes [bands] seen on the diff) or a developmental arrest suggesting primary hematologic disease. Following are pictures of the disease processes associated with increases and decreases in the proportions of the various specific leukocyte types reported on the diff. **An erythrocyte is shown on the right in images 2–5 for size comparison.**

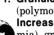

1. **Granulocytes**
   (polymorphonuclear [PMN])
   Increase consistent with infections (endocarditis, pneumonia, septicemia), granulocytic leukemia, burns, eclampsia, RBC destruction.
   Decrease consistent with drugs, viral infections, bone marrow invasion or aplasia.

2. **Lymphocytes**
   Increase consistent with infections (mononucleosis, infectious hepatitis, and other viral infections), TB, lymphocytic leukemias.

3. Monocytes
Increase consistent with monocytic leukemia, TB, myeloproliferative disorders, HD, lipid storage diseases, SBE, collagen disease (RA, SLE), chronic infection or inflammation.

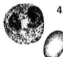

4. Eosinophils
Increase consistent with allergic disorders (asthma, hay fever), parasitic infection, collagen vascular disease, pernicious anemia, Addison's disease.
Decrease consistent with hypercortisolism, infections.

5. Basophils
Increase consistent with CML, polycythemia, myeloid metaplasia.

C. **Blood smear analysis.** While the WBC differential is concerned primarily with the association between disease processes and the **proportions** of various leukocytes seen in the blood, the blood smear analysis is concerned primarily with the association between disease processes and red and white blood cell **morphology.** Since the morphology of blood cells is a function of both **intracellular events** and **extracellular environment,** analysis of the peripheral smear is a simple and powerful screening test for assessing systemic disease as well as cellular metabolic pathology.

Following are images of the most significant abnormalities commonly noted in red cells and leukocytes (together with the pathophysiologic basis for these abnormalities) and the common differential diagnoses associated with them.

Abnormality	Significance	Seen In
1. Red cell abnormal forms **A.** Target cells	Increase in surface-volume ratio	Liver disease, hemoglobinopathies, thalassemia, Fe^{2+} deficiency anemia, postsplenectomy states
B. Spherocytes	Decrease in surface-volume ratio	Hereditary spherocytosis, autoimmune hemolytic anemia
C. Siderocytes (need Fe^{2+} stain)	Cells with deposits of iron-containing granules	Postsplenectomy states, severe hemolysis, sideroblastic anemia
D. Basophilic stippling	Aggregations of defective ribosomes	Lead poisoning
E. Howell-Jolly bodies	Nuclear fragments	Postsplenectomy states, megaloblastic anemia
F. Macroovalocyte	Defective RBC maturation	Megaloblastic anemia, bone marrow failure

Abnormality	Significance	Seen In
G. Polychromatophilic and immature erythroid forms in peripheral blood	Immature red cells	Any stress erythropoiesis (e.g., hemolysis, chronic hemorrhage)
H. Sickled cells	Molecular defect in hemoglobin beta-chain	Sickle cell anemias
I. Helmet cells	Sheared and traumatized erythrocytes	Microangiopathic hemolytic anemias (e.g., DIC), malignant hypertension, uremia, burns
J. Teardrop cells	Deformed RBC membrane	Marrow infiltration, myeloproliferative syndromes, extramedullary hematopoiesis
K. Reticulocytes (need special stain)	RNA network visible in very young RBC	Any state of high erythropoietic activity, e.g., post-bleed, post-Fe^{2+} treatment for anemia
2. White cell abnormal forms		
A. Toxic granules in PMN	Reaction to sepsis	Infection or inflammatory disease
B. Dohle bodies in PMN	Ribosome-containing immature granules	Infection, burns
C. Hypersegmented PMN	Abnormality of nuclear division or chromatin	Folate or B_{12} deficiency, marrow failure
D. Auer rods (in myeloblasts)	Clumped granule material	AML, AMoL
E. Atypical lymphocytes (vacuolated cytoplasm; lobulated monocytoid nucleus; nucleoli)	Activated T cells or lymphoblasts	Infectious mononucleosis, viral infections, immunologic reactions
F. Immature granulocytes in peripheral blood	Immature granulocytes	Infections, leukemoid reaction, leukoerythroblastic reactions, AML, CML
G. Bacteria in PMN	Phagocytosed bacteria	Severe infection

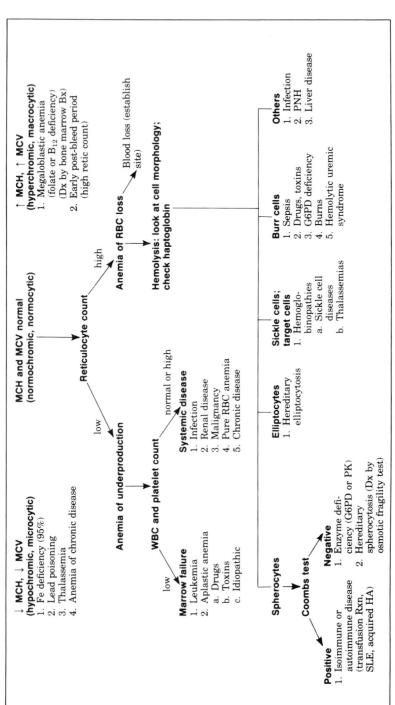

Fig. 7-1. Approach to the diagnosis of anemia on the basis of red cell indices. HA = hemolytic anemia; PK = pyruvate kinase; PNH = paroxysmal nocturnal hemoglobinuria; Rxn = reaction.

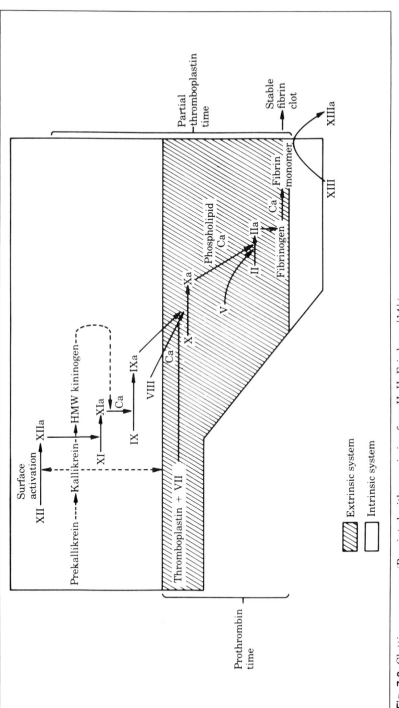

Fig. 7-2. Clotting sequence. (Reprinted with permission from H. H. Friedman [14].)

D. Platelet count and clotting indices. The platelet count and clotting indices are reflections of the state of the patient's hemostatic systems. Fig. 7-2 reviews the classic model of the coagulation cascade and illustrates which factors are measured by the PT and PTT. Recent evidence shows that the actual workings of coagulation are more complex than this simple cascade model, with positive and negative feedback loops between many of the factors. See Broze [6] for more details.

1. **Abnormal platelet counts**

   a. **Increased** with malignancy, myeloproliferative diseases, postsurgery or postsplenectomy states, collagen disorders (rheumatoid arthritis), Fe^{2+} deficiency anemia, bleeding, acute infection, primary thrombocytosis.

   b. **Note:** platelet is an acute phase reactant.

   c. **Decreased** with idiopathic thrombocytopenic purpura (ITP), marrow invasion or aplasia, hypersplenism, cytotoxic therapy.

E. Erythrocyte sedimentation rate. Because it is so nonspecific, the ESR is most useful in deciding between sets of disease states that may have similar presentations but different degrees of inflammatory reaction and antibody formation. For instance, the ESR may be useful in deciding between rheumatoid arthritis (increased) and degenerative joint disease (normal).

1. **Abnormal ESR values**

   a. **Increased** with acute MI, infection, rheumatic fever, malignancy, myeloma, collagen diseases (RA, systemic lupus erythematosis [SLE]), pregnancy, tuberculosis, active hepatitis, inflammatory necrosis.

   b. **Decreased** with sickle cell anemia, polycythemia, congestive heart failure (CHF), diabetes insipidus (DI), trichinosis.

B **Practical Points Concerning Hematologic Tests**

I. **Complete blood count and indices**

A. Remember that the red cell indices are mechanically calculated as the average of a great many cells. **Look at the smear** to confirm that the erythrocytes are morphologically homogenous. Multiple erythrocyte populations with mathematically compensatory abnormalities may result in falsely normal results.

B. You can get a good estimate of the hematocrit by multiplying the hemoglobin by three (e.g., a Hgb of 10 predicts a Hct of 30). Also note that, because the MCHC depends on these interlinked Hgb and Hct values, it will almost always be approximately 33 (and is therefore relatively useless).

C. When discussing a patient's problems, always state the **type of anemia** (e.g., microcytic hypochromic). Strictly speaking, anemia is not a disease; it is a family of diseases. You must specify the nature of the anemia.

D. Remember that the most common etiology of anemia is **iron deficiency,** which results in microcytic hypochromic erythrocytes. This is a very common finding, especially among menstruating women.

E. **Bleeding** can produce either a normochromic normocytic or hyperchromic macrocytic picture. In a patient with a normal hematocrit who becomes anemic over the course of a few hours, always think about an acute bleed.

F. In working up an anemia of unknown etiology, always guaiac the stool to rule out **gastrointestinal bleeding.**

II. Differential white cell count

A. The differential is a relatively expensive test and is probably overordered in most hospitals. You can perform your own minidifferential simply by looking at the smear and quickly scanning the field for **PMN band forms.** If the smear shows more than a few percent bands, the sample is probably left-shifted.

B. Remember to look at the **eosinophil count** in patients with allergic disorders. (A mnemonic for remembering which problems are associated with high eosinophil levels: **worms, wheezes, weird diseases.**)

III. Blood smear analysis

A. It is worth learning to do a **Wright stain** of the peripheral blood; it will be useful for some patients you work up. The best way to learn how to do this is to watch a technician or hematologist a few times. It is impossible to interpret a poorly made smear.

B. Learn to scan the microscopic field with an eye to four parameters: (1) **cell size,** (2) **cell shape,** (3) **nuclear shape,** and (4) **cytoplasmic inclusions.** As in all lab tests, you should think about the patient's clinical history while looking at the smear. (Is there a history of liver disease? If so, does the peripheral smear show acanthocytosis?) Ask yourself not only, "What do I see?," but also, "What do I not see?"

C. Make friends with the **technicians** in the hematology lab. You should try to look at each smear you order (or at least the interesting ones) with the technicians—it is a great way to learn more about your patients' diseases.

IV. Platelet count and clotting indices

A. Specific factor deficiency tests are expensive and should not be ordered routinely. Remember that abnormalities on clotting screens are more commonly due to **systemic disease** (e.g., liver failure) than to congenital factor deficiencies.

B. Because the platelets are important in the **primary hemostatic reaction** but play virtually no role in clotting, a hemophiliac with normal platelet levels will usually have a normal bleeding time.

V. Erythrocyte sedimentation rate.
There are three different ways to test the ESR: the Wintrobe and Landsberg, the Westergren, and the zeta methods. The normal values differ for each method, as well as for men and women. Always check what the technicians in your hospital lab consider a normal ESR.

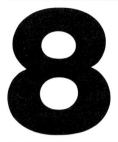

Serum Chemistry Tests

> *Time can be a physician's ally and a legitimate diagnostic test.* The desire to reach a rapid diagnosis is often medically and economically justifiable. But in many instances, when the answer is not readily revealed, the pressure to find the diagnosis need not force the clinician to obtain more and more tests and to engage in ever more invasive procedures. Time allows a disease process to "declare itself" (or go away). The physician working in close communication with the patient can use time with little risk.
>
> **Thomas P. Stossel, M.D.**

A

Outline of Serum Chemistry Tests

I. **Indications for ordering serum chemistry tests.** Serum chemistry tests have become an important part of modern medical management. In general, they are ordered for four reasons:

1. To aid in medical **diagnosis.**
2. To allow the physician to **follow the course** of a problem or treatment regimen.
3. To monitor **fluid and electrolyte balance.**
4. To **screen for occult disease.**

   Chemistry tests are usually run in batteries of 6 to 20, which are run at the same time on a single machine. One such battery is the SMA-7, which consists of a set of electrolytes (Na, K, Cl, HCO_3), BUN (blood urea nitrogen), serum creatinine, and serum glucose. Though many clinicians routinely order these batteries both on admission and at times during a patient's hospitalization, you should always ask yourself why you are ordering each test, and what you would do with abnormal results.

   This chapter covers 20 of the most important serum tests, providing short lists of common diseases associated with abnormal values for these tests, and some essential points related to their interpretation. Further clinical points related to serum chemistries in general are included in Part B of this chapter.

II. **Interpreting serum chemistry tests.** The following lists of physiologic and pathologic conditions associated with lab abnormalities include only some of the more common serum chemistry correlates. For a more complete treatment of the general subject, see Wallach's *Interpretation of Diagnostic Tests* [25]. The numbers in parentheses indicate normal ranges for these tests.

A. **Sodium** (136–145 mEq/L)

1. **Increase:** dehydration, diabetes insipidus (DI), Cushing's syndrome, hyperaldosteronism.

   2. **Decrease:** congestive heart failure (CHF), diuretic use, syndrome of inappropriate antidiuretic hormone (SIADH).

   3. **Note:**

      a. Hyperlipidemia and hyperglycemia are causes of spurious hyponatremia. For each 100mg/dl increase in blood glucose above normal, you should correct the serum sodium by adding 1.6 mEq/L. For example, in a patient with a glucose of 700 and sodium of 130, the corrected sodium would be $130 + (1.6 \times 6) = 140$.

      b. Most hyponatremia is secondary to free water retention (in excess of retained sodium) rather than to sodium loss.

B. Potassium (3.5–5.2 mEq/L)

   1. **Increase:** renal failure, acidosis, iatrogenic cause, mineralocorticoid deficiency.

   2. **Decrease:** metabolic alkalosis, diuretic use, mineralocorticoid excess.

   3. **Note:**

      a. RBC hemolysis in blood sample acquisition can spuriously increase serum potassium.

      b. Thrombocytosis spuriously elevates serum potassium.

      c. Alterations in serum potassium may produce ECG changes, including peaked T waves, wide QRS, and loss of P wave in hyperkalemia; and flattening of T wave and presence of U waves in hypokalemia.

C. Chloride (96–108 mEq/L)

   1. **Increase:** dehydration, non–anion gap metabolic acidosis, hyperalimentation, mineralocorticoid deficiency.

   2. **Decrease:** diuretic use, CHF, SIADH, compensated respiratory acidosis, vomiting.

   3. **Note:**

      a. Hypochloremia is the most common cause of metabolic alkalosis.

      b. The laboratory method for measuring chloride is a nonspecific test for halides; hence, bromides and iodides may spuriously elevate serum chloride.

D. Bicarbonate (24–30 mEq/L)

   1. **Increase:** dehydration ("concentration alkalosis"), compensated respiratory acidosis.

   2. **Decrease:** metabolic acidosis, compensated respiratory alkalosis.

E. Anion gap (10–12 mEq). The anion gap represents unmeasured anions and is calculated as the difference, in milliequivalents, between serum sodium and the sum of serum chloride and bicarbonate.

   1. **Increase:** renal failure, lactic acidosis, ketoacidosis, salicylate toxicity, ethylene glycol ingestion, methanol ingestion.

   2. **Decrease:** multiple myeloma, bromide ingestion, polycythemia vera, disseminated intravascular coagulation (DIC), pregnancy.

   3. **Note:**

      a. Use of the anion gap helps to distinguish between two types of metabolic acidosis: hyperchloremic metabolic acidosis (the type associated with a *normal* anion gap) and high–anion gap metabolic acidosis.

    b. Some people define the anion gap as the difference, in milliequivalents, between the sum of sodium *and potassium* (rather than sodium alone) and the sum of chloride and bicarbonate; from a practical standpoint, either method may be used.

F. BUN (6–26 mg/dl)

    1. Increase: renal failure of all types, accelerated protein catabolism (e.g., GI bleed), dehydration.

    2. Decrease: liver damage, protein deficiency states.

G. Creatinine (0.7–1.3 mg/dl) Affected by muscle mass and turnover as well as renal function.

    1. Increase: renal failure, muscle disease, increased muscle mass.

    2. Decrease: rarely clinically significant.

    3. Note:

        a. Creatinine is a more specific indicator of renal disease than BUN.

        b. The BUN-creatinine ratio is sometimes helpful in distinguishing prerenal azotemia (>20) from intrinsic renal disease producing azotemia (<20).

        c. Hemodialysis of patients with chronic renal failure (CRF) usually normalizes BUN; creatinine, however, may not change at all with dialysis.

H. Glucose (fasting, 65–110 mg/dl)

    1. Increase: diabetes mellitus (DM), pregnancy, stress, pancreatic disease.

    2. Decrease: reactive hypoglycemia, pancreatic islet-cell tumors, starvation, liver disease.

    3. Note:

        a. Measuring the fasting blood sugar (FBS) is the best method, short of a formal oral glucose tolerance test, to document DM.

        b. Be careful of spuriously high readings from blood drawn from a site above an IV line containing dextrose.

I. Calcium (9.0–11.0 mg/dl)

    1. Increase: malignancies, primary hyperparathyroidism.

    2. Decrease: hypoparathyroidism, CRF, malabsorption syndromes, vitamin D deficiency, hypoalbuminemia.

    3. Note:

        a. Free ionized calcium is the physiologically important form of the cation; hence, correction must be made for the concentration of the major calcium-binding protein, albumin. (Correction = 0.8 mg/1.0 mg change in albumin.)

        b. Changes in serum calcium are reflected in the ECG. An increase in calcium shortens the Q–T interval while a decrease in serum calcium lengthens the Q–T interval.

J. Phosphorus (2.5–4.2 mg/dl)

    1. Increase: CRF, hypoparathyroidism, vitamin D excess, bone disease.

    2. Decrease: alcoholism, nutritional deficiency states, hyperparathyroidism, diabetes, gout, antacid use.

   3. **Note:** Hypophosphatemia can decrease myocardial contractility and effective tissue oxygenation (through decreased production of 2,3-DPG).

K. Albumin (3.5–5.5 gm/dl)

   1. **Increase:** rarely clinically significant.

   2. **Decrease:** chronic disease, nutritional deficiency states, protein-losing enteropathy.

L. Total protein (6.0–8.5 gm/dl)

   1. **Increase:** multiple myeloma.

   2. **Decrease:** chronic disease, protein-losing enteropathy.

   3. **Note:** The difference between the levels of total protein and albumin is the amount of globulin.

M. Amylase (5–75 IU/L)

   1. **Increase:** pancreatitis, mumps, parotitis, duodenal ulcer, ectopic pregnancy, diabetic ketoacidosis, biliary tract disease, peritonitis, macroamylasemia.

   2. **Decrease:** pancreatic destruction.

   3. **Note:**

      a. Almost any intraabdominal process can elevate serum amylase.

      b. Salivary gland amylase and pancreatic amylase are different isozymes and can be distinguished by electrophoretic analysis.

      c. The amylase-to-creatinine clearance ratio may be useful in distinguishing macroamylasemia (<1%) and other causes of increased amylase from pancreatitis (>5%).

N. Uric acid (1.5–8.0 mg/dl)

   1. **Increase:** gout, asymptomatic hyperuricemia, renal failure, cancer with rapid tumor cell turnover, use of thiazide diuretics.

   2. **Decrease:** allopurinol use, uricosuric-agent use, Hodgkin's disease, Wilson's disease, aspirin ingestion.

   3. **Note:** The greatest acute risk in elevated uric acid is the development of uric acid nephropathy, particularly in patients receiving chemotherapy. This can be avoided by adequate hydration, allopurinol therapy, and urinary alkalinization.

O. Cholesterol (desirable total cholesterol 140–240; see **3.c**)

   1. **Increase:** hypercholesterolemia, hyperlipidemia, biliary tract obstruction, pancreatitis, hypothyroidism.

   2. **Decrease:** starvation, chronic disease, hyperthyroidism.

   3. **Note:**

      a. Cholesterol levels increase postprandially.

      b. Elevated total cholesterol levels are a risk factor for coronary heart disease (CHD), and thus this is an important screening test for the general population. Other related risk factors for CHD include elevated low-density lipoproteins (LDLs) and triglycerides, as well as low high-density lipoprotein (HDL) cholesterol.

      c. For adults more than 65 years old, total cholesterol under 200 is considered desirable; 200–239 is borderline high; and 240 and up is considered high. In persons with high total cholesterol, fasting triglycerides and HDL levels should be measured, and then the LDL fraction calculated (total cholesterol = [HDL + LDL + triglycerides]/5). An LDL level under 130 is considered desirable; 130–159 is borderline high; and 160 and up is considered high. Patients with either high cholesterol, or borderline-high values in addition to other risk factors for heart disease should consider lifestyle changes or pharmacologic intervention (see Carleton et al. [7]).

P. Bilirubin (total 0.2–1.0 mg/dl; direct < 0.2 mg/dl; indirect < 0.8 mg/dl)

  1. **Increase: direct (conjugated) hyperbilirubinemia** (biliary obstruction, hepatitis), **indirect (unconjugated) hyperbilirubinemia** (hemolysis, Gilbert's syndrome).

  2. **Decrease:** rarely clinically significant.

  3. **Note:** The most prevalent cause of mild, asymptomatic unconjugated hyperbilirubinemia is Gilbert's syndrome.

Q. Alkaline phosphatase (30–115 units/L)

  1. **Increase:** biliary tract obstruction, bone disease (especially Paget's disease).

  2. **Decrease:** rarely clinically significant.

  3. **Note:** Heat fractionation helps distinguish alkaline phosphatase of hepatic origin from that of bone origin ("bone burns"). Electrophoretic analysis of isozymes is also available.

R. AST (8–20 U/L), and **ALT** (8–20 U/L). Aspartate aminotransferase (AST) was previously known as serum glutamic-oxaloacetic transaminase (SGOT), and alanine aminotransferase (ALT) was known as serum glutamic-pyruvic transaminase (SGPT). Generally, changes in these two enzymes parallel each other.

  1. **Increase:** myocardial infarction, hepatocellular disease, CHF, muscle disease, hemolysis.

  2. **Decrease:** rarely clinically significant.

  3. **Note:**

    a. Increased AST (SGOT) levels can help in diagnosis of myocardial infarction, when used in the context of other abnormal chemistries, for example, an elevated creatine phosphokinase (CPK). See Chap. 16 for further discussion.

    b. Elevations of AST, ALT, and lactate dehydrogenase (LDH) suggest hepatocellular disease, whereas elevations of alkaline phosphatase and bilirubin suggest obstructive liver disease.

    c. ALT (SGPT) is more elevated than AST (SGOT) in viral hepatitis, and AST is elevated more than ALT in alcoholic hepatitis.

S. LDH (lactate dehydrogenase; 45–100 units/L)

  1. **Increase:** myocardial infarction, CHF, hepatitis, pulmonary embolus, muscle disease, neoplasia, hemolysis.

  2. **Decrease:** rarely clinically significant.

  3. **Note:** There are five isozymes of LDH, which can be electrophoretically fractionated. This fractionation is useful in distinguishing LDH elevations of myocardial origin (isoenzymes I and II) from that of other sources. An LDH_1-LDH_2 ratio greater than 1 may be used to help predict recent myocardial infarction (within the past 3–5 days); LDH_5 is greater than LDH_4 in liver diseases.

T. CPK (creatine phosphokinase; in women 50–60 IU/L, in men 50–180 IU/L)

   1. Increase: myocardial infarction, striated muscle necrosis, cerebrovascular accident, hypothyroidism.

   2. Decrease: rarely clinically significant.

   3. Note:

   a. Isozyme fractionation of CPK produces three bands: MM (striated muscle), MB (cardiac muscle), and BB (brain). The MB band (normally less than 6 percent) is elevated in an acute myocardial infarction, but other sources of MB-band CPK include tongue and diaphragm. The BB band is elevated in cerebrovascular accidents only if the blood-brain barrier is interrupted. See Chap. 16 for a diagram of the time course of elevation after MI.

   b. CPK is increased in hypothyroidism and renal failure because of decreased renal clearance.

B   **Practical Points Concerning the Serum Chemistries**

I. Ordering serum chemistry tests

   A. At many hospitals, you can **order just one test,** even though tests are done as automated batteries. If all you really care about is the potassium concentration, try ordering just that test rather than a full electrolyte panel. Also, because lab tests are generally done as automated batteries, you often can call the lab and get results of lab tests not originally requested.

   B. Learn to think of serum chemistry tests in **groups:**

   1. The electrolytes (K, Na, Cl, HCO_3).

   2. Kidney function tests (BUN, creatinine). Also helpful in assessing fluid status.

   3. Liver function tests (AST, ALT, albumin, total protein, bilirubin, alkaline phosphatase).

   4. Acute myocardial infarction enzymes (CPK, AST, LDH).

   5. Metabolic bone disease tests (Ca, P, alkaline phosphatase).

   C. Know the status of each lab test that you have ordered (i.e., keep track of whether it has been officially ordered, drawn, received in the lab, and finished). Know the results for patients you are following; remember that you may call the lab to learn the results if they have not yet made it back to the ward. A big part of learning to be an effective and efficient clinical clerk is knowing how to keep track of the progress of your patient's work-up.

   D. Note that the electrolytes, BUN, creatinine, and glucose are often recorded quickly using a "standardized" lattice pattern:

$$\begin{array}{c|c} Na & Cl \\ \hline K & HCO_3 \end{array}\Big\langle \begin{array}{l} BUN \\ glucose \\ creatinine \end{array}$$

II. Interpreting serum chemistry tests

A. While it is easy to learn a simple collection of common variations in serum chemistries and their causes, it is not very practical. On the wards, you usually will not be faced with an isolated abnormal lab value (except for alkaline phosphatase or glucose); more often you will be confronted with a group of abnormal values derived from all the tests done in your test battery. For this reason, it is more helpful to learn to recognize **common clinical patterns of abnormal routine serum chemistries,** such as those shown below. Note that in these examples the combination of values helps suggest a more limited and directed diagnosis than would any single abnormal value.

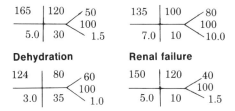

Dehydration   Renal failure

Excessive diuretic use   Diabetic ketoacidosis

B. Remember that **lab or measurement error** is a common explanation for abnormal serum chemistry results. A wise clinician will try to repeat a lab test or confirm an abnormal result by some other test (e.g., an ECG can help confirm a high serum potassium) before acting on a lab result that does not seem appropriate for the clinical picture.

C. When prescribing any **medication,** keep in mind which lab tests you would expect to be altered by the administration of the drug. Watch these test results carefully over the following few days, and use them to assess the efficacy or toxicity of your regimen. For example, diuretics commonly lead to hypokalemia.

Colorplates

Though detailed compilations of colorplates may be found in most comprehensive specialty texts, a smaller number of core illustrations is appropriate for an introductory manual. Colorplates A and B demonstrate the routine Gram stain procedure (see detailed explanation of these in the following paragraphs), and Colorplate C displays the characteristic Gram stain appearance of the most commonly encountered microorganisms. Colorplate D demonstrates the actual appearance of many of these organisms under $1,000 \times$ (oil-immersion) magnification. They are identified in the table following the colorplates. Similarly, Colorplates E-I display some basic dermatologic lesions with which every student should be familiar.

Colorplate A. The Gram stain reaction is of primary importance in the morphologic and taxonomic classification of bacteria. A simplified, brief version is presented here. **The smear should be thin, air-dried, and gently heat-fixed.**

1. Flood the slide with **crystal violet** — 10 seconds. (Wash with running tap water.)
2. Flood with **Gram's iodine** (brown) — 10 seconds. (Wash with water.)
3. Carefully **decolorize with 95% ethanol or ethanol-acetone mixture** until the thinnest parts of the smear are colorless. (Wash with water.)
4. Flood with **safranin** (red) — 10 seconds or longer if hard-to-see gram-negative organisms such as *Bacteroides* or *Haemophilus* are suspected.
5. **Results.** Organisms that retain the violet-iodine complex after washing in ethanol will stain **purple (gram-positive)**; those that lose this complex will stain **red (gram-negative)** from the safranin counterstain. Although the mechanism of this reaction is not completely understood, a plausible explanation is that the cell walls of gram-positive bacteria contain less lipid than the cell walls of gram-negative organisms and therefore are less permeable to organic solvents. This enables gram-positive bacteria to retain the violet-iodine complex. In a properly executed Gram-stained smear, **cellular elements and most background material stain pink to red.**

Colorplate B. The clinician can quickly assess the adequacy of the Gram stain by comparing several different areas of the slide, using the oil-immersion lens. Granulocyte nuclei and gram-negative organisms in a thin area of the smear should stain red, and gram-positive organisms should stain purple (see # 3). Finding red bacteria near slightly purple (marginally decolorized) cellular elements in a thicker part of the smear can confirm that bona fide gram-negative organisms are present (see # 2) rather than over-decolorized gram-positive bacteria (see # 4). Fields wholly under-decolorized (see # 1) indicate only the presence of the bacteria but not necessarily their staining characteristics.

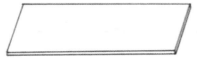

Prepare thin smear. Air-dry and heat-fix.

1. Flood with crystal violet 10 seconds. Rinse with tap water.

2. Flood with Gram's iodine 10 seconds. Rinse.

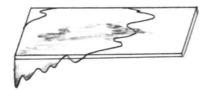

3. Critical step: Decolorize and rinse.

4. Flood with safranin counterstain 10 seconds or more. Rinse. Blot or air-dry.

A. Gram-stain method.

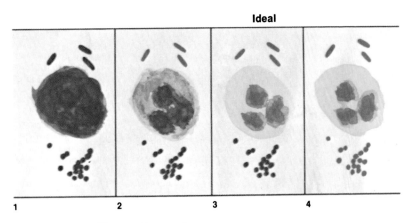

B. Variations possible on a Gram stain.

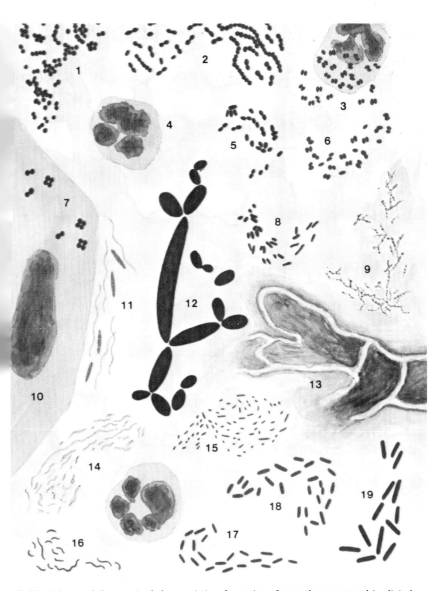

C. Morphology and Gram-stained characteristics of organisms frequently encountered in clinical specimens. Average-sized organisms, shown here in scale and as they appear under optimal conditions, are usually seen at 1,000× (oil-immersion lens).

1. *Staphylococcus*
2. *Streptococcus* and Pneumococcus
3. *Neisseria*
4. Polymorphonuclear leukocyte
5. *Listeria*
6. *Acinetobacter (Mima, Herellea)*
7. *Micrococcus*
8. *Corynebacterium* (diphtheroids)
9. *Nocardia* or *Actinomyces*
10. Epithelial cell
11. *Fusobacterium* and *Borrelia*
12. *Candida*
13. *Aspergillus* (higher fungi usually do not take up Gram stain)
14. *Bacteroides*
15. *Haemophilus* (and other often rare organisms such as *Pasteurella*)
16. *Vibrio*
17. *Pseudomonas*
18. Enterobacteriaceae (*Escherichia coli*, *Proteus*, *Salmonella*, etc.)
19. *Clostridium*, *Bacillus*, or *Lactobacillus*

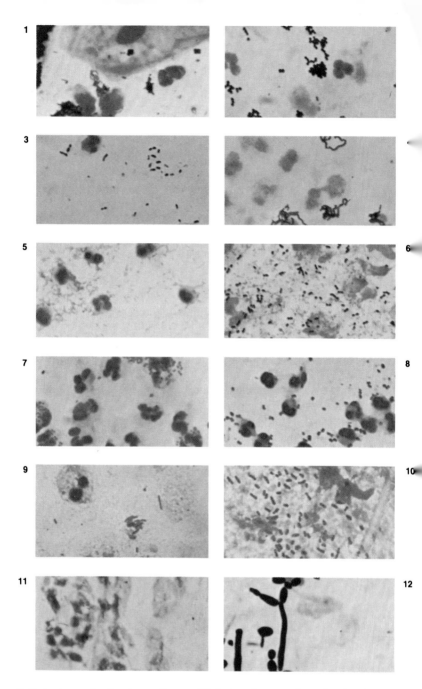

D. Photomicrographs of various pathogens. All photographs were taken using the oil-immersion lens (×1,000) and are Gram-stained specimens, with the exception of number 11, which was stained by the Ziehl-Neelsen method. Descriptions of these organisms are given in the table following colorplate I.

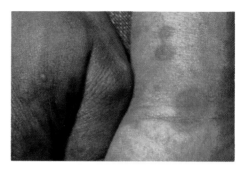

E. Erythema multiforme—iris (target) lesions.

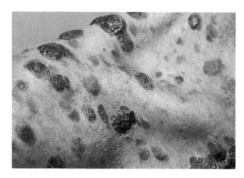

F. Seborrheic keratoses.

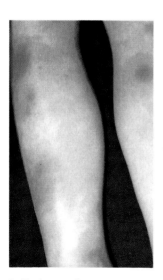

G. Erythema nodosum.

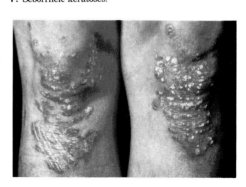

H. Psoriasis.

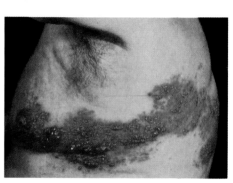

I. Herpes zoster.

Descriptions of the organisms in Colorplate D

Number	Specimen	Observation	Likely possibility	Culture report	Comment
1	Throat	Epithelial cell, gram-positive and gram-negative cocci, small gram-positive rods, thin gram-negative rods	Variety of organisms—normal throat flora	Normal throat flora	No inflammatory cells, wide variety of organisms. Specimen not indicative of infection.
2	Sputum	Gram-positive cocci in singles, pairs, and clusters; neutrophils	Staphylococcus	*Staphylococcus aureus*	Classic smear of staphylococcal pneumonia.
3	CSF	Gram-positive and gram-variable cocci in pairs and short chains; PMNs	Pneumococci or streptococci	Pneumococcus (*Streptococcus pneumoniae*)	Neutrophils are stained correctly; nearby organism is nicely gram-positive. Since only one kind of organism usually causes meningitis, and gram-positive organisms may become gram-negative with age, etc., it is likely that all these organisms are gram-positive cocci.
4	Knee joint fluid	Gram-positive cocci in very long chains	Streptococci	Group A streptococcus (*Streptococcus pyogenes*)	Gram-positive cocci in very long chains, although conceivably pneumococci, are most likely to be streptococci.
5	CSF	Small gram-negative coccobacilli and rods	*Haemophilus*, remote chance of other small gram-negative organism such as *Pasteurella*	*Haemophilus influenzae*	Small gram-negative cocci, coccobacilli, and relatively slender rod forms are typical of *H. influenzae*.

6	Sputum	Gram-positive cocci in pairs, small gram-negative coccobacilli, hints of neutrophils	Pneumococci, *Haemophilus*	Sputum from patients with chronic bronchitis often contains *H. influenzae*—here, an active infection of pneumococci is superimposed. Gram-negative organisms can be especially hard to see in mixed infections. Always carefully examine the background!	Pneumococcus, *Haemophilus influenzae*
7	Urethra	Gram-negative intracellular diplococci (GNID)	*Neisseria* spp.	Classic smear of gonococci—abundant intracellular organisms in many, but not all, PMNs. Although *Acinetobacter (Mima, Herellea)* organisms may be morphologically similar to *Neisseria*, they usually do not evoke such a neutrophil response and normally occur in a different clinical setting.	Gonococcus (*Neisseria gonorrhoeae*)
8	CSF	Gram-negative diplococci, neutrophils	*Neisseria*, remote chance *Acinetobacter*	Classic *Neisseria*—note coffee-bean shape and snug "belly-to-belly" alignment, different from paired pneumococci, which do not have adjacent sides flattened. Organisms in CSF do not have to be intracellular to be considered significant.	Meningococcus (*Neisseria meningitidis*)

Descriptions of the organisms in Colorplate D (Continued)

Number	Specimen	Observation	Likely possibility	Culture report	Comment
9	Unspun urine	Gram-negative rods, neutrophil	Enteric gram-negative rod	*Escherichia coli*	Presence of one or more organisms per oil-immersion field of unspun urine indicates 10^5 or more bacteria per milliliter. Note that the enteric gram-negative rods tend to be larger and plumper than those of *H. influenzae.*
10	Sputum	Plump, beaded, gram-negative rods	Enteric gram-negative rod such as *Klebsiella*	*Klebsiella*	Although *Klebsiella* often appears as large, plump, beaded rods with a hint of capsule, it has no monopoly on these characteristics and need not exhibit them.
11	Sputum	Small red bacilli, many with granules (Ziehl-Neelsen stain)	Acid-fast bacilli	*Mycobacterium tuberculosis*	Gram's stain typically revealed no organisms. Acid-fast stain obligatory.
12	Sputum	Budding yeasts with pseudohyphae	*Candida* spp.	*Candida albicans*	Although budding yeast forms are indistinguishable from one another, abundant pseudohyphae in tissue suggest *Candida* spp.

Source: Adapted from P. Gardner and H. T. Provine, *Manual of Acute Bacterial Infections* (2nd ed.). Boston: Little, Brown, 1984. Pp. 183–190.

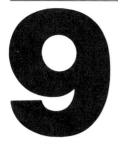

Urinalysis

For the patient with renal disease, the evaluation of the *urinary sediment* is not a laboratory procedure but rather an integral part of the physical examination to be performed by the physician, like listening to the chest or palpating the abdomen. Only then can the physician appreciate the often inconspicuous admixtures of cells and casts that define parenchymal disease: *red cell casts* indicating proliferative glomerular disease, *hyaline casts* indicating proteinuria, *white cell casts* indicating interstitial disease, *broad casts* indicating tubular atrophy, *waxy casts* indicating nephron death.

Warren E. Grupe, M.D.

A   Annotated Outline of the Urinalysis

I. Indications for the urinalysis

A. The urinalysis (U/A) is useful for patients with diseases of the urinary tract or certain metabolic diseases, such as diabetes mellitus (DM). Because urinary tract infections are so common, serial urinalyses are also done on patients with sepsis or fever of unknown origin.

B. An **admission urinalysis** will be done on most patients. This urine sample may have been collected and sent to the hospital lab before the patient arrives on the hospital floor. In this situation, it is not uncommon for the medical student or house officer to perform a second urinalysis as part of the initial patient work-up. Centrifuge, microscope, and stains are usually provided on the wards for this purpose.

II. Parts of the urinalysis. There are nine basic parts to a complete urinalysis. A test marked with an asterisk (*) is done by dipstick:

1. Specific gravity
2. Appearance
3. pH*
4. Protein*
5. Glucose*
6. Ketones*
7. Blood*
8. Sediment analysis
9. Gram stain for bacteria (see Colorplates A, B, and C)

Fig. 9-1 is a flow diagram of the entire urinalysis, which can be done in 10 to 15 minutes.

In instances where urinary tract infection is suspected, a bacterial **culture and sensitivity** screen is added to the above list.

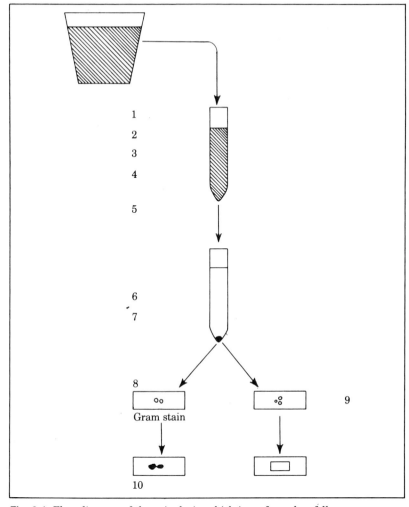

Fig. 9-1. Flow diagram of the urinalysis, which is performed as follows:

1. Pour 5–10 ml into a conical test tube.
2. Check specific gravity in remainder.
3. Using dipstick, check for pH, protein, sugar, ketones, and heme in remainder as well.
4. If UTI is suspected, check Gram stain of *unspun* specimen.
5. Spin at 1,000–2,000 rpm for 3–5 min.
6. Pour off supernatant.
7. Resuspend pellet in the 1–2 drops of urine that will remain after decanting by flicking bottom of test tube several times with your fingers or by knocking it against countertop.
8. Place 2 drops on a glass slide to dry for Gram stain.
9. While Gram stain preparation dries, place 2–3 drops of sediment on another glass slide; cover the second slide immediately with cover slip.
10. Examine sediment under high-dry power (never oil). Examine Gram stain slide under oil.

III. Interpreting the urinalysis

A. Specific gravity

1. **Normal range** 1.001–1.035, with urine isotonic to plasma (285–295 mOsm) 1.010–1.012. The specific gravity (SG) is used as an indirect measure of the kidney's ability to concentrate the urine. If a first morning specimen is SG 1.025 or greater, it is generally taken as evidence of adequate concentrating ability.

2. **Elevated in:** dehydration, excessive fluid loss (vomiting, diarrhea, fever), DM, congestive heart failure (CHF), syndrome of inappropriate antidiuretic hormone (SIADH), adrenal insufficiency, decreased fluid intake.

3. **False elevations** of SG may occur with iodinated contrast material, excessive glucose, and massive proteinuria.

4. **Decreased in:** diabetes insipidus (DI), renal disease (glomerulonephritis or pyelonephritis), excessive fluid intake or IV hydration.

B. Appearance.
Urine is often described as "straw" or "yellow." Following are common causes of **abnormal color or turbidity:**

Red-brown: hemoglobin, myoglobin, bile pigments, blood, food dyes
Yellow-red: pyridium, vegetable or phenolphthalein cathartics
Blue or green: beets, methylene blue in IV
Dark or black: porphyrins, melanin
Turbid: frequently secondary to urates or phosphates (benign), RBCs, WBCs
Foamy: protein, bile acids

C. pH

1. **Normal range** of urine pH is **4.5–8.5.**

2. **Elevated in:** bacteriuria, renal failure with inability to form ammonia, presence of certain drugs (antibiotics, sodium bicarbonate, acetazolamide).

3. **Decreased in:** acidosis (metabolic or respiratory), presence of certain drugs (ammonium chloride, methenamine mandelate), DM, starvation, diarrhea.

D. Protein

1. **Normal amount** of urine protein is less than 50 mg/day. Persistent proteinuria is a highly significant finding.

2. **Elevated in:** renal disease (glomerular, tubular, interstitial), CHF, hypertension, neoplasms of the renal pelvis and bladder, multiple myeloma, Waldenström's macroglobulinemia

   a. Note that protein in urine may be either **normal** serum proteins (indicating glomerular permeability or renal tubular disorders) or **abnormal** serum proteins (suggesting possible plasma cell dyscrasia). In multiple myeloma, Bence Jones (BJ) proteins will give a negative dipstick result about 50 percent of the time.

E. Glucose

1. A **normal** result is no detectable glucose (negative dipstick).

2. This test is the main method for diagnosis of the common disease **diabetes mellitus.** The dipstick is extremely sensitive and specific for glucose, since the reaction relies on the enzyme glucose oxidase. However, the results are qualitative. Other causes of glucose in the urine

are renal glycosuria (decreased renal threshold for glucose) and glucose intolerance.

In situations where a quantitative assessment of urine glucose is desirable (for example, to monitor how much glucose your patient with diabetes is spilling—an indirect way of assessing the efficacy of insulin therapy), use the Clinitest tablets and follow bottle directions for dilution.

F. Ketones

The dipstick (and the Acetest tablets that are sometimes used) measure only acetoacetic acid and acetone (*not* beta-hydroxybutyrate).

Recall that ketosis is seen in cases of **diabetic ketoacidosis, alcoholic ketoacidosis,** and **starvation.**

G. Blood. Hematuria is virtually always significant, except in a patient with a recent history of catheterization. (See Table 9-1 for a discussion of RBCs in urine.)

H. Sediment.

    1. Preparation (see Fig. 9-1)

        a. Turn condenser down to distance it farther from slide. Use reduced light.

        b. Use lower power first.

Table 9-1. Cell types in the urine sediment

Cell type	Normal range	Clinical points
RBC	0–3/HPF	**Cystitis** is the most frequent cause of hematuria, although slight hematuria often occurs secondary to exertion, trauma, or febrile illness. **Yeast cells** may be confused with RBCs. To distinguish between the two, RBCs may be lysed with 2–3 drops of acetic acid under cover slip (yeast cells will not lyse). Tumors, kidney stones, and glomerulonephritis are also common causes of elevated RBCs.
WBC	0–5/HPF	**Polymorphonuclear leukocytes** are the most common form of WBCs observed. If seen, and routine cultures × 2 are negative, send culture to be tested for tubercle bacilli.
Epithelial	0–2/HPF	**Epithelial cells** increase with tubular damage or heavy proteinuria.
Bacteria (see Colorplate D, 9)		Presence of bacteria on Gram stain of *un*spun specimen correlates well with culture growth of $\geq 10^5$ organisms (i.e., indicates presence of urinary tract infection). Send specimen for "culture and sensitivity" if suspicious. If culture comes back with between 10^4 and 10^5 organisms of a single type, reculture it; you must culture specimen at least twice to obtain >90% chance of documenting infection.

HPF = high-power field; 40× magnification.

c. Examine near the four edges of the cover slip, where casts accumulate.

d. Go to high power for cell counts and identification of casts and debris.

e. If the urine specimen is purulent or bloody, remember to look at an unspun specimen first.

f. You may want to stain the sediment to visualize better the various elements present. The most useful stain for this purpose is the Sternheimer-Malbin stain (crystal violet-Safarin 0); use 2 drops for each 0.5 ml sediment.

2. Common errors leading to unsatisfactory urine sediment examination:

  a. Contamination of collecting vessel with foreign material.

  b. Inadequately resuspended sediment.

  c. Failure to use both high- and low-power magnification.

  d. Too much light.

  e. Dried specimen.

3. Sediment analysis

  a. Cells in the urine sediment.

   (1) Cell counts. Count RBCs, WBCs, epithelial cells, and bacterial cells present in a typical high-power field (HPF).

   (2) Interpretation of cellular sediment. Table 9-1 lists cell types found in urine sediment and their significance.

Table 9-2. Casts in urine sediment

Cast type	Clinical points
Hyaline (translucent albumin) cast	The majority of casts seen in normal urine are hyaline. Since their refractile index is close to that of water, they are difficult to see unless light is reduced. A few hyaline casts/HPF may be normal.
WBC cast	Use acetic acid to prove that these are not RBC casts (acetic acid will lyse RBCs). WBC casts indicate inflammation in kidney parenchyma (often pyelonephritis).
RBC cast	Must search entire perimeter of cover glass if you suspect RBC casts. They are most consistent with glomerular inflammation or ischemic injury.
Granular-waxy cast	Granular casts are so named because of their granular appearance under microscope. They are thought to be degenerating cellular casts, usually epithelial in origin. If they have a red tinge, R/O RBC casts.
Broad cast	Broad casts probably originate in wide collecting duct. They are formed when flow rate is low. They often have ominous prognostic significance.

HPF = high-power field.

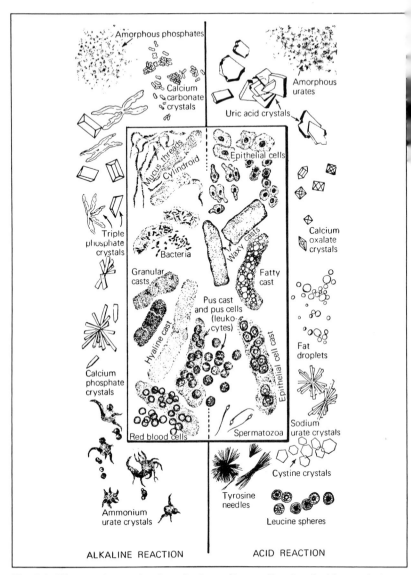

Fig. 9-2. Microscopic examination of urine sediment. (Reprinted with permission from M. A. Krupp et al., *Physician's Handbook* [19th ed.]. Los Altos, Calif.: Lange, 1979.)

b. **Casts in the urine sediment** are often difficult to interpret. Remember that no casts are pathognomonic for a specific renal parenchymal change, and that they may be absent in any of a number of nephropathies.

Casts are so named because they are casts of the nephron. They are distinguished from other debris by **smooth, parallel sides** (which may show the trapezoidal narrowing of the collecting system). Table 9-2 lists the various types of casts found in the urine and their clinical significance. These casts are illustrated in Fig. 9-2.

c. **Crystals in the urine sediment** are due to precipated chemicals and cellular debris. Some of the more common types of crystals are illustrated in Fig. 9-2. Their interpretation depends on the clinical presentation involved.

B   **Practical Points Concerning the Urinalysis**

I. **Ordering and performing the urinalysis**

A. Since a urinalysis takes only about 10 minutes to perform, do a urinalysis virtually every day on your patients who have active **renal disease.** You will be able to follow the course of the disease more closely and present the case more forcefully in rounds if you can correlate the clinical history with the urinalysis findings.

B. Beware of assuming that urine samples indicate urinary tract disease if they are entirely normal except for **large numbers of red blood cells.** Menstruating women often contaminate their urine sample accidentally, and Foley catheters commonly cause hematuria, while individuals seeking narcotics may deliberately mix blood into their urine to feign a kidney stone and receive pain medication. If you are suspicious about a urine sample, supervise its collection yourself.

C. Always Gram stain and culture the urine if your patient develops a **fever of unknown origin.** Surgical patients or any patients who have had urethral instrumentation often develop urinary tract infections.

II. **Interpreting the urinalysis results**

A. If you are having trouble identifying cells in the urine sediment, take a buccal scraping from your mouth and suspend it in a drop of the urine. Observing this sample should give you an idea of the size and appearance of epithelial cells at whatever magnification you are using.

B. In a patient with diabetes that is not well controlled, you will want to dipstick each urine sample and attempt to correlate the urine sugars with the blood sugars and other changes in the patient's clinical condition. It is extremely useful to discover a reasonable correlation between blood sugar and urine dipstick sugar.

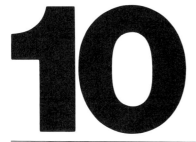

Electrocardiography

Outline of Electrocardiography

I. Indications for ordering an electrocardiogram. Many patients you work up will need an ECG. In the patient with cardiac disease, the ECG will add to your growing understanding of the altered cardiovascular system, complementing the history and physical exam. In the noncardiac patient, the ECG screens for occult cardiac abnormalities and helps ensure the absence of acute disease. In both cardiac and noncardiac patients, the ECG provides a baseline picture of the heart and its conducting system with which future changes in cardiac status may be compared.

II. Patterns analyzed in electrocardiographic analysis. The best way to analyze the ECG, especially at first, is to systematically look at:

A. Rate and rhythm

B. Axis

C. P-R, QRS, and Q-T intervals

D. QRS morphology

E. S-T segment and T wave changes

F. Comparison with previous tracings

Table 10-1 is a quick checklist for analyzing the ECG.

III. Analyzing and interpreting the electrocardiogram

A. Rate and rhythm

1. Every ECG should be inspected to determine the heart's rate and rhythm. Rhythm is often not easily deciphered until the other basic patterns are considered. Decide first whether the ECG shows a normal sinus rhythm or an arrhythmia.

2. Determining rates

a. Regular rate. Recall that you can learn the rate quickly from the R-R interval. For a normal tracing (2.5 cm/sec or 5 large spaces marked by the heavier black line), an R-R interval of:

1 large box = rate 300
2 large boxes = rate 150
3 large boxes = rate 100
4 large boxes = rate 75
5 large boxes = rate 60
6 large boxes = rate 50

Table 10-1. Quick checklist for the ECG

1. **Rate** (bradycardia? tachycardia? regular or irregular?)
2. **Axis** (RAD? LAD?)
3. **P wave morphology** (constant? saw-toothed? notched?)
4. **P-R interval** (<0.12? 0.12–0.20? >0.20?)
5. **QRS interval** (0.08–0.10? >0.10?)
6. **Q-T interval** (within range 0.32–0.40?)
7. **QRS morphology** (shape? height? depth? Q waves?)
8. **S-T segment** (elevated or depressed?)
9. **T wave** (upright or inverted? peaked or flattened?)
10. **Rhythm**
    a. Regular or irregular
    b. P/QRS relationship (1 : 1? extra P waves? extra QRS?)
    c. Reconsider P wave and QRS morphologies
11. **Previous tracing** (change in any lead? How recent?)

RAD = right axis deviation; LAD – left axis deviation

For example, look at the first two ECGs in Table 10-4. In the first tracing, the adjacent R peaks are between 5 and 6 large boxes apart, giving a rate between 50 and 60. In the second, the RR interval spans between 2 to 3 large boxes, giving a rate between 100 and 150.

  b. **Irregular or slow rate.** Note the small black marks at the very top of the ECG paper. At normal chart speed, these marks fall 3 seconds apart. Therefore, to find the rate of an irregular or slow rhythm, count out the number of beats in 2 consecutive 3-second spaces and multiply by 10.

  c. Always **check the atrial and ventricular rates separately.** Usually they will be the same; if they are not, a second- or third-degree heart block may be present.

B. **Axis.** Determine the axis for every cardiogram you read. To do this quickly, look at limb leads I, II, and aVF, noting whether the major direction of the QRS complex's deflection is positive or negative. Now recall the axis diagrams, as shown in Fig. 10-1. There are only three possibilities for axis that you need consider (+ represents upright QRS complex; − represents negative QRS complex deflection):

	Look for
Upright or inverted	Changes in leads I, II, and V_4–V_6, where T waves usually upright.
Peaked or flattened	T waves peaking in the presence of ↑ K^+
	T waves flattening as K^+ ↓ below normal range
	T waves altering their morphology as ischemic damage to the myocardium occurs

If right axis deviation (RAD) is present, you must exclude right ventricular hypertrophy (RVH). If left axis deviation (LAD) is present, you must consider that left anterior fascicular block (LAFB) or left ventricular hypertrophy (LVH) is present. **If the axis is normal, it does not contribute significantly to the differential diagnosis, unless it has changed significantly from prior tracings.**

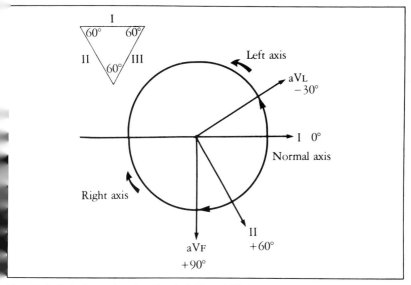

Fig. 10-1. Axis determination. Leads I, II, and III form a hypothetic equilateral triangle, with 60-degree angles as shown. Depolarization moving toward the left arm, parallel to lead I, is designated 0 degrees. Lead aVF, perpendicular to I, is thus labeled 90 degrees, and II is designated 60 degrees. Since aVL is perpendicular to II, forming a 90-degree angle, it is designated +30 degrees. (Reprinted with permission from G. H. Mudge, Jr. [21].)

   C. Intervals. Measure three intervals and record them:

      1. Interval P-R: measure onset of P wave to onset of QRS complex.

         a. Normal range: 0.12–0.20 sec.

         b. Physiologic correlate: time spent between sinoatrial (SA) node depolarization to the initiation of ventricular depolarization, including conduction through the atrioventricular (AV) node.

         c. If the P-R interval is >0.2 sec or is variable, a type of heart block is present. If it is <0.12 sec, this variant may be normal or it may be due either to a rhythm whose atrial focus is quite close to the AV node or to a preexcitation syndrome such as the Wolff-Parkinson-White or Lown-Ganong-Levine syndrome.

      2. Interval QRS: measure onset to end of QRS.

         a. Normal range: 0.08–0.10 sec.

         b. Physiologic correlate: time required for the spread of the electrical impulse through the ventricular muscle.

         c. The abnormal QRS duration is important in two instances. First, it will be prolonged in intraventricular conduction defects (IVCD), as outlined in Table 10-2. Second, in arrhythmia analysis a wide QRS may indicate aberrant conduction of a supraventricular impulse or a ventricular ectopic focus (see the footnote to Table 10-4).

      3. Interval Q-T: measure onset of QRS to end of T wave.

         a. Normal range: rate dependent, but usually 0.32–0.40 sec.

Table 10-2. Intraventricular conduction defects (IVCDs)

IVCD	QRS duration	V_1 morphology	V_6 morphology
Right bundle branch block (RBBB)	≥0.12 sec	R′ in V_1	Deep S in V_6
Left bundle branch block (LBBB)*	≥0.12 sec	Wide S in V_1	Large R in V_6 often with jagged up-stroke
Left anterior fascicular block (LAFB)	Diagnosis suggested by presence of axis ≤ ⁻30 degrees		
Left posterior fascicular block (LPFB)	Diagnosed by *newly* developed rightward shift in axis in the appropriate clinical setting (e.g., shift from + 80 to + 160 degrees in setting of an acute posterior MI or by extreme rightward axis)		

*In the presence of LBBB, no other conclusions may be read from the QRS morphology: hypertrophy, ischemia, and infarction are not reliably interpretable because of the abnormal pathway to ventricular depolarization.

   b. Physiologic correlate: time required for complete depolarization and repolarization.

   c. The Q-T interval varies with heart rate. The corrected Q-T interval is $(Q-T)_c$ = Q-T (measured) ÷ (R-R interval)$^{1/2}$ and equals 0.42 sec. Usually the uncorrected Q-T interval is 0.32–0.40 sec. Instances to be aware of that will significantly alter the Q-T interval include:

Quinidine	↑ Q-T	by increasing T wave duration
Hypocalcemia	↑ Q-T	by increasing length of S-T segment
Hypokalemia	↑ Q-T	by prolonging T wave with U wave formation
Hypercalcemia	↓ Q-T	by decreasing length of S-T segment

D. QRS morphology. The QRS complex is the most important configuration of the ECG. In addition to the duration of the QRS interval, carefully analyze its morphology with respect to:

   1. General shape. Are there notches? Is the upstroke jagged or smooth? This is helpful in differential diagnosis of IVCD.

   2. Height of R waves and depth of S waves, especially in leads I, II, V_2, V_5. Helpful in determining presence of ventricular hypertrophy.

   3. Presence of Q waves, which are defined as an initial downward deflection in the QRS lasting >0.4 sec (1 small box) or 25 percent of the height of the associated R wave. This is a criterion for Q wave myocardial infarction.

E. S-T segment and T wave changes. One of the mistakes made by beginning electrocardiographers is to focus on the S-T and T wave changes without fully interpreting the QRS complex. The S-T segment and T wave should be analyzed once the QRS complex is evaluated. The S-T segment is most helpful in determining the presence of ischemic changes (see Table 10-3 and Fig. 10-2). Remember that it may vary in normal individuals and

Table 10-3. ECG criteria for atrial abnormalities and ventricular hypertrophy

	P wave morphology		Major limb lead	Major precordial criteria	S-T and T wave changes
	II	V_2			
Left atrial abnormality	See Fig. 10-2	See Fig. 10-2	—	—	None
Right atrial abnormality	See Fig. 10-2	See Fig. 10-2	—	—	None
LVH (with or without strain)	—	—	R in I + S in III ≥ 20 mm	R in V_5 or V_6 + S in V_1 or V_2 ≥ 35 mm	S-T segment unchanged; T wave may be taller (without strain) S-T segment depressed; T wave inverted in leads V_4–V_6 (with strain)
RVH (with or without strain)	R/S ratio ≥ 1.0 in V_1 R/S ratio ≤ 1.0 in V_6		Right axis deviation (≥ + 90 degrees)		S-T segment unchanged; T wave may be taller (without strain) S-T segment depressed; T wave inverted in leads V_1, V_2 (with strain)

LVH = left ventricular hypertrophy; RVH = right ventricular hypertrophy.

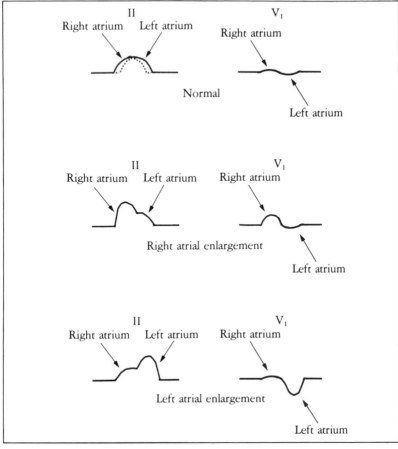

Fig. 10-2. P wave configuration. (Reprinted with permission from G. H. Mudge, Jr. [21].)

is easily affected by drugs (especially digitalis) and electrolyte imbalance. Determine:

1. **Whether S-T segment is elevated or depressed.** Note elevation ≥1 mm or depression ≥0.5 mm; clinical correlates of ischemia; any drugs patient may be taking.

2. **Relation of T wave to S-T segment.** Elevated S-T segment with T wave incorporated into S-T elevation is suggestive of ischemia; T wave that remains discernible from S-T segment elevation is more consistent with normal variant (early repolarization).

3. The **T wave** is often a labile entity, and changes in its morphology can be difficult to interpret. However, the presence of T wave inversion is often associated with three clinical situations: ischemia, digitalis, and strain (a pattern associated with ventricular hypertrophy). Determine whether the T wave is:

   a. **Upright or inverted.** Note changes in leads I, II, and V_4–V_6, where T waves are usually upright.

     b. Peaked or flattened. Note T waves peaking in the presence of ↑ K[1]; T waves flattening as K[1] ↓ below normal range; T waves altering their morphology as ischemic damage to the myocardium occurs.

F. Comparison with previous tracings. It is important to compare the admitting ECG with previous tracings on record. The six basics of ECG analysis mentioned in sec. **II** (see also Table 10-2) should be compared in detail and any changes noted in the write-up. If there is no significant change, that fact should be specifically mentioned.

G. Arrhythmias. Although the teaching of arrhythmia analysis is beyond the scope of this book, you can move a long way toward diagnosis by making this crucial distinction first: **is the rhythm in question regular or irregular?** Note the following diagnostic possibilities for these categories.

Regular rhythm	Irregular rhythm
Sinus tachycardia	Multifocal atrial tachycardia (MAT)
Paroxysmal atrial tachycardia	Atrial fibrillation
(PAT)	Regular rhythm with variable block
PAT with block	
Atrial flutter	
Ventricular tachycardia	

Once you have determined the category in which the rhythm in question belongs, there are several ways to analyze the rhythm further. For instance, the response to carotid sinus pressure (see **Part B**), the P wave morphology, and the QRS morphology may all be helpful. Further information regarding the analysis of several of the more common arrhythmias is presented in Table 10-4.

B   **Practical Points Concerning Electrocardiography**

I. **Performing the electrocardiographic test.** Within the first few weeks of your clinical rotations, learn how to perform a **12-lead ECG.** The key here is to aim for consistency in lead placement and a flat baseline. Remember to obtain a rhythm strip. The rhythm strip is usually done with lead V_2.

II. **Patterns analyzed in electrocardiographic analysis**

    A. It is important to become comfortable enough with ECGs to be able to peruse them quickly and to detect abnormal features. The key task at this point is to pay attention to the basics of analysis and to begin to train yourself to **recognize patterns**—that is, to "eyeball" the tracing, first taking in the overall picture, and then delving into the details of the tracing.

    B. It is crucial to analyze the ECG within the **clinical setting.** This point may seem trivial, but it is in fact the most important consideration in ECG interpretation. The ECG has meaning for you as a clinician only in the context of the patient for whom you are caring.

III. **Analyzing and interpreting the electrocardiogram**

    A. In preparation for learning ECG analysis, refamiliarize yourself with the anatomy and physiology of the **His-Purkinje system.** Also relearn the course and distribution of the **coronary arteries** if you have forgotten them.

    B. Review a normal 12-lead ECG with particular attention to limb lead II and precordial lead V_2. Analyze the normal tracing step by step, in the manner detailed in **Part A.III,** as a "warm-up" for the wards.

Table 10-4. Arrhythmias

Rhythms	Atrial rate	Ventricular rate	P wave morphology	CSP response	QRS morphology	Clinical points
Regular rhythms Sinus bradycardia	<60	<60	Normal	(Not used)	Normal	Often normal variant, especially in athletes. May accompany obstructive jaundice with ↑ serum bilirubin; ↑ intracranial pressure; digitalis; or acute inferior MIs. Most common cause at present is probably use of beta blocking drugs.
Sinus tachycardia	>100	>100	Normal	Gradual slowing; change to tachycardia when CSP released	Normal	Especially associated with fever, infections, hemorrhage, hyperthyroidism.

Paroxysmal atrial tachycardia	140–220	140–220	Usually obscured by preceding T wave Theoretically abnormal (focus other than SA node)	No change or abrupt termination of arrhythmia	Normal	May see S-T segment depression associated with PAT.
PAT with block	140–220	Fixed fraction of the atrial rate (e.g., ½)	Abnormal morphology	No change or ↑ in degree of block (e.g., from ½ to ¼)	Normal	May indicate digitalis toxicity.

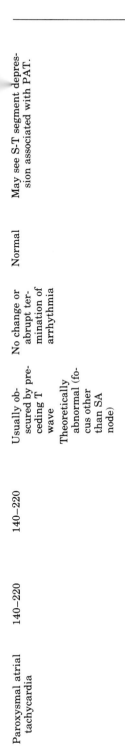

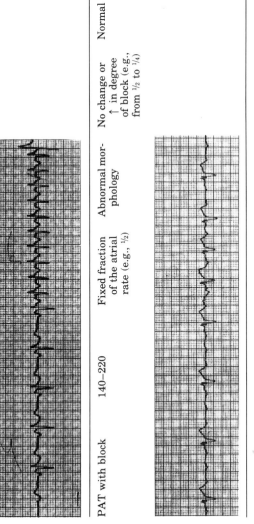

Rhythms	Atrial rate	Ventricular rate	P wave morphology	CSP response	QRS morphology	Clinical points
Atrial flutter	220–320 (300–320 most common)	Fixed fraction of atrial rate (e.g., ½ or ¼, so called 2 : 1 or 4 : 1 block)	Saw-toothed "flutter" waves	Usually no change or ↑ in block	Normal	Look for flutter waves in II, III, aVꜰ, V₁, and V₂.
Junctional tachycardia	>75	>75	**None** often; may be present in close proximity to QRS (either preceding or following); see Clinical points	No change or termination	Normal	Must exclude digitalis toxicity. Look for inverted P waves (from retrograde conduction) in II, III, and aVꜰ. P waves may arrive at atria after QRS is inscribed and thus follow QRS on ECG.

Ventricular tachycardia	P waves rarely seen (occasionally retrograde P waves appear)	140–280	Rare	No change If retrograde P waves present, CSP may block them out ("V-A" block)	Wide, irregular	Converts at low DC cardioversion energies (≤10 watt-seconds 90 percent of the time).
Ventricular flutter	None seen	>300	None	No help	Bizarre shape, ↑ duration	Ventricular tachycardia with faster rate. An ominous rhythm that may progress to ventricular fibrillation and death.

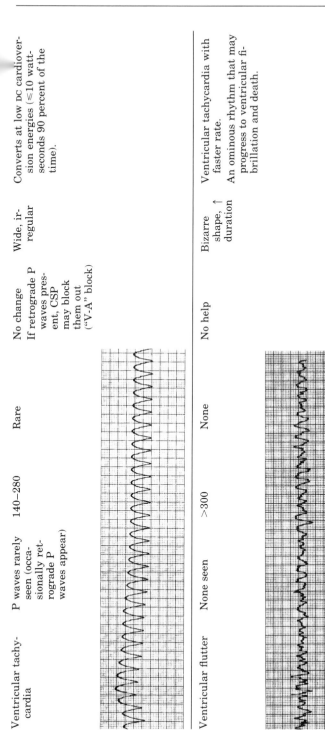

Table 10-4 (continued).

Rhythms	Atrial rate	Ventricular rate	P wave morphology	CSP response	QRS morphology	Clinical points
Irregular rhythms Multifocal atrial tachycardia (MAT)	>100	>100	≥3 different P wave morphologies	No change or transient slowing	Normal	Present in patients with COPD or pulmonary processes. Often must treat the primary process (not the arrhythmia).
Atrial fibrillation	None seen (flat or undulating baseline between Q waves)	40–300 (variable)	None	Usually no change; occasionally ↑ block	Normal	May be confused with atrial flutter. Classically associated with mitral stenosis and chronic mitral regurgitation; also present in CHF and coronary artery disease.

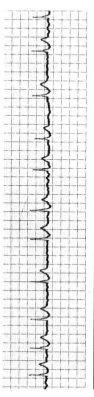

Regular rhythm with variable block (not pictured)	140–220	Varying fraction of atrial rate (e.g., 2 : 1 block alternating with 4 : 1 block)	Abnormal	See PAT with block and Atrial flutter, above	Normal	This is **not an irregularly irregular rhythm** like atrial fibrillation.

Note: A widened QRS may be due to either (1) conduction of an impulse that originates in the atria but encounters refractory conduction tissue in the ventricular His-Purkinje system **(aberrant conduction)** or (2) an impulse that originates in ventricular tissue **(ventricular ectopic activity)**. In either case the widened QRS is due to electrical spread **directly** through ventricular muscle (outside the conducting system). Both mechanisms will lead to QRS interval prolongation, and making the distinction between them is often difficult. At this point it is sufficient to know that these two possibilities exist.

CSP = carotid sinus pressure; PAT = paroxysmal atrial tachycardia; COPD = chronic obstructive pulmonary disease; CHF = congestive heart failure.

IV. Using carotid sinus pressure (CSP). This is a useful technique that employs the physiologic response of increased vagal tone to the AV node by stimulating the afferent limb of the carotid reflex. Two warnings, however, should always be remembered. First, it is important to avoid CSP in patients who have a history of transient ischemic attack (TIA) or stroke or who have known carotid disease on exam. Second, performing this technique can have complications even if you are cautious; it **must** be done in the presence of an experienced house officer and with ECG monitoring.

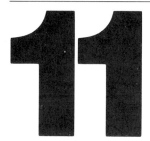

Chest Radiology

Annotated Outline
of Chest Radiology

I. **Indications for ordering chest roentgenographs.** Chest radiology is a vital tool in the work-up of pulmonary, cardiovascular, and systemic problems. There are many indications for ordering a chest film series, which usually includes both posteroanterior (PA) and lateral views:

A. **Admission chest x-rays** used to be a standard part of the admission test battery at virtually all hospitals. Today, however, many experienced clinicians believe that doing routine chest x-rays (CXRs) on every patient is not beneficial, wastes scarce resources, and exposes many patients to unnecessary radiation. Always ask yourself why you are ordering an x-ray and what you will do with the results, before you order it.

B. **Sepsis and fever** work-ups almost always include a chest x-ray, even if there are no obvious respiratory symptoms.

C. **Cardiovascular** pathologic processes are often accompanied by changes in the cardiac silhouette, the appearance of the great vessels, or the pattern of pulmonary vascular distribution.

D. **Pulmonary disease** processes as diverse as infection and neoplasm may be indistinguishable on the basis of the physical exam, and the CXR interpreted in the context of the clinical history is often the sine qua non of pulmonary diagnosis.

E. **Chest pain,** whenever thought to be due to musculoskeletal processes, routinely involves a chest x-ray as part of the diagnostic work-up. The CXR is especially indicated in patients with "atypical chest pain" syndromes, where one must decide between cardiovascular or noncardiovascular etiologies.

F. **Systemic diseases** often result in roentgenologic changes that, while rarely pathognomonic, are useful in diagnosis.

G. All of the pathologic processes mentioned in **B–F** can be followed with **serial chest x-ray studies,** although the radiologic picture may "lag behind" the clinical exam as a process resolves.

H. **Interventional procedures** such as thoracenteses and central line placements are often concluded with a CXR to assess the efficacy of the procedure (e.g., what is the position of a central line?) and to rule out complications (e.g., is there a pneumothorax?).

II. **General approach to chest x-ray interpretation.** Unlike many lab tests that can be successfully interpreted without any knowledge of the actual test methodology, the interpretation of all radiologic studies requires that the interpreter understand some basic radiologic principles. Most of these principles are intuitively obvious and follow from the concept that roentgenographs are actually **transilluminations of body structures,** similar to the transillumination of the cheek produced with a flashlight when one is investigating an oral lesion.

A. **Radiologic densities and images.** The x-ray is a two-dimensional composite shadow produced by transmission of x-ray photons through three-dimensional structures that differ in their ability to attenuate the photons. It gives two types of information: shape and density. There are several important corollaries to this concept.

   1. All shapes except a sphere will show dramatic changes in their **shadow profiles,** depending on how the objects are positioned and rotated in front of the x-ray beam. Conversely, an object that looks circular on both the PA and lateral views is almost certainly spherical.

   2. An object will have a distinct **silhouette border** only if it differs significantly in density from the objects around it (the **silhouette sign;** see **III.A.2**). For the purposes of this chapter, there are **four basic densities:** (1) air, (2) fat, (3) tissue-fluid, and (4) bone. Because it is the most dense, bone will cause high levels of photon attenuation (and hence low photon transmission) and will appear to be the whitest on the x-ray. Conversely, the air in the lungs will allow high photon transmission and will show up as black or dark gray.

   3. A single image on the x-ray may involve the superimposition of multiple shadows. One must learn to use the PA and lateral views together to break down composite shadows into shapes of individual objects.

B. **Systematic roentgenographic interpretation.** Like the physical exam, x-ray interpretation is best done in a systematic way, following the same sequence of analysis every time. Although the more experienced interpreter may "gestalt" a film, making an almost instant diagnosis after observing the integrated pattern for a few seconds (much like the snap diagnosis that an experienced clinician may be able to make), the novice radiologist should choose a certain sequence of analysis and stick to it. One useful method is to begin with the least prominent information on the film and gradually move toward the most prominent findings. For example, such an analysis sequence might be (1) introductory background information, (2) bones, (3) pulmonary vasculature, (4) pulmonary parenchyma and lung fields, and (5) cardiac silhouette and mediastinum. Each of these areas will be discussed. Fig. 11-1 shows reproductions of a normal PA and lateral chest x-ray, with diagrams of the heart and great vessels superimposed to indicate their positions.

   1. **Introductory background information.** Much information about the context of an x-ray study can be found on the film or the film folder. Always check this information first to ensure that you are looking at the correct CXR and that you understand the technique of the study. In particular, note:

      a. **Patient name and number.** Films are often placed in the wrong file.

      b. **Date of study.** Check the film itself, not just the envelope.

      c. **PA or anteroposterior (AP) projection.** Standard films are PA, while portable films are AP. AP views make the heart appear enlarged and thus make true cardiac size difficult to assess.

      d. **Supine or upright patient position.** Check stomach bubble position. Supine position causes increased prominence of pulmonary vasculature.

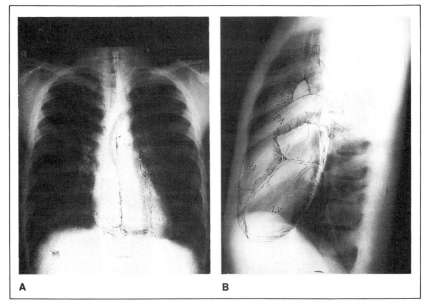

Fig. 11-1. Normal CXR patterns with superimposed diagrams of heart and great vessels. **A.** PA view. **B.** Lateral view.

    e. Patient rotation. Check the clavicles for symmetry. If the patient is rotated, the film will be harder to interpret and to compare with other studies.

    f. Film penetration. An underpenetrated film makes pulmonary vasculature more prominent.

    g. Dates of previous CXR studies. Are old films available for comparison?

2. Bone radiology in the chest x-ray. Most CXR studies are not ordered to investigate the thoracic bones, but it is important to make a habit of looking at the bones every time you analyze a CXR, both because the bones themselves may provide valuable diagnostic information about a patient's condition (especially in cases of systemic disease) and because the bones provide a kind of grid or coordinate system, which will be useful in the identification, comparison, and description of the soft tissue.

An investigation of the bones often begins with the clavicles, whose symmetry allows an assessment of patient rotation. It then proceeds to the shoulders, where one checks the appearance and relationships of the various elements of each joint and the general symmetry of the two shoulder joints. Although an appreciation for the texture and the limits of normal in the appearance of the skeletal system is difficult to acquire, the novice may make many diagnoses by paying special attention to any cortical breaks, fissures, "moth-eaten" areas, or areas that seem to have increased or decreased radiolucency when compared with the other bones and with the mirror-image area on the other side of the body.

Finally, every rib may be individually located, mentally numbered, and visually inspected along the length of its spiral course. Once again, the clinical history is of paramount importance. A patient complaining of localized chest pain should have a very careful CXR rib analysis to rule out skeletal pathology, while the asymptomatic patient needs only a quick scan.

3. **Pulmonary vasculature.** One of the most important clinical questions encountered in chest radiology is whether or not a patient is in congestive heart failure (CHF). Although the pulmonary vascular pattern is useful in assessing other types of cardiopulmonary pathology, it is in the clinical setting of heart failure that the novice radiologist will most often be concerned with these patterns. In addition to the appearance of the heart itself, three features of the pulmonary vasculature's appearance are important in making this diagnosis: (1) the pattern of vascular prominence and redistribution, (2) the existence of pulmonary edema, and (3) the finding of pleural effusion.

   a. **Vascular patterns.** The vasculature is most prominent in the medial lower lung (75 percent of total perfusion is normally to the lower lobes, due to the mass of lung parenchyma and to gravitational effects).

   The ratio of upper to lower vasculature is approximately 1 to 3 in the normal CXR. Vascular prominence can represent engorgement of arteries, veins, lymphatics, or all three. In general, pulmonary arteries run vertically, while pulmonary veins empty lower and course horizontally. Lymphatics are normally not visible. Although it is often difficult to decide between the arteries and veins on the basis of the x-ray alone, it is useful to remember that the backup or regurgitation of blood from the left ventricle to the lungs (c/w mitral stenosis, CHF, myocardial infarction, mitral regurgitation) will lead to venous prominence, while arterial engorgement will result from increased right-sided flow, as in left-to-right shunts (c/w patent ductus arteriosus, septal defects, etc.).

   b. **Pulmonary edema.** Pulmonary edema is the result of pulmonic vascular congestion to the point that the oncotic pressure of the blood is no longer able to maintain the integrity of the vascular system. The resulting edema fluid is taken up by the pulmonary lymphatics, which increase in radiologic prominence due to the increased flow.

   When the edema becomes severe, it is associated with **horizontal linear densities** known as **Kerley's lines.** Probably the most important of these are **Kerley's B lines,** which are assumed to represent engorgement of interlobular septa and are often observed in cases of CHF as well as tumor, fibrosis, and so forth (see Fig. 11-3).

   c. **Pleural effusion.** The costophrenic angles should be sharp and free of fluid on the normal CXR. If the patient has made a good inspiratory effort, the diaphragm should be visible at the level of rib 10 or 11.

   Because pleural fluid collects in the costophrenic recess, in the upright patient it first fills up the deeper **posterior** part of the recess; practically, this means that the **lateral view** will show evidence of an effusion before the PA view will. A caveat here: fluid may accumulate between the lung pleura and the diaphragm. In this case, the subpulmonic effusion may be difficult to distinguish from an elevated diaphragm or a consolidated left lower lobe. Repeating the lung exam after looking at the x-ray often helps to resolve this confusion.

4. **Radiologic patterns.** The vascular shadows associated with normal and pathologic perfusion patterns are schematically illustrated in Fig. 11-2.

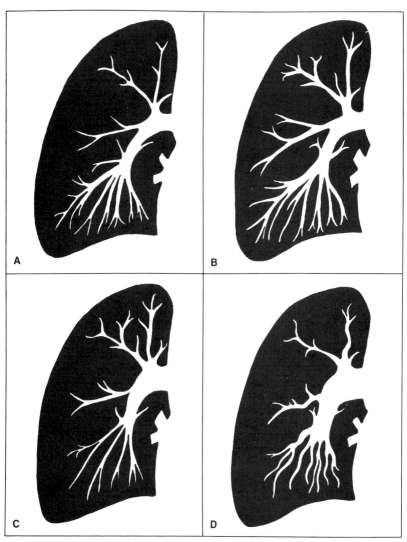

Fig. 11-2. Pulmonary vascular patterns in the right lung (PA film). In the normal lung, the majority of pulmonary perfusion is directed to the lower lobes, resulting in the CXR pattern seen in **A**. Generally increased vascular prominence without significant vascular redistribution is shown in **B**; this pattern represents the CXR of a patient with a high-output state, such as left-to-right shunt, anemia, or pregnancy. Vascular redistribution, as seen in congestive heart failure, results in upper lobe engorgement and the pattern shown in **C. D** illustrates the central engorgement and peripheral vascular "pruning" seen in cases in which high peripheral pulmonary resistance due to lung disease results in pulmonary hypertension. (Modified from *The Merck Manual* [20].)

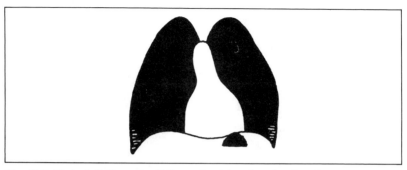

Fig. 11-3. Kerley's B lines. Small linear densities often found at the lung periphery, Kerley's B lines are assumed to represent engorgement of lymphatics due to pulmonary edema.

Fig. 11-3 shows Kerley's B lines associated with pulmonary edema. While these diagrams are simplified and more obvious than the actual appearance of these findings on real chest x-rays, the student who remembers these basic patterns and realizes that the pulmonary congestion found in congestive heart failure results in (1) venous engorgement with resultant increase in upper-lobe vascular radiologic prominence, (2) pulmonary edema with Kerley's B lines, and (3) bilateral pleural effusions will already be able to comment usefully on many chest x-rays seen on a general medical service.

III. **Pulmonary parenchyma and lung field infiltrates.** While vascular problems present radiographically as linear densities, the roentgenographic changes that suggest disease in the pulmonary air-space compartment involve space-occupying, often "patchy" densities. Such findings are called **infiltrates,** and are associated with many types of disease processes, notably infections, neoplasms, and hemorrhage. The patient's clinical history and physical exam are very important in the interpretation of infiltrates; an infiltrate without a history of fever might suggest a hemorrhage or neoplasm, whereas a clinical history suggesting infection would place pneumonia much higher on the differential list.

A. **Infiltrate localization.** The first step in analyzing an infiltrate is to attempt to determine exactly where it is. For the novice, there are three basic ways to locate an infiltrate.

1. Using the PA and lateral views together, an attempt is made to identify the three-dimensional location of the infiltrate. This is especially important in the analysis of small densities that may seem to represent coin lesions on the PA view but, when sought on the lateral, often turn out to signify either superficial structures (e.g., nipples, buttons) or collections of interlobular fluid **(pseudotumors).**

2. If an infiltrate is large enough to occupy a significant part of a lobe, it may result in the disappearance of the silhouette of an adjacent structure. This phenomenon is called the **silhouette sign,** and is actually nothing more than an application of the general principle that distinct outlines are visible on the x-ray only when there is a difference in density between adjacent structures. When lung tissue is replaced by blood, pus, or tumor, the radiographic outlines of the mediastinal or diaphragmatic organs superimposed on these infiltrated areas will dis-

appear. By paying attention to exactly which outlines are obscured by the infiltrate, and by using both the PA and lateral films, one can usually establish which lobes are involved and gain insight into the etiology and extent of the infiltrate.

Fig. 11-4 illustrates the x-ray changes associated with consolidation in each of the pulmonary lobes. Note, for instance, that involvement of the right lower lobe, which is posterior, will lighten but will not totally obscure the right heart outline because the heart is anteriorly placed. By contrast, a right middle lobe infiltrate often obliterates the right side of the cardiac shadow.

3. The presence of some degree of **mediastinal shift** is a third key to deciding where a lesion is located. The mediastinum is normally a set of roughly midline structures. Note that these appear superimposed on the vertebral column in the normal PA film in Fig. 11-1. Consider especially the positions of the column of air in the trachea, the aortic arch, and the right heart border; these serve as reference points to the upper, middle, and lower mediastinum.

If the mediastinal structures appear to bow to one side, this may suggest either a **vacuum effect** caused by lung collapse or a **mass effect** caused by neoplasm, exudate, or hyperinflation. Once again, the specific pulmonary lobes affected may be deduced from the mediastinal borders that are shifted. For instance, if only the right lower lobe is collapsed, the cardiac border will shift to the right while the trachea and the aortic arch may remain in their usual positions. **The mediastinum will be shifted toward the side of lung collapse and away from the side of lung overexpansion** (e.g., as in emphysematous change) and thoracic masses (e.g., as in pleural effusions, tumors). Shifts in the positions of the major and minor pulmonary fissures may be used in the same way. These are probably somewhat more revealing, although slightly more difficult to recognize.

B. **Infiltrate identification.** The radiologic differential diagnosis of pulmonary infiltrates is difficult and is dependent on the hints given by the clinical history. Often the most useful approach is to think in terms of broad categories of disease (e.g., infectious, neoplastic, collagen vascular, hemorrhagic) and then to use the clinical history to determine the most likely specific diagnosis. For instance, a right lower lobe infiltrate may suggest pneumonia, while the production of thick sputum with gram-positive diplococci would make the diagnosis of pneumococcal pneumonia virtually certain.

One very important question in the identification of a lung-field density is whether the density is simply a collection of fluid located outside the alveoli or whether there is actual **consolidation** of the air spaces. A useful sign to look for is the presence of the **air bronchogram** pattern, which basically is nothing more than the air in the bronchial tree made visible by increased density of the surrounding structures. Normally, the bronchi are not well seen because there is not enough contrast in radiologic density; they consist of a tubelike arrangement of air spaces surrounded by a very thin wrapping of tissue. However, under conditions of lobar consolidation, due to tumor or pneumonia, the radiologic density surrounding these air spaces is much greater, and the contrast makes the bronchial markings visible.

Table 11-1 summarizes some of the classic findings useful in the differential diagnosis of pulmonary infiltrate.

IV. **Cardiac silhouette.** An analysis of the cardiac silhouette on the chest roentgenograph extends the information acquired during the physical exam. For

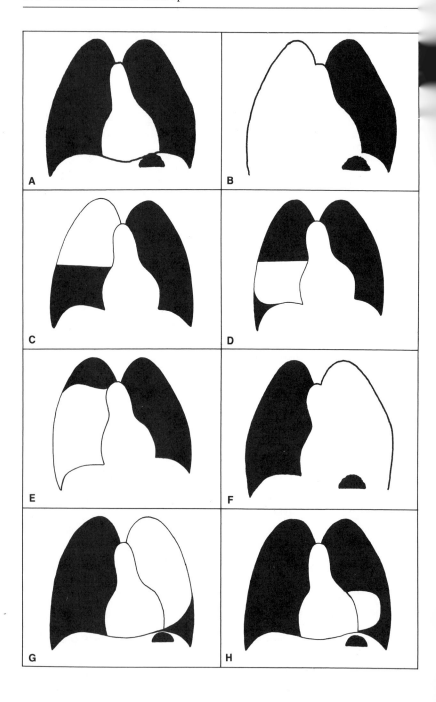

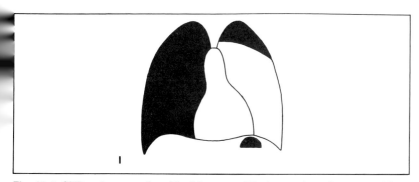

Fig. 11-4. CXR patterns produced by lobar consolidations such as those caused by pneumonia or tumor. Note the disappearance of various parts of the cardiac and diaphragmatic borders due to the increased density of the consolidated lung tissue. This loss of density contrast borders is called the *silhouette sign.* **A.** Normal CXR. **B.** Total R lung consolidation with obliteration of the R heart border. **C.** R upper lobe consolidation. **D.** R middle lobe consolidation. **E.** R lower lobe consolidation. **F.** Total L lung consolidation with obliteration of the L heart border. **G.** L upper lobe consolidation. **H.** L upper lobe lingular consolidation with disappearance of the L heart border. **I.** L lower lobe consolidation; L heart border still faintly visible due to air in lingula. (Modified from L. Squire and R. A. Novelline [24].)

example, a soft S_3 coupled with an enlarged ventricle on CXR strongly suggests the possibility of congestive failure.

The key to interpreting a patient's cardiovascular status via the CXR lies in the recognition of **specific chamber abnormalities.** Deciding that "the heart looks abnormal" is much less useful than deciding that there is dilatation of the left atrium and straightening of the left heart border, suggestive of mitral valve disease.

A. Components of the cardiac silhouette. The borders of the cardiac shadow can be broken down into a series of nine overlapping arcs (Fig. 11-5). The systematic analysis of the cardiac shadow involves breaking the shadow down into these arcs and determining which, if any, are abnormal. Once you memorize the information in Fig. 11-5, it will be much easier to apply knowledge of cardiovascular pathophysiology to the interpretation of the chest film.

B. Cardiothoracic ratio. A specific example of the use of cardiac chamber appearance in radiologic diagnosis is the cardiothoracic ratio. This concept, illustrated in Fig. 11-6, is based on the rule of thumb that, in the PA exposure, the extreme right and left borders of the cardiac outline (segment A-B) should be no farther apart than one-half the width of the chest at its widest point (segment C-D). Because an enlarged left ventricle is most often the cause of an enlarged cardiothoracic ratio, this rule is most useful in the diagnosis of heart failure associated with ventricular dilatation or hypertrophy.

Fig. 11-7, a reproduction of the lateral CXR of a patient who has undergone triple valve replacement, clarifies the position of the cardiac valves and outflow tracts.

See Table 11-1 for a summary of some of the common CXR findings associated with specific cardiovascular problems.

Table 11-1. Summary of roentgenographic findings associated with disease processes of various organ systems

Disease process	Roentgenographic findings
Cardiovascular*	
1. Atrial septal defect	RA and RV prominence with normal LA; prominent lung vascularity
2. Tricuspid regurgitation	RA enlargement; cardiac enlargement
3. Tricuspid stenosis	RA enlargement
4. Pulmonic regurgitation	No good CXR findings
5. Pulmonic stenosis	May be normal; otherwise, RV and outflow prominence; PA poststenotic dilatation
6. Pulmonary hypertension	RA and RV enlargement; prominent central pulmonary vessels near hilum; rapid tapering; avascular peripheral lung fields
7. Mitral regurgitation	LA and LV enlargement; mitral valve calcification; pulmonary congestion if chronic
8. Mitral stenosis	LA enlargement; prominent pulmonary venous system; mitral calcification; Kerley's B lines
9. Aortic regurgitation	LV enlargement; more prominent if chronic aortic dilatation
10. Aortic stenosis	Calcified aortic valve. LV enlargement; prominent ascending aorta
11. Hypertension	LV hypertrophy; prominent tortuous aorta
12. Congestive heart failure	LV enlargement and pulmonary congestion; Kerley's B lines
13. Constrictive pericarditis	Small or slightly enlarged heart; pericardial calcification
14. Coarctation of aorta	Notching of lower rib borders
Pulmonary infiltrates: infectious	
1. Viral pneumonia	Nodular infiltrate; diffuse involvement
2. Pneumococcal pneumonia	Lobar or bronchopneumonic infiltrates and consolidation; air bronchograms; pleural effusion
3. Tuberculosis	Apical infiltrate; parenchymal calcification
4. Granulomas (due to tuberculosis, histoplasmosis, coccidiodosis, etc.)	Fibrosis; calcifications; satellite densities
Neoplasms	
1. Bronchogenic carcinoma	Solitary lesions without calcifications
2. Bronchoalveolar cell cancer	Segmental distribution; can mimic infiltrate
3. Metastatic cancer	Often multiple lesions
4. Hodgkin's disease, lymphoma, leukemia	Parenchymal infiltrate; hilar node enlargement; mediastinal widening
Pulmonary	
1. Foreign body	Foreign body may be obvious on CXR; may cause "check valve" hyperinflation
2. Atelectasis	Plate-like densities
3. Bronchiectasis	Basilar patchy densities
4. Emphysema	Overexpanded lungs; low diaphragms; increased radiolucency of lungs; heart may seem small
5. Interstitial lung disease (due to inhalants, drugs, collagen vascular disease, etc.)	Diffuse infiltrate
6. Pneumothorax	Visceral pleural line visible on x-ray

*Cardiac enlargement is usually a late finding in cardiovascular diseases.

LA = left atrium; LV = left ventricle; PA = posteroanterior; RA = right atrium; RV = right ventricle.

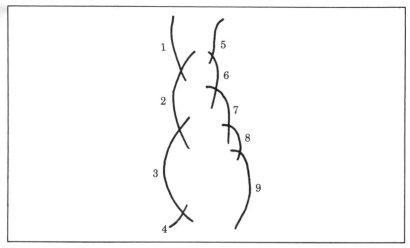

Fig. 11-5. The normal mediastinal profiles are all vascular and resolve into a series of nine intersecting arcs: (1) superior vena cava; (2) ascending aorta; (3) right atrium; (4) inferior vena cava and cardiac fat pad; (5) left subclavian vein and artery, left common carotid artery; (6) aortic arch; (7) pulmonary artery; (8) left atrium; (9) left ventricle. (Reprinted with permission from L. Squire and R. A. Novelline [24].)

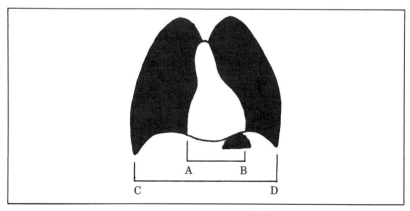

Fig. 11-6. Cardiothoracic ratio. In a routine PA CXR, the width of the cardiac shadow (segment A-B) should be no more than half the width of the thoracic cavity (segment C-D). This is a rough rule of thumb, and it should be used together with an analysis of the cardiac chamber configuration to obtain a reasonable estimate of heart size.

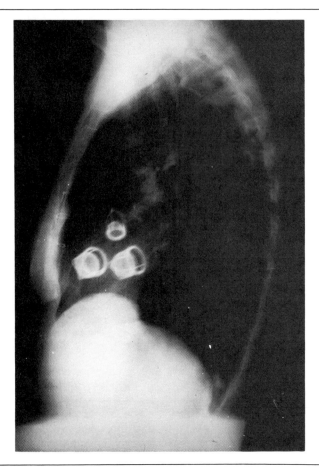

Fig. 11-7. Lateral CXR of patient who has undergone aortic, mitral, and tricuspid valve replacement, demonstrating the position of these valves and their outflow tracts (compare with Fig. 11-1).

B   **Practical Points Concerning**
                                        Chest Radiology

I. Ordering the chest roentgenograph

   A. The **requisition form** for a CXR usually includes a space for you to provide **clinical information** to be used in the radiologist's interpretation of the film. It is important that you provide the radiologist with two types of information:

   1. The clinical history that relates to your **specific questions** (e.g., "55-year-old male with long smoking history, recent weight loss, and chronic fever; rule out cancer.").

2. Clinical details relating to known **x-ray findings** that might otherwise confuse the radiologist (e.g., "Patient has history of pulmonary radiation treatment 2 years prior to admission.").

The better your clinical summary, the better your radiology reports will be.

B. Every radiology department has its own set of **protocols** for working up specific problems. It is worth your while to talk to a radiologist about the department's preferences (e.g., "Should this suspicious CXR be followed by MRI or by a CT scan of the chest?"). Try to use the radiologist as a diagnostic consultant as well as a film interpreter. In the process you will learn a lot of medicine.

II. General approach to chest x-ray interpretation

A. Before attempting to interpret chest x-rays, you should review the gross anatomy of the **thorax** concentrating especially on:

1. The relations of the internal organs in the thorax, especially the mediastinal structures around the T_4 level (e.g., determine the relation of the heart to the tracheal bifurcation and the esophagus).

2. The exact position of the heart and its chamber in the thorax. Think about possible pathophysiologic changes in the shape of the heart. For instance, where on the cardiac margin would you see the protruding atrium in an instance of left atrial dilatation? What diseases might cause this change?

3. The lobes of the lungs and the approximate positions of the pulmonary fissures. Which fissures would you expect to see from the PA perspective? Which from the lateral?

B. Commonsense principles are of the utmost importance in attempting to learn CXR interpretation. Keep the following general principles in mind:

1. With certain obvious exceptions, the human body is a bilaterally symmetric structure. Consequently, an area on one of the lungs that appears to demonstrate vascular prominence may be profitably compared to the mirror-image area on the other lung (bearing in mind, of course, that the lungs themselves are not perfectly symmetric).

2. **Changes** in serial x-ray studies are of the utmost importance, especially if the changes occur around the time that the patient's clinical history changes. Try to review the patient's x-ray files to find when the films first began to deviate from normal. To develop the ability to recognize changes, you will have to study many normal films and pay careful attention to serial films taken on your patients. For patients who receive a film daily, take the time every so often to compare that day's film with one taken a week earlier; changes may be more obvious.

3. Although it is often a good teaching exercise to try to interpret an x-ray before you read the clinical history, you should always think about your patients' films in relation to their clinical conditions. Could you hear rales in the patient whose chest films suggest pulmonary edema? Was there the sudden onset of pleuritic pain or dyspnea just before the patient's films began to show a segmental lower lobe infiltrate consistent with a pulmonary embolus? You should constantly recheck old films as the clinical story evolves; often an old x-ray finding can be reinterpreted in light of new information. You should learn to use the x-rays to sharpen your physical examination skills; the **listen-look-listen** method (listen to the lungs; look at the x-ray; listen to the lungs again) is an excellent self-teaching device.

4. **Pathophysiologic processes** that are very different clinically may look very similar on the x-ray (for instance, bronchoalveolar cell carcinoma may appear identical on x-ray to lobar pneumonia). Therefore, the vocabulary with which you speak of and think about the roentgenograph should be that of radiologic appearance ("nodule," "opacity," "infiltrate") and not diagnosis ("tumor," "granuloma," "pneumonia"). First describe what you see; then attempt to interpret it in light of the facts of the case. The essence of radiology is shrewd pattern recognition coupled with a knowledge of radiologic differential diagnosis.

5. **Straight lines** usually belong in the province of physics, not biology. Differentiate between discrete lines, such as a fibrotic strand, and a straight interface, such as a pleural effusion. If you see an anomalous straight line cutting across a film, consider the possibility that it is caused by fluid collecting under the force of gravity or by something extrinsic to the thorax. Tilting the patient often causes a change in the fluid level, which may help in your interpretation. The gas-fluid interface in the stomach (stomach bubble) helps determine if the patient was standing up or lying down when the film was taken.

6. **Displaced organs** and anatomic structures generally suggest that something is either pushing or pulling them out of normal position, even though the deforming agent or process may not be visible on the x-ray. (A 16-year-old girl with a history of Hodgkin's disease, whose chest film shows progressively increased splaying of the carina, would therefore be investigated carefully for possible relapse.)

III. **Chest x-ray interpretation.** As a medical student doing core clinical rotations, you will be confronted with two different scenarios during which you will be asked to interpret the CXR.

A. **Reviewing your patients' roentgenographs** before you have obtained an "official" interpretation from a radiologist should be a routine part of your work-up, just like looking at the urine sediment or interpreting the ECG. Though you may wish to consult a radiologist before deciding on further diagnostic or treatment plans, you should formulate your own opinion of the CXR findings before asking for an expert opinion. Moreover, radiologists are often excellent teachers and will spend much more time with a student who seems to have some idea of basic radiologic principles than with one who simply puts a CXR on the viewbox and asks, "Is this normal?" Table 11-2 is a quick checklist for the review of a CXR.

B. When presenting roentgenographs as part of formal case presentations, it is best to **be systematic and complete.** Many radiologists use the following algorithm:

1. Describe what you see in very general terms.

2. Describe the pertinent findings that you do **not** see.

3. Give the radiologic differential diagnosis.

4. Now use the clinical history to defend your top diagnosis or group of diagnoses.

5. Finally, suggest what further studies should be done to arrive at a definitive diagnosis.

An example of a formal CXR interpretation follows:

There is a patchy wedge-shaped density in the right lung field, best seen on the lateral view. The hemidiaphragms are flat and there is some linear scarring at the bases. The heart and great vessels appear normal. I do **not** see any evidence of pleural effusion, and there are no air bronchograms. The top differential diagnosis would be right middle lobe pneumo-

Table 11-2. Quick checklist for the CXR

PA views
1. Clavicles (rotation?)
2. Bones (lesions?)
3. Breasts, soft tissue
4. Costophrenic angles (inspiratory effort? pleural effusion?)
5. Lung markings (engorgement? redistribution? hydrothorax or pneumothorax?)
6. Lung fields (coin lesions? consolidation? hilar adenopathy?)
7. Mediastinal shift
8. Cardiac shadow (cardiothoracic ratio? pericardial effusion?)
9. Specific cardiac chamber profiles (dilatation or hypertrophy? aortic profile?)

Lateral views
1. Right and left diaphragm outlines
2. Posterior sulci (pleural effusion?)
3. Thoracic vertebrae
4. Hilar markings
5. Trachea (air column position?)
6. Anterior and posterior clear spaces
7. Cardiac shadow (profile? specific chamber enlargement?)

nia superimposed on a picture of chronic bronchitis versus a tumor. The clinical history of acute-onset cough and green sputum production favors the diagnosis of pneumonia, but in a man with a 75 pack-year smoking history, a tumor must be vigorously excluded. The trial of antibiotics that you are presently undertaking will be informative. Bronchoscopy would probably be the next step in the evaluation of the infiltrate if no response to the antibiotic course is noted.

C. The **spot analysis** of a CXR is a frequent part of teaching rounds. A student will be asked to give an off-the-cuff analysis of a CXR that he or she has never seen before and knows nothing about. The best approach here is to be systematic. *Spend about 20 seconds looking at the CXR without saying anything.* If you want to, you can gain time by saying something such as, "I would have to know a bit of clinical history before being able to make a reasonable statement." (You may not get it, but you can always ask.) The first determination you must make is the organ system or systems involved in the abnormality. Once you have decided on the **type of process** going on, you can then refine your statements by zeroing in on the **exact findings.** A typical student-level spot analysis might be, "These lung fields look congested. There is a moderate degree of pulmonary vascular redistribution bilaterally. I don't see any Kerley's B lines, but there is a small pleural effusion on the right, seen best in the lateral. The heart looks big, and the profile suggests left ventricular dilatation. I don't see any infiltrates or bony lesions. Overall, I would call this a picture of moderate congestive heart failure."

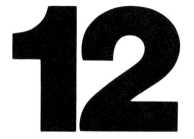

Arterial Blood Gases and Acid-Base Disorders

Annotated Outline of Arterial Blood Gas Indications and Interpretations

I. **Indications for testing arterial blood gas.** The arterial blood gas (ABG) is a test used to assess acid-base status and the ability of the cardiopulmonary system to oxygenate blood. Because a sample of arterial blood is somewhat difficult to collect and painful for the patient, an ABG is obtained only when there is reason to believe that hypoxemia, hypocapnia, hypercapnia, or a pH disturbance is present, or when there has been a serious alteration in the patient's cardiac or ventilatory status. Common clinical situations in which these disturbances are encountered include:

A. Suspected **myocardial infarction** or **cardiac arrest.**

B. **Respiratory distress** secondary to asthma or chronic obstructive pulmonary disease.

C. **Stroke** with altered level of consciousness.

D. **Right-to-left circulatory shunt.**

E. **Suspected acid-base disturbance.**

F. **Poisoning** or **trauma** with cardiopulmonary depression.

II. **Normal blood gas values.** The results of an ABG are given as pH, PO_2, PCO_2, HCO_3^-, base difference (excess or deficit), and percent oxygen saturation. pH, PCO_2, HCO_3^-, and base difference give information about acid-base homeostasis, while PO_2 and O_2 saturation give information on blood oxygenation.

A. Partial pressure of oxygen **(PO_2: normal 80–100 mm Hg).**

B. Oxygen saturation **(SaO_2: normal >95 percent).**

C. Partial pressure of CO_2 **(PCO_2: normal 35–45 mm Hg).**

D. CO_2 content **([HCO_3^-]: normal 22–26 mEq/L).**

E. Arterial pH **(pH: normal 7.40).**

F. All of these tests are usually performed together with an automated blood gas analyzer. The analyzer directly measures the pH, PCO_2, PO_2, and SaO_2, and calculates the HCO_3^- from the Henderson-Hasselbalch equation:

$$pH = pKa + \frac{\log[HCO_3^-] \text{ in mEq/L}}{0.03 \times PCO_2 \text{ in mm Hg}}$$

III. Defining acid-base disorders

A. The basics of acid-base disorders

1. Acid-base disorders can be divided into two types: **acidosis (pH <7.40)** and **alkalosis (pH >7.40)**. Acid-base disturbances occur due to abnormalities in the respiratory system, the metabolic-renal system, or both.

2. **For any primary disturbance in acid-base homeostasis there is a normal compensatory response.** A primary metabolic disorder leads to a respiratory compensation; a primary respiratory disorder leads to an acute metabolic response, due to the buffering capacity of body fluids, **and** a more chronic compensation, due to alterations in renal function.

3. In a normal patient, the **degree of compensation for a given primary disturbance has been well defined** and can be expressed in terms of the given primary disturbance. Table 12-1 lists the four major categories of primary acid-base disorders, the primary disturbance, the secondary compensatory response, and the expected degree of compensation in terms of the magnitude of the primary disturbance.

B. Simple versus mixed acid-base disorders

1. Most acid-base disorders result from a single primary disturbance and its normal physiologic compensatory response; these are called **simple acid-base disorders.** Fig. 12-1 is a nomogram that allows rapid systematic interpretation of ABG results to define simple acid-base disorders.

2. Sometimes, in particularly ill patients, two or more different primary disturbances may occur simultaneously, resulting in a **mixed acid-base disorder.** The net effect of mixed disorders may be additive (metabolic acidosis and respiratory acidosis) and result in extreme alterations in acid-base homeostasis, or may be opposite (respiratory acidosis and metabolic alkalosis) and cancel each other's effects.

   a. **Additive mixed acid-base disorder.** Consider a patient who has just suffered an acute myocardial infarction and has gone into respiratory arrest. The tissues of the patient are not being perfused, and a metabolic acidosis due to the buildup of lactic acid will develop quickly. Because the lungs of the patient are not functioning, the patient will also retain CO_2, resulting in a respiratory acidosis as well. The patient's disorder is thus a mixed **metabolic acidosis and respiratory acidosis,** and the pH of the patient may be extraordinarily low, requiring immediate HCO_3^- treatment and mechanical ventilation.

Table 12-1. Simple acid-base disturbances

Acid-base disorder	Primary abnormality	Secondary response	Expected degree of compensatory response
Metabolic acidosis	↓ $[HCO_3^-]$	↓ PCO_2	$PCO_2 = (1.5 \times [HCO_3^-]) + 8$
Metabolic alkalosis	↑ $[HCO_3^-]$	↑ PCO_2	$PCO_2 = (0.9 \times [HCO_3^-]) + 9$
Respiratory acidosis	↑ PCO_2	↑ $[HCO_3^-]$	$\Delta [HCO_3^-] = 0.35 \times \Delta PCO_2$
Respiratory alkalosis	↓ PCO_2	↓ $[HCO_3^-]$	$\Delta [HCO_3^-] = 0.50 \times \Delta PCO_2$

Reproduced with permission from L. G. Gomella [15].

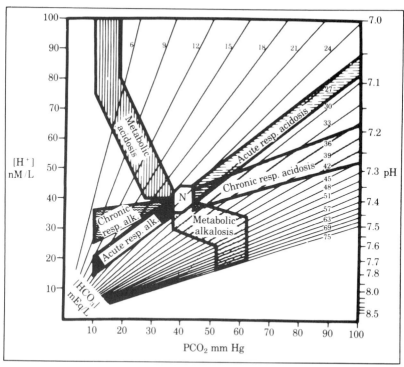

Fig. 12-1. Acid-base map showing the usual compensatory range of pH, PCO$_2$, and plasma HCO$_3^-$ concentrations in simple acid-base disorders. Values on the vertical axis represent plasma H$^+$ concentration (left) in nanomoles per liter, or pH (right). Values on the horizontal axis represent PCO$_2$ in mm Hg. Diagonal lines are isopleths for the plasma HCO$_3^-$ concentration in mEq/L. Clear area in the center of the graph is the range of normal (N). Note that the metabolic component (plasma HCO$_3^-$ concentration) and the respiratory component (arterial blood PCO$_2$) of the acid-base equation always change in the same direction. (Reprinted by permission from M. Goldberg et al., Computer-based instruction and diagnosis of acid-base disorders: A systemic approach. *J.A.M.A.* 223:269, 1973. Copyright © 1973, American Medical Association.)

    b. Nullifying mixed acid-base disorder. Consider a patient who has emphysema and is being treated for congestive heart failure (CHF) with high-dose diuretics. Due to the emphysema, the patient will suffer from a respiratory acidosis (increased PCO$_2$), and due to the diuretic, the patient will suffer from a metabolic alkalosis (increased [HCO$_3^-$]). In this case the pH of the patient may be normal, as the two acid-base disturbances cancel each other's effects on pH.

IV. Arterial blood gas interpretation. The easiest way to interpret a blood gas result is to ask yourself four questions, first about the primary disturbance, and then about any compensatory mechanisms.

    A. Question 1: Is the primary disturbance an acidosis (pH < 7.40) **or an alkalosis** (pH > 7.40)?

B. **Question 2: Is the primary disturbance metabolic or respiratory in nature?** The best way to answer this is to determine **which component, respiratory or metabolic, is altered in the same direction as the pH.** For instance, in the case where the blood gas pH > 7.40 (an alkalosis):

1. If the PCO_2 < 40 mm Hg and $[HCO_3^-]$ < 24 mEq/L, then the acid-base disturbance is a respiratory alkalosis.

2. If the PCO_2 > 40 mm Hg and $[HCO_3^-]$ > 24 mEq/L, then the acid-base disturbance is a metabolic alkalosis.

3. If both $[HCO_3^-]$ and PCO_2 are changed in the same direction, then there is a mixed acid-base disorder present. For example, if the PCO_2 < 40 mm Hg and $[HCO_3^-]$ > 24 mEq/L, then the acid-base disorder is a mixed respiratory alkalosis and metabolic alkalosis.

4. Refer to Table 12-1, and make sure you understand this logic.

C. **Question 3: Is the degree of compensation adequate?** Given the primary disturbance identified in question 2, use the equations in Table 12-1 to calculate the expected compensatory response. If this expected response is significantly different from what is observed, then a mixed acid-base disturbance is present. As an alternative to remembering the exact equations for the four acid-base derangements given in Table 12-1, there are two guidelines that follow from the Henderson-Hasselbalch equation that are helpful in discerning simple versus mixed acid-base disorders:

1. A change in PCO_2 equal to 10 mm Hg results in a change in pH equal to 0.08 units.

2. A pH change of 0.15 results in a change in $[HCO_3^-]$ of 10 mEq/L.

D. **Question 4: What is causing the disorder?** Each type of simple or mixed acid-base disturbance has its own differential diagnosis, as described in sec. **V.** The final step in interpreting a blood gas is to correlate the whole of the patient's clinical presentation with the acid-base disorder you have determined, come up with a diagnosis, and then plan for treatment.

Note: If ABG values do not seem possible, assume there is human or mechanical error and draw a new arterial blood sample.

V. **Differential diagnoses of acid-base derangements**

A. **Metabolic acidosis: pH < 7.40, PCO_2 < 40 mm Hg, $[HCO_3^-]$ < 24 mEq/L.** Metabolic acidosis is caused by an increase in acid in body fluids, which results in a decrease in $[HCO_3^-]$ as it attempts to buffer the new acid load, and a compensatory decrease in PCO_2 as the lungs attempt to blow off CO_2. Causes of metabolic acidosis are classified as either an anion gap acidosis or a non-anion gap acidosis.

The **anion gap = $[Na^+]$ − ($[Cl^-]$ + $[HCO_3^-]$)**; normal range: 8–12 mEq/L.

1. **Anion gap acidosis:** anion gap > 12 mEq/L. Caused by a decrease in $[HCO_3^-]$ that results from the buffering of unmeasured acid ion from either endogenous production or exogenous ingestion (normochloremic acidosis).

2. **Non-anion gap acidosis:** anion gap = 8–12 mEq/L. Caused by a decrease in $[HCO_3^-]$. The anion gap is not increased here, because of an increase in chloride (hyperchloremic acidosis).

Fig. 12-2 outlines the causes of anion gap and non-anion gap acidosis. A useful mnemonic to remember the causes of anion gap acidosis is

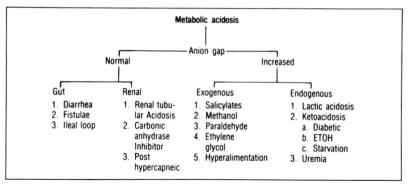

Fig. 12-2. Differential diagnosis of metabolic acidosis. ETOH = ethyl alcohol. (Reproduced with permission from L. G. Gomella [15].)

SLUMPED:

Salicylates
Lactic acid
Uremia
Methanol
Paraldehyde
Ethylene glycol/**E**thanol
Diabetic ketoacidosis

B. Metabolic alkalosis: pH > 7.40, PCO₂ > 40 mm Hg, [HCO₃⁻] > 24 mEq/L.
Metabolic alkalosis results from a primary increase in [HCO₃⁻] with a compensatory increase in PCO₂.

There are two mechanisms by which the kidneys retain [HCO₃⁻]. They can be differentiated by the level of urinary [Cl⁻] and the way in which they respond to NaCl treatment.

  1. Chloride-responsive metabolic alkalosis: urinary [Cl⁻] < 10 mEq/L. The initial problem is a sustained loss of chloride out of proportion to the loss of sodium (either by renal or gastrointestinal losses). This chloride depletion results in renal sodium conservation leading to a corresponding reabsorption of [HCO₃⁻] by the kidney. These disorders **respond to treatment with intravenous NaCl.**

  2. Chloride-resistant metabolic alkalosis: urinary [Cl⁻] > 10 mEq/L. Results from direct stimulation of the kidneys to retain bicarbonate, irrespective of electrolyte intake or losses. These disorders **do not respond to treatment with intravenous NaCl.**

  3. Chloride-responsive metabolic acidosis is far more common than the resistant form. Fig. 12-3 outlines the causes of chloride responsive and resistant metabolic alkalosis.

C. Respiratory acidosis: pH < 7.40, PCO₂ > 40 mm Hg, [HCO₃⁻] > 24 mEq/L.
Respiratory acidosis results from an increase in PCO₂ with a compensatory elevation in plasma [HCO₃⁻]. Increased PCO₂ occurs when alveolar ventilation is decreased. Conditions in which respiratory acidosis occurs include:

  1. Neuromuscular abnormalities with ventilatory failure

    a. Defects in the muscles of respiration (mysthenia gravis, muscular dystrophy).

    b. Depression of respiratory center (due to anesthesia, narcotics, tran-

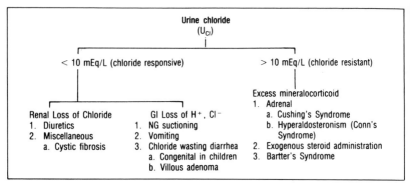

Fig. 12-3. Differential diagnosis of metabolic alkalosis. (Reproduced with permission from L. G. Gomella [15].)

quilizers, sedatives, vertebral artery embolism or thrombosis, increased intracranial pressure).

c. Defects in peripheral nervous system (ALS, poliomyelitis, Guillain-Barré syndrome, botulism, tetanus, organophosphate poisoning, spinal cord injury).

2. Airway obstruction

    a. Chronic (chronic obstructive pulmonary disease [COPD]).

    b. Acute (due to asthma, foreign body, laryngospasm).

3. Thoracic-pulmonary disorders

    a. Thoracic cage disorders (flail chest, rib fractures, pneumothorax, kyphoscoliosis).

    b. Pulmonary disease (pneumothorax, severe pulmonary edema, severe pneumonia, interstitial fibrosis).

D. Respiratory alkalosis: pH > 7.40, PCO_2 < 40 mm Hg, [HCO_3^-] < 24 mEq/L. Respiratory alkalosis results from a decrease in PCO_2 with a compensatory decrease in plasma [HCO_3^-]. Decreased PCO_2 occurs when alveolar ventilation is increased. Conditions in which respiratory alkalosis occurs include:

1. Central stimulation

    a. Hyperventilation syndrome (anxiety, pain, hysteria).

    b. Head trauma or cerebrovascular accident (CVA) with neurogenic hyperventilation.

    c. Tumors.

    d. Drugs (salicylate, xanthines, progesterone, epinephrine, thyroxin, nicotine).

    e. Gram-negative sepsis.

    f. Hyponatremia.

2. Peripheral stimulation

    a. Congestive heart failure.

    b. Interstitial lung disease.

    c. Hypoxemia (pneumonia, pulmonary embolus, atelectasis, high altitude).

3. Miscellaneous

  a. Hepatic encephalopathy.

  b. Pregnancy.

  c. Iatrogenic overventilation.

B
Practical Points Concerning the Arterial Blood Gas

I. Performing the arterial blood gas determination

A. The order of preference for **ABG puncture site** is radial artery, then brachial artery, and finally femoral artery. You should familiarize yourself with the exact location of these arteries and practice palpating them on yourself. Learn to feel for these arteries in a way that lets you "see" their course underneath your fingertips.

B. **Allen's test** is a procedure for evaluating the collateral circulation in patients in whom arterial puncture might result in severe hypoperfusion of the hand if the collateral circulation were inadequate. First, have the patient make a tight fist to expel the blood from the surface vessels of the palm, and use your finger to occlude either the radial or ulnar artery. Then have the patient open his or her hand and check to see if the blood returns to the palm and fingers (indicated by the return of a pink hue to the surface). If this pink hue is delayed, then you should suspect obstruction to the blood flow in the artery that you did not compress.

C. Take opportunities to practice your arterial puncture technique in nonemergency situations so that you will be able to act quickly, safely, and competently when speed is necessary. Being able to obtain a sample of arterial blood without unduly traumatizing your patient is an important clinical skill.

II. Interpreting arterial blood gas results

A. Recall that **the oxygen saturation curve for hemoglobin has a steep sigmoid shape** that starts to level off near a PO_2 of 70 mm Hg. This means that a patient may have a PO_2 of 65 mm Hg and still have an O_2 saturation > 90 percent. Conversely, the difference between a PO_2 of 50 mm Hg and a PO_2 of 60 mm Hg is very significant clinically, because it lies on the steep slope of the curve.

B. Always **note whether an ABG was drawn while the patient was receiving oxygen therapy.** This fact is often forgotten in the heat of the moment and obviously affects the PO_2 and oxygen saturation.

C. Always **analyze the ABG results together with the serum electrolytes and the anion gap.** If the patient is acidotic, the anion gap becomes the next step in constructing the differential diagnosis.

D. In analyzing the clinical status of a patient who has undergone an ABG, you must **know what baseline values are normal for your patient.** Many patients with chronic pulmonary disease exist quite happily with a PO_2 of 60 mm Hg, and it would be futile and dangerous to attempt to improve respiratory status much beyond this level.

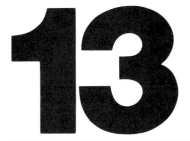

The Medical Write-up and Progress Notes

Life and death crises actually occupy a reasonably small portion of clinical medicine, and an even smaller portion of the patient's concern over the quality of life. We must recognize that *when a patient feels a problem is an emergency, it is, by definition, an emergency* to the patient, whether or not the physician views the problem as life threatening. Even the highest quality of scientific medical management will not satisfy the patient unless these underlying concerns are answered.

Harley A. Haynes, M.D.

A. Annotated Outline and Example of the Medical Write-up and Progress Notes

I. **General points concerning the medical write-up**

  A. **Purpose.** The write-up has three major purposes.

    1. **To convey information to consultants,** who are not as familiar with the case as the responsible house officer, and to **covering house officers,** who may be asked to make a decision in the middle of the night concerning a patient with whom they are not familiar.

    2. **To document and clarify the impression and approaches** of the medical team for future medical reference and medicolegal inquiries.

    3. To force the writer **to quantify and organize** his or her own impressions in order to gain a better understanding of the case.

    The student write-up, for better or worse, has an additional purpose: to show the student's preceptors how thoroughly the student has investigated and analyzed the case, and how familiar he or she is with the differential diagnoses and the various management options that exist.

  B. **Format.** Two major formats are currently in use for teaching hospital write-ups.

    1. The first, sometimes called the **traditional write-up,** is by far the most widely used. Its outline is shown in the sample write-up following Part A of this chapter. Its major advantage is that it is issue-oriented: within a general framework, its complexity expands and contracts in relation to the complexity of the medical case. Its major disadvantage is that information may be recorded and organized in a rather haphazard way. Information pertaining to multiple separate medical problems, for instance, may be grouped in a single long paragraph, making future chart review more difficult.

2. The second write-up format is the **problem-oriented medical record (POMR).** Its chief advantage is its comprehensiveness and the ease with which the current status of any medical problem can be assessed. Its chief disadvantage is that it is somewhat more cumbersome and difficult to use than the traditional format. A complete description of the problem-oriented system is beyond the scope of this chapter; essentially it involves the recording of all medical data as entries under the headings of specific medical problems.

Although the problem-oriented system may be used with increasing frequency as medical records become computerized, its use at present is still the exception rather than the rule. Many physicians, however, are starting to incorporate certain elements of the POMR into a traditional write-up framework (e.g., an "active problem list" is now a standard part of many hospital charts), and hybrids of the two systems are now common. Students beginning their clinical rotations should check with their preceptors to determine which specific write-up format is preferred within their hospital system.

C. **Stance.** The good write-up is not simply an organized rehashing of the information collected in the process of the work-up. It is a structured narrative in which the writer walks the delicate line between objective recording and subjective interpreting; it **takes a stance and persuades as well as informs.** The good write-up organizes the details of the case into a coherent whole that explicitly reflects the writer's impression of which issues are central and which are more peripheral. It should contain all the relevant data necessary for the reader to form an independent opinion concerning the case, but it should arrange the data in a way that lets the reader understand what has led the student to draw the conclusions that are offered. A common pitfall in student write-ups is an attempt to be overly "evenhanded"; to record objectively every bit of information obtained in the work-up, and to avoid deliberately taking any stance until the assessment portion of the write-up. While this evenhandedness may seem admirable, it often results in a sort of laundry list of patient complaints and lab data that leaves the reader with little sense of the actual crucial issues. Although the student may be expected to produce a long differential diagnosis list in the assessment section, the entire write-up should be geared toward differentiating between the two or three most likely possibilities.

II. Progress notes

A. **Purpose.** Once the initial admission write-up is completed, the student or house officer is expected to write a brief progress note every day. As the name implies, these notes summarize what progress has been made in the case since the previous note. The central issues of the progress note address the following questions:

1. What are the patient's **current symptoms and complaints?** Are there **any changes?**

2. Is there any **change in the physical exam?**

3. Are there any **new lab data?**

4. Is there any **change in the formulation of the case** or in the relationship of the patient's various medical problems to one another?

5. What are the **current diagnostic and therapeutic plans** for the patient?

B. **Format.** As with the initial admission write-up, there are two main formats for progress notes: the **traditional format,** which is simply a set of paragraphs summarizing the progress, and the **problem-oriented format,** in which entries for each medical problem are divided into four sections:

1. **Subjective data:** the patient's impressions of current symptoms.

2. **Objective data:** the clinical exam and lab data.

3. **Assessment:** the writer's impression of the data and their relation to the case.

4. **Plan:** both diagnostic and therapeutic.

A progress note with information arranged in the order subjective-objective-assessment-plan is often referred to as a **SOAP note.** No matter whether the initial write-up follows the traditional or the problem-oriented format, many clinicians believe that all progress notes should be written in some variant of the SOAP note format, because it makes chart review much easier.

C. **Off-service notes.** The off-service note is a specialized version of the progress note. Above all, it should be **brief,** usually one page or less in length, and it should contain:

1. A short **summary of the patient's case,** usually one paragraph.

2. A short **summary of the hospital course,** again usually one paragraph.

3. A **problem list** that details ongoing, active problems and any outstanding diagnostic tests or work-up.

4. A list of **current medications and dosages.**

Remember that the purpose of the off-service note is to allow the physician who is coming on-service to orient himself to the patient's case in an expeditious way.

III. **Sample write-up and progress notes**

A. Reproduced on pp. 134–151 is a good second-year student's admission write-up, together with two progress notes from the same case. Note that the write-up, while primarily organized in the traditional format, contains elements of the problem-oriented system. The chief complaint and the present illness essentially become problem no. 1 on the patient's problem list, while the past medical history comprises the rest of the patient's active medical problems. Part B of this chapter is keyed to the following sample write-up and contains specific practical points about the format and content of each section. As is usually the case with medical notes, many abbreviations and acronyms are used. The Abbreviations and Acronyms List on the inside cover includes most of these standard terms.

B. While the sample write-up represents a better than average second-year write-up, it would be considered inappropriately wordy and compulsively thorough by third- or fourth-year standards. In particular, note that the review of systems (ROS) is written out in its entirety. While most second-year students are required to describe the complete ROS, the third-year student is generally permitted to record a shorter list of pertinent positives and negatives, while the fourth-year student may simply record the essential ones and note that the "remainder of the ROS was negative in detail." Also note that the Assessment and Plan section is too brief and could be fleshed out.

C. The first progress note (pp. 148–149) is organized in the traditional style, while the second (pp. 150–151) is written as a SOAP note. In a complicated case, with many consultants writing notes, it is not unusual to see multiple styles being used on the same case, and a student should become comfortable with all of them. Note that whether or not a formal SOAP note is written, all notes organize information in the same order—subjective, objective, assessment, and plan—and so the acronym is useful regardless of the style used.

PROGRESS NOTES

INPATIENT

— Medical Student Admission Note —
3/3/87

Source: pt, who seems reliable, and old chart.

This is the second admission for Mrs. Elsa Jones, a 55 y.o. black seamstress who enters with C.C: "weakness," "cough," and "feverish feeling" of several days duration

H.P.I: Mrs. Jones was in her usual state of health until this past Friday (2/28/87) when she noted fatigue during her work-day and in the evening, without other associated symptoms. The following morning this tired feeling persisted and the pt. confined herself to her home "to rest" for the majority of Saturday. She slept well Saturday night but awoke with nasal stuffiness and an occasional cough productive of clear mucoid sputum. As the day progressed nausea accompanied by 3 to 4 episodes of vomiting occured, as did several mild chills without overt shaking. The pt. first recalls feeling feverish at approximately this time, though she did not take her own temperature.

PROGRESS NOTES

INPATIENT

She recalls a ® temporal HA and sub/periorbital aching as well. Sunday evening the pt's general malaise increased and she noted weakness, dizziness and a change of sputum produced from clear to brown in color. At this time she denies any h/o dyspnea, sore throat, pain associated with respiration or frank hemoptysis. Mrs Jones was brought to the hospital this morning at her son's insistence.

The pt. denies a h/o viral syndrome, pleuritic pain, myalgias, or illness concurrently in a family member. There is no previous h/o chronic sputum production, sinusitis, bronchitis, pneumonia, TB exposure or respiratory illness, $\bar{x}$ for an occasional UTI. There is no h/o rheumatic fever or heart ⓜ. The pt. has a smoking h/o < 2 pack years.

PMH:

② Diabetes: first diagnosed in 1963 following complications of a peptic ulcer that eroded into pancreatic tissue. She underwent surgical Rx for this event at that time and developed polyuria/polydipsia ≈ 6 months later. She was placed on insulin at that

PROGRESS NOTES

INPATIENT

time and currently is on 80u NPH, 15 CZI qd, which maintains her serum glucose / urine S+A's under good control.

③ HTN: dx'ed 7 yrs ago on clinic visit, well controlled (< 150/96) on 50 mg Guanethidine qd from then until present.

④ Hyperlipoproteinemia: dx'ed in 1972 on routine lab studies. Noted to have chol 442 mg%, TG 750 mg%; was re-evaluated the following year c̄ Chol 368, TG's 5,900 and dx'ed c̄ Type I hyperlipoproteinemia. Placed on Atromid-S subsequently c̄ reasonable control (TG of 411 mg% reported 9/79). Presently taking Atromid qid; without recent TG in chart.

⑤ R.A.: Mrs. Foxes has a 30 yr h/o Rheumatoid arthritis, dx'ed at MGH clinic. History vague; symptomatic relief c̄ ASA since that time and pt reports not a problem currently (see ROS)

Childhood illness(es): 3 significant, Pt. recalls a Kidney infection ~ 20 yrs ago but few other

PROGRESS NOTES

INPATIENT

details. No h/o freq., sore throats, TB, rheumatic
fever.

Allergies. Sulfa drugs → diffuse rash

Previous Admissions :

admission	year	hospital
Pregnancy, hysterectomy	1961	MGH
ulcer complications, Pancreatectomy ≗ 1963		MGH
Dental Work	1977	PBBH

Other PMH : No h/o accidents/trauma or broken bones.

FHX

gassed, WWI [41] ─────── (56) Ht disease
                              Stroke

multiple (61)   (55)   (58)   [65] pneumonia X1
MI   multiple
                          MI
                        repeated
                        ~~Kidney~~
                        infections

No family h/o AODM, Ca, TB; No h/o HTN, sickle
cell disease

⊕ CAD, MI as noted in diagram

Social Hx:

Widow of 6 yrs, Mrs. Jones' husband died
of an MI. Lives with her son, age 26. States

PROGRESS NOTES

INPATIENT

they are extremely close.
Has worked as a sticher for 38 yrs ot Sharon
Dress Co. in Roxbury. Pt makes her own hours
and enjoys her job a great deal. No h/o toxic
exposures ot work.
Describes herself as generally happy/content
person.

Current meds: Etoh ⊖ Tobacco Hx: <2pk-yrs.
Insulin NPH 80u + CZI 15u SC qAm
Guanethidine 50 mg po qd
Atromid S ī tab po qid

ROS
Constitutional: fatigue often; onset of present
fatigue notable. No recent wt change,
night sweats, chills, ō insomnia.
Integument: ⊕ itching, nightly; localized to
back, of 1-yr. duration. ↑ thinning hair
X 3 yrs. ō rash (x̄ ē sulfa drugs), sores,
bruising/bleeding.
Head: ō h/a x̄ ē present illness (see HPI). ō
fainting, LOC; seizures or h/o trauma.
Eyes: glasses x 10-12 yrs. Last eye exam 3 weeks
ago (frequent excessive tearing, ō apparent
agg/allev factors). Notes blurred vision often,

PROGRESS NOTES

INPATIENT

but improved since eye exam. Occasional Ⓡside pain in region of ext. canthus - "like a knife going through my eye" - relieved by sleep.

Ears: hearing "pretty good." ⊖ pain, discharge, vertigo.

Resp: see HPI

Breasts: no masses, pain, discharge. Does self-exam

CV: ⊕ ankle edema at end of day. No h/o palpitations, dyspnea, PNO, chest pain or discomfort cyanosis, varicose veins. ⊕DM, smoking presently; hyperlipoproteinemia as noted.

GI: dental plate, top teeth; partial on bottom. ⊕ vomiting c̄ present illness - clear, fluid, less than 3-4 tablespoons each time. No h/o heartburn, hematemesis, Abd pain/discomfort since ulcer difficulties in 1963, food intolerance, jaundice, hematochezia. No recent Δ in stool (normal frequency, color, consistency).

GU:

1. Urinary ⊕ nocturia, 2-3 x/night; has had nocturia "as long as I can remember." No h/o dysuria, pyuria, stones, flank pain, urgency/frequency.

2. Menstrual: menopause c̄ hysterectomy in 1961, accompanied by hot flushes, depression. Reports reason for hysterectomy was "tumor" discovered at time of son's birth. Last pap smear 3 months

PROGRESS NOTES

INPATIENT

ago (neg) No present c/o vag. discharge, itching.
Endocrine: hirsutism c̄ androgens p̄ hysterectomy.
No present problems c̄ polyuria, polydipsia.
MS: ⊕ occasional calve "pulls" - Rx c̄ hot soaks.
⊕ arthritis c̄ "all joints," accompanied by
warmth, soreness, morning stiffness most
mornings, Rx c̄ Ben-Gay® hot soaks q AM,
ASA c̄ good relief.

Neuro:
motor: s̄ atrophy, involuntary movements
Sensory: ⊕ numbness in toes often. s̄ anesthesia/
hyperesthesia.
mental status: mentation s̄ Δ, memory
writing intact.

Physical Exam:
Mrs Jones is a moderately obese middle-aged
black woman who is resting quietly in her
chair s̄ apparent distress. She holds a
tissue with several streaks of blood visible
in her hand.
VS: Temp 102.8°   weight: 61.2 kg
    Pulse 94, regular, strong
    BP 122/72 Ⓛ ® arm
       110/70 o— ® arm
    Resp. 25, somewhat shallow

PROGRESS NOTES

INPATIENT

Integument: Skin warm, dry, s̄ bruises, rashes, cyanosis. Nails nl.

HEENT:

Head: normocephalic, s̄ evidence of trauma or scalp lesions. Hair thin, oily.

Eyes Visual acuity c̄ glasses ≈20/40 each eye. Conjunctiva nl PERRLA. Palpebral fissures ≈ equal. EOM's intact. (L) Fundus: clear, c̄ sharp disc, ⊖ hemorrhage or exudate. (R) Fundus: not visualized - ? Cataract (R) eye.

Ears: Hearing intact. Minimal cerumen. TM clear c̄ good light reflex.

Nose: nares patent, septum midline, ⊖ sinus tenderness/discharge.

mouth/throat: dental plate - upper teeth, lower molars. Tongue well papillated, moist. Uvula midline. Throat s̄ injection/exudate

Lymphadenopathy: s̄ cervical, axillary or inguinal.

Neck: trachea midline; ⊕ slt ↑ in thyroid size (easily palpated); s̄ nodules/tenderness.

Back: Spine s̄ curvatures; ⊖ CVA tenderness.

Lungs: Chest symmetrical ↓ respiratory excursion evident, (R)⟨L⟩ symmetry preserved. percussion: nl, s̄ dull areas. Diaphragm

PROGRESS NOTES

INPATIENT

descends 1-2 cm > on ℗

auscultation: ⊕ end inspiratory rales, ℗ axilla.
⊖ tactile fremitus, egophony, whispered
pectoriloquy.

Breasts pendulous, symmetric, s̄ masses,
discharge or tenderness.

CV: JVP 7-8 cm
PMI - not visible or palpable. s̄ lift or
impulse palpable.
S₁: nl intensity S₂: nl intensity, nl split
c̄ inspiration. ⊕ soft S₄ ⊖ S₃.
Grade 2/6 SEM at LLSB s̄ radiation to
axilla or neck.

pulses:

	Carotid	radial	femoral	popliteal	D.P.	P.T.
ℝ	2+, nl upstroke, s̄ bruits	2+	1+, s̄ bruits	1+	2+	s̄
ℒ	2+, nl upstroke, s̄ bruits	2+	1+, s̄ bruits	1+	2+	s̄

Abdomen:
s̄ liver, spleen edge

obese, bowel sounds ⊕
liver: 10-11 cm by
percussion

cecum
palpable

25-30 cm scar
c̄ keloid
(ulcer surgery)

10-15 cm scar
(hysterectomy)

PROGRESS NOTES

INPATIENT

Genital Exam:
external: ∅ discharge, lesions
pelvic: deferred to private gynecologist. Last pap 12/87, negative.
Rectal Exam: sphincter good tone. Guaiac neg.
MS. nl. ROM all 4 extremities. Feet slt ↓ temperature; color nl; hair present on toes.
⊕ joint hypertrophy - DIP's ⊖ tenderness, ⊖ subcutaneous nodules. muscular strength 4+/5+ all four limbs.

Neuro:
Motor: (see MS) F →N√√, H→s√√. Rhomberg ⊖. Gait slow, slt shuffling
Sensory: pinprick ↓ in both feet, nl position, vibration
CN: II → XII √√
Reflexes:

⊖ babinski as illustrated

Mental status: oriented x3; serial 7's intact; pt is alert.

PROGRESS NOTES

INPATIENT

Laboratory data

CBC: HCT 35.7

WBC: 11.8 (79 polys, 6 Bd, 7 ly, 7 mo, 1 baso)

PT.   11.3/12.5   PTT 25/25.3   ESR 24

U/A: straw/yellow ; SG 1.020 ; pH 6.0

 Prot 3+ Heme 1+   O-1 RBC/HPF

 Gm $\ominus$ Rods in unspun specimen

 analysis ; 3-5 WBC/HPF

 S/A - 1+/$\ominus$

Serum Chems: $142 | 102 \big\langle{}^{12}_{18} \big\rangle{}^{}_{7}$ Ca/PO$_4$ 9.6/3.8

 $3.7 | 29 \big\rangle 1.0$ Cholesterol 210

 UA 6.8

 TG's - not checked

EKG: Axis - 20°   .14/.08/.90   ?LVH (V$_1$+V$_5$ = 36mm)

 Rate 120, NSR   insignificant Q in II, F

 Remainder $\bar{s}$ abnormality

CXR: $\oplus$ RLL superior segment alveolar

 infitrate.   Borderline cardiomegaly.

 $\ominus$ effusions

Sputum gm stain : 4+ polys, numerous gm $\oplus$

 diplococci

urine, sputum cultures : pending.

Assessment/Plan

 Summary: This 55 yo. black $\female$ presents $\bar{c}$

 fever, productive cough and progressive

PROGRESS NOTES

INPATIENT

malaise of 3-4 days duration.

① Productive cough: Recent onset of cough, productive of sputum which changed from mucoid → brown, fever, nausea, vomiting are all c/w dx of pneumonia. PE data includes presence of ℞ axillary rales but no signs suggestive of consolidation. There was no evidence from Hx or PE supporting obstruction (acute or insidious) → no wt. Δ, h/o aspiration, other evidence of cachexia; also no wheezing or rhonchi on lung exam. There was no evidence for non-pulmonary etiology (mitral stenosis, e.g.) Lab data increases the likelihood that this is a bacterial pneumonia: sputum c̄ 4+ polys and gm ⊕ diplococci; CXR c̄ ℞ LL infiltrate.

    Important to R/o obstruction, and TB as other common possibilities. Pul. embolism, uncommon infections cause are less likely.

Plan: ① Place TB test c̄ mumps/candida control
② Begin antibiotics with Ampicillin 500mg q6h IV (see below for discussion of antibiotic choice)

PROGRESS NOTES

INPATIENT

③ blood cultures × 2

② Asymptomatic Bacteriuria – discovered during laboratory work-up. Though pt $\bar{s}$ symptoms will choose antibiotics for presumptive pneumonia that covers typical gm ⊖ rods causing UTI (generally enteric organisms). Note that pt. is predisposed to UTI's if her diabetes is not well controlled (see below).

Plan : ① send urine for definitive culture/
    sensitivities
  ② begin Ampicillin 500 mg Q6h IV
  ③ check urine S+A's

③ Opacity, ® eye : pt $\bar{c}$ numerous visual complaints but $\bar{s}$ marked loss of ® eye vision; also last eye exam 3 weeks ago. However, $\bar{c}$ hx/of diabetes, ↑ incidence of cataract. Will therefore:

Plan : ① attempt to contact ophthalmologist
  ② in-house ophthalmology consult

④ AODM. Will assess degree of control while pt. in hospital. Note that infection likely to increase insulin requirement and thus may show some ↑ in BS (may account for asymptomatic bacteriuria noted above).

PROGRESS NOTES

INPATIENT

Plan: ① urine S+A's
② ✓ FBS
③ 1800 cal/day diet (ADA)

⑤ Type IV Hyperlipoproteinemia: Last triglyceride recorded in chart was 9/94
Plan: ① check TG level
② Continue Atromid-S

⑥ Hypertension: Under good control with BP 122/72 sitting; 110/70 supine. Ophthalmology consult planned (see ③ above)

⑦ Rheumatoid arthritis: though pt says currently not a problem, she also states arthritis is present in "all" joints, accompanied by warmth, soreness; also morning stiffness most mornings. Rx c̄ ASA at present. Will
Plan: ① Rheumatology consult to evaluate Rx.

Overall Impression: a 55 year old woman with pneumococcal pneumonia and possible UTI.

John Smith
2nd Year Medical Student

PROGRESS NOTES

INPATIENT

3/4/87 Medical Student Progress Note

Hx. No real change in Sx. Still c̄ cough and fever. Still bringing up small amounts of brown sputum.

PE: T 101° P 90, regular BP 120/70 ℞ and o—
RR: 24 Weight: 61.7 Kg (+0.2 Kg)
Exam: S change. Still c̄ expiratory râles ®>Ⓛ
T.B. Test PPD Ⓝ at 24 hrs.
Candida control⊕

Lab. CBC   34.2
      15.7⟩──── Diff (61 p 25 B 8 L 5 m 1 Eo)
         187 k

U/A S.g. 1.015   pH 6.0
     2+ protein 1+ heme 1+ sugar -acetone
     0-1 RBC/2-5 WBC per HPF
     few gram Ⓝ rods per HPF in unspun
              specimen

Chemistry   140 | 100 ⟨ 15
            3.8 | 26   205
                         1.1
     triglyceride: pending
Sputum Gram Stain 4+ polys, gram ⊕ diplococci
Sputum Cultures ⊕ Pneumococcus sensitive to
                  Ampicillin
Urine Cultures: pending

PROGRESS NOTES

INPATIENT

THE CHILDREN'S HOSPITAL MEDICAL CENTER, BOSTON, MASSACHUSETTS

03706 50M 6/77

Impression: ①Pneumococcal Pneumonia: Temp now ↓ but WBC ↑; will continue Ampicillin 500 mg IV q6h. CBC and CXR tomorrow.
② UTI: No Sx; cultures pending
James Smith
Medical Student II

PROGRESS NOTES

INPATIENT

3/5/87   Medical Student Progress note
VS: Temp 99.2 P 85, regular BP 120/70 ♀ and ♂
    RR 20   Weight 62.0 Kg

Problem #1: Pneumococcal Pneumonia:
  S: Feels better. No more cough, very little
     sputum.
  O: Exam: still $\bar{c}$ scattered expiratory wheezes.
     TB Test PPD ⊖ at 48 hours.
     CBC   34.8
          12.1/221K   diff (68p 18B 9L 5M)
     Sputum Gram Stain: 2+ polys; +diplococci
     CXR: Still $\bar{c}$ RLL infiltrate.
  A: Symptomatically improved, Temp and WBC ↓
  P: Continue Ampicillin

Problem #2: UTI
  S: Still $\bar{s}$ Sx
  O: Urine culture from 3/3/87:
     >10⁵ Klebsiella sensitive to ampicillin
     U/A: ↓ change from 3/4/87, still
          $\bar{c}$ gram ⊖ rods in unspun; 2+ polys
  A: Klebsiella UTI sensitive to current antibiotics
  P: Continue Ampicillin; repeat urine
     cultures tomorrow.

Problem #3 AODM:
  S: No new Sx or c/o
  O: Urine S+A: 1+/⊖

PROGRESS NOTES

INPATIENT

Blood sugar 172 this AM
A and P : Well controlled.
Other Problems s̄ change.

— James Smith
Medical Student II

B   **Practical Points Concerning
                                             the Medical Write-up and
                                             Progress Notes**

I. Introductory information and chief complaint

A. All chart notes should be written on **hospital progress-note paper** that has been marked or stamped with the patient's name and number. You may find it useful to prepare a supply of this stamped paper when you are first assigned a patient, so that you can carry it around on your clipboard and work on notes when you are away from the chart. Of course, **all entries must be dated and signed.**

B. It is customary to **title each note with the level of seniority of the writer** (e.g., "Medical Student Admission Note" or "Heme Attending Note"). Consultants who review the chart can thus identify critical entries.

C. Record your source if you derive any of the information in your note from a source other than the patient or the old chart. Although a reliability caveat may be appropriate here (e.g., "patient appeared confused and vague"), it should never be humorous or flippant.

D. The introductory sentence and chief complaint (given with its duration) should provide a **10-second sketch of the patient** and the patient's reason for seeking medical help. A word or two about the patient's past medical history may be appropriate here as well (e.g., "a 55 y.o. black seamstress with a long history of hypertension"). You will often use this introductory sentence to refer to the patient in discussions with those not familiar with the case.

II. History of the present illness

A. Chronologic organization is the key to a well-written history of the present illness (HPI). Begin with a sentence describing the onset of the constellation of symptoms that you perceive as the present illness. If the present illness is simply the latest episode in a long-standing medical problem, begin with a sentence about how long the patient has suffered from the disease (e.g., "The patient has a 20-year history of asthma usually involving 1 or 2 attacks each spring."). Then organize the salient features of the case, always noting the dates on which the features appeared. For a long-standing problem, this will require a careful chart review, with dates of hospitalizations, surgical procedures, therapies, and definitive diagnostic tests all highlighted. The goal here is to give the reader a feeling for the tempo of the disease process.

B. All pertinent positives and **some pertinent negatives** from the ROS of the organ system(s) involved in the present illness belong in the HPI. Often it is not clear whether a certain pertinent negative is really important enough to note in the HPI. In these cases a good rule of thumb is to ask yourself whether the information in question helps exclude a possible diagnosis that has entered your mind while considering the patient's symptoms. If it does, then the information belongs in the HPI.

III. Past medical history

A. All **active** and **significant inactive medical problems** should be listed in the past medical history (PMH). This section can be anywhere from a few sentences to a few pages in length, depending on the severity and the significance of the problems. For each problem, the significant issues that you should concentrate on include:

1. The **date on which the problem was diagnosed.**

2. The **results of definitive tests** that will indicate to the reader the severity of the problem (e.g., "cardiac cath in 1989 showed a 38% ejection fraction").

3. The dates of any **surgeries or hospitalizations** for the problem.

4. **Current treatment regimens.**

5. An assessment of the **problem's significance at present,** and its potential for interacting with the present illness.

B. **Other parts of the medical history** included in the PMH include:

1. **Current medications.** The medication list should document all significant, pharmacologically active substances used by the patient. These include all medicines, vitamins, skin creams, laxatives, and sleeping medications. List each of these substances with the dosage and route of administration. It is customary to use the Latin acronyms for dosage frequency, for example, "bid" (*bis in die*) for "2 times/day." (See Abbreviations and Acronyms, inside covers.)

2. **Allergies** and the nature of the allergic reaction.

3. A list of **past hospitalizations and surgical procedures** (even if mentioned elsewhere).

4. A list of significant **childhood illnesses.**

5. **Habits.** History of tobacco, ethanol, and recreational drug use should be obtained, as well as diet and exercise information. The smoking history should be listed in pack-years. Drinking history may be quantitated in familiar units (six-packs, quarts).

6. A list of **exposures** to radiation, toxins, poisons, chemicals, and so on. Patient should be questioned about possible occupational exposures.

IV. **Family history**

A. The family history (FHx) is usually presented in a standard **pedigree format.** For example:

   (30) = female, 30 years old
  MI ⬛ = male, died at age 42 of myocardial infarct
  → (55) = patient, female, 55 years old

For most cases, you will want to list the patient, the patient's siblings, and the patient's parents and children.

B. Any family history of **diabetes, cancer, cardiovascular problems,** or other disease with significant genetic penetration should also be listed in the FHx. A family history of the disease (or symptoms) that the patient has presented with should always be sought.

V. **Social history.** The social history (SHx) should be very brief unless a lengthy description would be of crucial importance to the case. The goal is to give the reader an idea of the patient as a person. For most patients, this section of the write-up will involve a few words about the patient's **living situation and work.** Names and telephone numbers of close family members can also be listed here. Recall from Chap. 1 the instances in which this section would assume a larger role, such as cases of occupational exposure or pulmonary disease.

VI. **Review of systems.** The ROS should be **listed by organ system.** Once again, the length of this list will depend on the complexity of the case and the level of the writer. Experienced clinicians may simply write "ROS negative." When first beginning your clinical training you should list, at a minimum, all the ROS positives and enough of the pertinent negatives to show the reader that you did a complete ROS and that all the important facets of the case are listed. List the ROS telegraphically. For example: "GI: Nausea, vomiting, diarrhea, constipation, abd. pain."

VII. Physical examination

A. Introductory information and vital signs. Begin with a statement describing the overall appearance of the patient. The vital signs (including orthostatic changes in blood pressure and pulse) should be listed before the rest of the exam. For most patients with cardiovascular or renal problems, the admission weight should be listed with the vital signs.

B. Organ system examination. Starting with a description of the integument and then proceeding in a generally head-to-toe direction (leaving the neurologic exam results for last), transcribe the results of your physical exam. Just as in the ROS, the second-year student should include all significant positive and negative findings, while the more advanced student can concentrate on the major positive findings, listing only the most fundamental pertinent negatives.

C. One key to a good physical exam write-up is **specificity.** Always quantitate and localize (e.g., "a 6 × 6-cm round erythematous patch on the left buttock"). Draw **diagrams** whenever they are helpful. Specifically, the dermatologic exam, breast exam, abdominal exam, and neurologic exam are often illustrated with diagrams and stick figures to indicate the exact location of the findings.

VIII. Laboratory data (see also Chaps. 7–12).

A. Hematologic studies are usually listed together in shorthand form, as follows:

HEME: WBC $\diagdown$ Hgb $\diagup$ Plts   MCV _____ PT _____ PTT _____
        $\diagup$ Hct $\diagdown$

diff: (____ P____ B____ L____ M____ Eo)   ESR _____

Any special hematologic tests or comments on the blood smear, which should be examined whenever the differential is abnormal or suggestive, are recorded below these results.

B. Serum chemistry data can be divided into two groups:

1. Seven "core" tests, which are conveniently recorded in a lattice format:

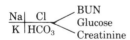

2. The remainder of the serum chemistry results, which are recorded underneath and beside this lattice. Often these other tests are best grouped by organ system (e.g., the liver function tests). You should circle lab values that are abnormal or significant for the diagnosis in question.

C. Urinalysis (U/A) data are recorded in tabular form: color and appearance; specific gravity; pH and dipstick results; sediment analysis; quantitation (number of cells or structures per high-power field). The time and conditions of collection (e.g., catheter or clean-voided specimen) and the total urine volume in a specified time period may also be recorded here. If you do one U/A and the lab does another, include both sets of data, noting the source of each.

D. Electrocardiographic data should be recorded in the following sequence:

1. Rate and rhythm.

2. Axis.

3. P-Q, QRS, and Q-T intervals.

4. Comments concerning the following areas:

    a. Q waves and S-T segment morphology.

    b. R wave progression.

    c. QRS morphology and conduction blocks.

    d. Evidence for drug effects.

    e. Other significant findings.

5. Overall impression, **including degree of change from the last recorded ECG.**

E. **Chest x-ray** results are recorded either verbally or by means of a labeled diagram. Always include a statement concerning the degree of change from the last chest film.

F. In a similarly telegraphic fashion, record the remainder of the lab data, including:

    1. **Arterial blood gas results** (record the FiO_2 together with the results and the time the sample was drawn).

    2. **Microbiologic data** (include antibiotic sensitivities if known).

    3. **Pathology reports.**

    4. **Other radiologic tests.**

    5. **Other special diagnostic tests.**

IX. **Assessment and Plan.** Up until this point in the write-up, the **analytic** portion of the work-up has been collected and organized. Now the history, physical exam, and lab data are considered together in the **synthetic** portion of the work-up, in which each problem is systematically assessed and a management plan for each is formulated. This section of the write-up may be considered in four parts: (1) a **summary** is written; (2) a complete **problem list** is generated; (3) an **assessment** is made of each problem on the list; and (4) a **plan**—for further diagnosis and for therapy—is formulated.

A. **Summary.** Write a **brief, two- to three-line** summary after the last piece of lab data is recorded and before the assessment and plan are made for each problem. Summarizing serves to refocus both your own and the reader's attention on the case at hand, emphasizing the central concern(s) of the HPI. See the sample write-up for an example.

B. **Problem list.** You will be familiar with the concept of a problem list from earlier medical studies, but several specific points are useful to remember here:

    1. A problem list is the **collected set of findings** that you believe need to be addressed as part of a patient's overall case. **Problems are derived from four general areas: the history, the physical exam, laboratory findings, and a synthesis of any or all of these three.** Thus findings such as chest pain, a supraclavicular node, and a low serum sodium value might all be possible entries in a case of pneumonia, a diagnosis arrived at by synthesizing data from the history, physical exam, and laboratory. As you gain experience, it will become clear that certain entries previously considered distinct from one another in fact may be subsumed under one new heading on your problem list. What is important at the outset is identifying all abnormalities or problems by methodically examining the data available. The problem

list should serve as an **overall outline** for thinking about the case; ideally it will consist of the fewest number of entries that together explain all your findings.

2. The construction of a problem list is not simply an academic exercise; it is the **initial step in management** of the patient. Therefore, if there is a problem that you have no intention of addressing (e.g., poor dentition), it probably does not belong on your problem list.

3. The problem that is central to the present illness usually occupies the number 1 spot on the problem list. Related and distinct problems from the history, physical exam, and laboratory data are then **ranked** in order of the importance you ascribe to them.

C. **Assessment.** Now that the problem list exists, you need to address each problem in turn, considering its significance and reflecting on diagnostic possibilities if the etiology is unclear. The analysis of each problem is at least partially put to paper in the form of the assessment. As is illustrated in the sample write-up, each problem is discussed in turn, and from this "thinking on paper" arises the logical sequence of further diagnostic steps and therapeutic interventions, which are listed after each problem as the **plan.** The assessment is usually written in the form of one paragraph for each problem.

1. Begin by stating the **diagnoses** that seem to be the most probable explanation for the problem in question (unless, of course, your heading is a diagnosis, such as "pneumonia").

2. Methodically mention the compelling **history, physical exam, and laboratory findings** that are related to the problem in question and that help support the conclusion you are drawing about the significance of a given problem.

3. Mention **other diagnostic possibilities** that you have entertained, and, again using data from the history, physical exam, and laboratory, state why they are unlikely or not yet excluded.

4. By this point the **further diagnostic studies** necessary to arrive at a decisive diagnosis will be fairly clear. These studies form the first part of your plan list.

5. Last, consider **conditions related to the problem in** question that may be important to explore. This part of the assessment requires experience and a firm knowledge of pathophysiology and clinical presentations of disease. For example, if a patient's pneumococcal pneumonia was his third such event in the past 18 months, it might be worthwhile to rule out the possibility of an underlying multiple myeloma (which predisposes to recurrent pneumonia, especially with encapsulated bacteria) by ordering a serum immunoelectrophoresis.

D. The **plan** logically proceeds from the reasoning presented in the paragraph following each problem on the problem list; it is simply a checklist of things to be done. The first entries are further **diagnostic** steps, as mentioned above **(C.4).** Following these are the **therapeutic interventions** on which you and your team have decided. To summarize and elaborate on the areas that the assessment and plan address, we have listed below topics to consider when formulating these sections:

1. **Definitive diagnoses.** For problems that are unsolved, try to narrow the diagnostic possibilities and decide what needs to be done to arrive at a final diagnosis. Consider the need for subspecialty consultations here.

2. **Correction or compensation of pathophysiology.** This subject is the cornerstone of medical management. Thinking about pathophysiology, try to understand what perturbation has caused the problem in question and what might be done to compensate for or correct that causative factor.

3. **Therapeutic measures.** In addition to correction or compensation, consider the following areas with respect to therapy:

   a. Pain relief.

   b. Specific medications useful for the problem in question.

   c. Ancillary help (e.g., physical or occupational therapist, nutritionist).

   d. Prevention of complications (e.g., bedsore prophylaxis for those who must be on their back constantly).

   e. Long-term care (e.g., potential need for outpatient assistance, nursing home, visiting nurse). As is evident from the sample write-up, each problem is addressed in turn, and a list of further steps is created.

E. **Conclusion.** As you come to the end of the assessment and plan, having addressed each problem, two measures are useful to help conclude your write-up. First, conclude with a brief impression of the case, as explained in sec. **X.** Second, and perhaps more important, define for yourself the **endpoint** for your patient's present hospitalization. Although you may revise the endpoint deliberately, if it is not considered from the day of admission, you will find that the reasons for the patient's hospitalization seem to shift and change emphasis, making the process of concluding the hospitalization very frustrating.

X. **Concluding information.** In a complicated case, it is sometimes useful to conclude the write-up with a few sentences that present your **overall impression,** in which the case priorities and the long-term goals and sequence of therapies that you suggest are briefly mentioned. This is a chance to integrate the patient's medical problems into a unified picture of the patient as a person rather than simply as a set of organ systems.

XI. **Progress notes**

A. Keep your progress notes **brief** and **telegraphic.** Concentrate on any new data that you have, and any change in clinical symptoms or signs. Even if the patient's chart has a separate lab result section in which the lab tests are routinely recorded, you should still summarize new results in your progress notes. If a test has been done but the results are not available, note that the test is "pending." No matter what format is used, a good progress note should enable the reader to skim the day's data in a minute or two and answer the following questions:

   1. Is there any **new diagnostic information?**

   2. Is the patient getting **better or worse?**

   3. Are the **chosen therapies** working?

   4. What **further diagnostic and therapeutic steps** are in progress or planned?

B. **Flowcharts** are extremely useful, especially for patients with multiple interrelated medical problems. For instance, a patient with severe renal failure might benefit from a flowchart that allows quick day-by-day comparisons of those clinical parameters affected by renal failure. Such a flow chart might be set up as follows:

Date: 7/1   7/2   7/3   7/4

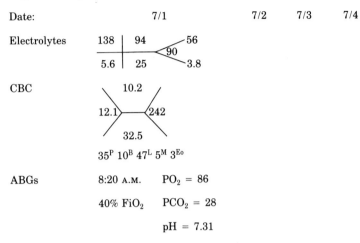

Electrolytes

$$\frac{138 \mid 94}{5.6 \mid 25} < \frac{56}{90} \atop 3.8$$

CBC

35^P 10^B 47^L 5^M 3^{Eo}

ABGs   8:20 A.M. $PO_2 = 86$

              40% FiO_2 $PCO_2 = 28$

                      pH $= 7.31$

Although this sort of chart does not take the place of daily notes, it can be an invaluable aid to consultants who see the patient only every few days, as well as to you and your intern, when you wish to summarize the case.

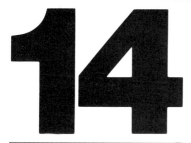

Medical Case Presentations

Perhaps the most difficult thing for medical students and house staff to learn and a lessson the experienced physician frequently relearns, often with discomfort but rarely with surprise, is that for everything we do, based upon sound rationales, for or to acutely ill patients, *there are often equally persuasive competing rationales as to why we should **not** choose a certain treatment* or intervention. Recognizing and dealing with those opposing issues constitutes a most challenging basis for developing clinical judgment. That developmental process begins with awareness of the issues and plans to detect and evaluate adverse effects at the earliest reasonable moment.

Roland H. Ingram, Jr., M.D.

In this chapter, Part A outlines the two types of presentations: the **brief presentation** on work rounds and the more **formal presentation** delivered to the attending physician. Part B provides a description of the teaching points emphasized during attending rounds and some of the general areas that need to be addressed when presenting cases.

Although practical information and hints have most often been confined to Part B in Chaps. 1 through 10, some can be found in Part A of this chapter as well. In fact, presenting a case is an art, and as such it can be described only partially and learned only with practice.

A — Annotated Outline of Medical Case Presentations

I. **Introductory points.** You will need to be familiar with two types of presentations:

  1. Short, 1–2 minute "**bullet**" **presentations.**
  2. More complete, 5–6 minute **formal presentations.**

The logical flow of the presentation emerges from a good **work-up (history and physical exam) and write-up (admission or transfer note).** The write-up is the template from which you prepare the presentation you will give to the team later that day or the next morning. Formal presentations should not exceed **5–6 minutes,** even for the most complicated cases.

II. **Preparing the data for presentation**

  A. **Note card.** A useful adjunct to every write-up, the note card allows the most important parts of the work-up to be summarized, organized, and recorded in a portable, accessible manner. Prepare the note card at the end of the work-up, when the case is still fresh in your mind, and use your write-up as a guide. Your note cards are vital to your success on the wards, for they function as your portable chart rack and memory prompt. This is true especially at the beginning of your clinical experience, when note cards may be used **to present,** unless you are specifically required to present without notes.

B. Information to note. At first, it is useful to have a number of facts on the note card. Later, when presenting from memory is less difficult, it is still useful to carry the following information on a note card. (Information that is especially important is marked with an asterisk.)

1. **Patient information.*** Use addressograph plate to stamp top of your card.

2. **Introductory sentence.*** Record necessary information from your write-up.

3. **Chief complaint** (CC) and its duration.*

4. **History of present illness.**

   a. Record salient points, using **single words** that jog your memory and allow you to tell the patient's story as you summarized it in your write-up.

   b. State pertinent negatives.

   c. State risk factors, positive family history.

5. **Past medical history.** Record only **active problems.**

6. **Allergies.*** Record all, and explain type of reaction if drug allergy.

7. **Medications.*** Note **all,** with dosages. Include ethanol and tobacco use.

8. **Review of systems.** Note **only** significant positives (usually you will have covered these in your HPI).

9. **Physical exam findings.**

   a. Introductory descriptive sentence.

   b. Vital signs.

   c. Pertinent positive findings only.

10. **Laboratory tests.*** State all **pertinent positive findings.**

11. **Problem list.*** Recorded from the assessment and plan section of the write-up.

C. The above information should fit on a 3-by-5-inch index card, unless the case is very complicated or you have large handwriting.

III. Presenting

A. The **bullet presentation** is a *quick,* 1–2 minute summary, most often delivered on work rounds in the morning. It is to be considered a **brief, orienting introduction** to those members of the team who do not know the patient at all. Think of the bullet presentation as a **summary of the note card** you have prepared: **it is the distillation of your first distillation.** A bullet presentation should include:

1. **Introductory sentence.***

2. **CC** and its duration.*

3. **HPI.** Often condensed in a bullet. Include it if your resident wants it; do not drone on. Summarize the HPI in a few sentences.

4. **Medications.***

5. **Physical exam findings.***

   a. Give the patient's **general condition** (good, fair, stable, guarded, critical).

   b. State "**vital signs** stable," or report those that are not.

   c. State definitive **positive findings.**

6. **Pertinent positive laboratory tests.***

7. **Summary.** If the case is complicated, give a one- or two-sentence summary.

   Be brief: if there are laboratory tests your team members want to know about, they will ask.

B. General principles concerning the bullet presentation:

   1. The presentation is a skeleton or framework that allows others to think about the person they are about to meet.

   2. Someone undoubtedly will ask whether anything important is missing from the bullet. So long as the basic information noted above is given, you have done your job.

   3. Speak decisively and distinctly.

   4. Mention **active** and **potential** problems: this is the time that team members who cover the patients at night hear about them.

C. Sample bullet

   I'll present Mrs. Jones's case formally during attending rounds, but to give all of you who haven't met her a brief introduction: she's a 55-year-old black woman with a history of well-controlled diabetes, hypertension, hyperlipidemia, and rheumatoid arthritis. She entered complaining of weakness, cough, and a feverish feeling of 2–3 days' duration. At home, she's been on 80 units of NPH and 15 of CZI insulin per day, she takes 50 mg of guanethidine per day and is on Atromid-S qid.

   On physical exam, she's in good condition now with stable vital signs, a temp of 103°F last night, a few rales in her right axilla, but nothing else on her last chest exam. The remainder of her physical exam was unremarkable.

   Pertinent labs included a CBC with 12,000 WBCs without a left shift, gram-negative rods on an unspun urine (but no UTI symptoms), and a right lower lobe infiltrate on her chest film. In addition, her sputum contained polys and gram-positive diplococci. We think she has pneumococcal pneumonia, and she has begun to defervesce on 500 mg ampicillin IV every 6 hours.

D. The **formal presentation** is essentially a presentation of the note card outlined in sec. **II.B.**

   1. **Patient information.** If the case is complicated, you may want to interject the phrase "with multiple medical problems."

   2. **Introductory sentence.**

   3. **CC** and its duration. In a presentation, unlike a write-up, **avoid using the patient's words.** Instead, give a description that allows the listeners to focus quickly on the problem at hand.

   4. **HPI.** Present a **succinct** version of the HPI. Give pertinent positive findings from the appropriate ROS section(s). Note pertinent risk factors and family history.

5. **PMH.** Mention **prior admissions.** Flesh out other active medical problems.

6. **Allergies.** Note any drug reactions.

7. **Medications.** State **all present medicines,** with dosages.

8. **Positive ROS findings.** State only pertinent positives other than those mentioned during the HPI.

9. **Physical exam findings.**

   a. **Introductory sentence,** describing general appearance and condition.

   b. **Vital signs** are stated for every patient.

   c. **Pertinent positive findings.** Some attending physicians may want you to describe the entire physical exam (PE), system by system, even if normal, but this is unnecessary unless specifically requested.

10. **Laboratory tests.**

    a. **Pertinent positives** from these categories, in "**CUBS**" order:

       C   Complete blood count
       U   Urinalysis
       B   Blood chemistries
       S   Specials, if done (ECG, CXR, ABGs, CT scan, MRI, and so on)

    b. **Pertinent negatives** if you believe they are significant.

11. **Summary.** Give a brief, **two-sentence summary** and then **pause.** The discussion of the case is initiated here, so make your summary useful and make it clear from your voice and expression that you are done. The attending physician will ask you what you and the team did for the patient therapeutically, and will begin discussing specific questions concerning the case.

B   **Practical Points Concerning
                                          Case Presentations**

I. **Areas often discussed during the presentation to the attending.** Rounds with an attending physician ("the visit") are often initiated by the case presentation of the previous night's admission and continue, time permitting, with discussions about the case. The purpose of visit rounds preparation is *not* to be able to anticipate and answer every question you will be asked. Spend time reflecting on the case, read what you can, and, first and foremost, understand the pathophysiology. Following are some of the frequently discussed areas; although there is rarely time to learn about all of these for each case, choose those subjects you believe are the most pertinent to the case in question.

   A. **Pathophysiologic mechanisms.**

   B. **Historical findings and symptoms** associated with the disease(s) in question.

   C. **Physical findings** associated with the disease(s) in question.

   D. **Differential diagnosis:** other diseases that might present in a similar manner and imporant differentiating features among those possibilities.

   E. **Complications** associated with the disease(s) under consideration.

F. Mechanism of action and side effects of any **medications** the patient is taking or was placed on during this admission.

II. Caveats of presenting

A. **Speed of presentation.** Do not dawdle, but do not roar through the presentation so quickly that you cannot be understood. Try to relax, and speak as though explaining a subject to friends.

B. **Tone.** Do not read your presentation. This is the most common cause of a monotonic delivery. Tell your listeners a dynamic, interesting story.

C. **Pauses and interruptions.** Roll with the punches here; if a discussion ensues while you are presenting, note where you left off, listen to and perhaps participate in the digression, and be ready to resume, **repeating** the sentence you last spoke as you begin again. The attending or resident will usually ask you to continue.

D. **Enunciation.** Speak precisely. Do not say, for example, "one hundred six" for a temperature of "one hundred point six."

E. **Brevity.** The bullet presentation is meant to be brief, but even the formal presentation should be short enough to maintain the interest of your listeners. Up to 5–6 minutes is a reasonable amount of time to expect people to listen; after that you will begin to lose your audience.

F. **Condensation.** When it is necessary to describe in detail one or two problems, it becomes necessary, as well, simply to mention other issues that you may have wished to elaborate on. Condensing the presentation is preferable to making it too long. Describe problems in further detail only in response to your audience's queries.

G. **Omissions.** You should describe only positive and negative findings pertinent to the differential diagnoses you are entertaining. In other words, omit details that are not relevant to the "argument" you are constructing.

H. **Physical exam findings.** It is natural at all stages of clinical experience, especially at the beginning, to have equivocal physical findings arise. Point out your findings, and if others have disagreed or differed, simply state, "Another observer thought . . . "

I. **Concluding.** At the end of the history, physical exam, and laboratory data presentations, summarize the case in one to two sentences for your listeners, focusing on the problem that is most relevant. For example, "In summary, Mrs. Jones is a 55-year-old black woman with a history of diabetes, hypertension, hyperlipidemia, and rheumatoid arthritis who presented last night with a probable pneumococcal pneumonia."

J. **Hospital course.** If the patient has been in the hospital for any length of time, most attending physicians will discuss certain features of the case before they ask about the patient's hospital course. It is reasonable to ask the attending at the end of your presentation whether he or she would like to hear what the patient's hospital course has been. For patients with multiple **active** problems, describe the hospital course in a problem-oriented manner; for example, "First, with respect to the patient's pneumonia. . . . Second, with respect to her elevated blood glucose on admission . . . ," and so on.

K. **Refutations by the bedside.** You will sometimes present by the bedside, and you will almost always see the patient after you present. Patients often refute the stories being told about them, or correct them in major or minor ways. This is not a personal attack; it happens frequently to everyone caring for patients, and it may provide a valuable new clue. Since you are at an advantage, having heard the patient's story previously, try to decipher what the patient has corrected. How was he or she misunderstood originally? Then consider any implications the refutation has for the way in which you have considered the case. Above all, **do not panic, and do not argue with the patient.** Accept this correction respectfully and perhaps take the opportunity to ask a few related questions.

Disease Pathophysiology Review

> The diagnosis is nearly always contained in *the patients' words and physical findings*. The physician must translate their words and the data obtained with the eyes, ears, and hands into a language that describes disorders of organ functions. Remember: the hand of disease can be quicker than the eye of the physician.
>
> **Kenneth H. Falchuk, M.D.**

The two hardest and yet most important parts of your introduction to clinical medicine are (1) learning how to do a directed history and physical, and (2) developing an assessment and a plan. To do either of these well, you need to be able to apply the pathophysiology you learned during the first two years of medical school to the problems of real patients. While you most likely learned a large amount of material in those preclinical years, the information may not be in a form immediately useful to you on the wards.

This section of the book reviews some important facets of disease pathophysiology, going through each of the most common diseases you will encounter on the wards, by organ system. For each disease, it describes:

1. A **definition** of the disease, and any important subtypes as well.
2. The **clinical manifestations**—that is, what you should ask for in the history and especially look for on the physical exam. Also included are common lab tests that are used in making the diagnosis.
3. **Differential diagnosis**—other diseases that can present like the disease being described, or how to differentiate between important subtypes of the given illness.
4. **Pathophysiology**—a concise review.

These descriptions should help you in several ways. You can use them as a review of pertinent clinical facts about the major diseases you will see on the wards, or you can refer to them during a work-up, to remind yourself what to ask for and look for in a more directed work-up. In addition, you can use them to review basic facts about each disease before writing your analysis and plan, as well as to help you to organize your thoughts before presenting your patient at rounds.

The descriptions of diseases here are certainly not a substitute for the more comprehensive discussions found in textbooks, such as *Harrison's* or *Cecil's* (see **Appendix D**). The best way to learn and remember pathophysiology during your clinical training years is to read about each disease you encounter on the wards in a textbook such as these. We do feel, however, that these disease summaries will be helpful for you as you start your clinical career on the wards.

Among the various diagnostic possibilities pertaining to any seriously ill patient, *the curable ones* ought to be pursued first and most vigorously, whatever the diagnostic probabilities.

Alexander S. Nadas, M.D.

Pulmonary Diseases

15

Asthma

I. Definition. Syndrome of reversible airway hyperreactivity in response to a number of known stimuli **(allergic asthma)** or nonidentifiable stimuli **(nonallergic asthma).**

II. Clinical manifestations

A. History

1. Progressively worsening dyspnea, cough, tachypnea, chest tightness, and wheezing over a period of hours to days.

2. Elicit **provocative factors,** which may include exposure to animal dander, pollen, salicylates, or nonsteroidal anti-inflammatory drugs; exercise; cold weather; and the presence of an upper respiratory infection.

B. Physical exam

1. Patient is generally sitting forward, is diaphoretic, and may be unable to speak due to severe dyspnea.

2. Signs of respiratory distress: **grunting** sound during inspiration, **flaring** of nostrils during inspiration, **retractions,** use of accessory respiratory muscles during inspiration.

3. Tachycardia and tachypnea.

4. Pulsus paradoxus, inspiratory decline in systolic blood pressure > 10 mm Hg; reflects large intrapleural pressure swings.

5. Lungs: inspiratory-expiratory rhonchi, hyperinflated chest, prolonged expiratory phase, frank wheezing, cyanosis in severe cases.

6. Signs of impending respiratory crisis:

    a. the absence of wheezing, or decreased wheezing, can indicate worsening obstruction.

    b. Paradoxical abdominal movement on inspiration (detected by palpation over the upper part of the abdomen in a semirecumbent position) indicates diaphragmatic fatigue.

7. Mental status changes: generally secondary to hypoxia and hypercapnea, and constitute an indication for emergent intubation.

C. Diagnostic tests

1. **Complete blood count** (CBC). Eosinophilia; ↑ WBC with "left shift" may indicate coexistence of bacterial pneumonia; most associated pneumonias are viral.

2. **Sputum.** Eosinophilia; bronchial casts; aspergillosis; ± Curschmann's spirals (distal airway casts composed of respiratory epithelial cells); ± Charcot-Leyden crystals.

3. **Chest x-ray** (CXR). Hyperinflation (flattening of diaphragm and increased volume in the retrosternal airspace); look for evidence of pneumonia.

4. **Arterial blood gases** (ABGs). Can be used in staging severity of asthmatic attack.

   a. Mild: decreased PO_2 and PCO_2, increased pH.

   b. Moderate: decreased PO_2, normal PCO_2, normal pH.

   c. Severe: markedly decreased PO_2, increased PCO_2, decreased pH.

5. **Pulmonary function tests** (PFTs). FEV_1 ↓ ↓ ; FVC ↓ ↓ ; RV ↑ ; TLC ↑ acutely; subtle similar abnormalities may persist chronically.

III. **Differential diagnosis.** Findings that differentiate the two asthmatic populations, **allergic asthma** and **nonallergic asthma,** are compared in Table 15-1.

IV. **Pathophysiology.** The causes of asthma are twofold, consisting of **acute bronchospasm** and **chronic inflammation.** The bronchial musculature of both the large and small airways is hyperreactive to various stimuli. Bronchospasm is manifested by the intermittent attacks of wheezing, dyspnea, and cough. The chronic inflammatory component results in the formation of an adherent exudate that plugs up the airways. Bronchiolar smooth muscle contractions, bronchial wall edema, and thickened secretions all lead to diminished airway diameter.

Bronchiolar hyperactivity is caused by two distinct mechanisms: the **local pathway** and the **reflex pathway.** The local pathway, an example of type I immune hypersensitivity, is mediated by IgE immunoglobulins bound to the surface of mast cells. When an allergen binds the IgE molecule, the mast cell degranulates, releasing histamine, prostaglandins, eosinophilic chemotactic factor of anaphylaxis, and leukotrienes, which cause bronchiolar smooth muscle constriction and increased vascular permeability. The reflex pathway is triggered by submucous irritant receptors. Bronchiolar constriction in this pathway is the result of stimuli carried by the parasympathetic nervous system (vagus nerve).

Table 15-1. Diagnosis of asthma

	Allergic	Nonallergic
Inciting agent	Pollen, animal dander	Upper respiratory infections, emotional factors, nonspecific irritants
Age	70% of asthmatics < 30 yr	70% of asthmatics > 30 yr
Historical points	Spring-fall hay fever, ± infantile eczema, FHx allergies	H/O ↑ in winter, chronic cough, H/O respiratory infections, subset with salicylate intolerance
Physical exam	Urticaria, eczema, chest exam findings (see **II.C**)	Rhinitis, nasal polyps, chest exam findings (see **II.C**)
Laboratory	↑ circulating IgE, skin tests positive	Normal IgE levels, skin tests negative

Chronic Obstructive Pulmonary Disease (COPD)

I. **Definition.** COPD is chronic airflow obstruction secondary to chronic bronchitis, emphysema, or both.

   A. **Chronic bronchitis** is a clinical diagnosis characterized by excessive tracheobronchial mucus secretion so as to produce cough with sputum production on most days for at least 3 months of the year, during 2 or more consecutive years. "**Blue bloaters**" is the term used to describe patients with chronic bronchitis, derived from the fact that patients with chronic bronchitis often have a bluish tinge to their skin (secondary to chronic hypoxemia and hypercapnea) and frequently have peripheral edema (secondary to cor pulmonale).

   B. **Emphysema** is a pathological diagnosis characterized histologically by distention of the air spaces distal to the terminal bronchiole with destruction of alveolar walls. "**Pink puffers**" is the term used to describe patients with emphysema, derived from the fact that patients with emphysema often are cachectic and have a pink skin color (adequate O_2 saturation) and "puff" when they breathe. They assume a tripod position, purse their lips, and use accessory muscles to breathe.

II. **Clinical manifestations and differential diagnosis**

   COPD is rarely pure; more often it is a mixture of chronic bronchitis and emphysematous disease. Tables 15-2 through 15-4 provide differentiating features of these two types of COPD.

III. **Pathophysiology**

   A. **Cigarette smoking** plays a central part in etiology of both emphysema and chronic bronchitis by promoting the breakdown of elastin in the lung. In

Table 15-2. History and physical exam findings in COPD

Finding	Type A: emphysema (pink puffer)	Type B: chronic bronchitis (blue bloater)
Dyspnea	Insidious onset; often becomes severe	Mild to severe
Cough	Follows dyspnea	Precedes dyspnea
Sputum	Scant, mucoid	Copious, purulent
Symptoms at rest	Marked	Milder
Weight change	Often marked loss	Slight loss to moderate gain
Bronchial infections	Less frequent	More frequent
Respiratory insufficiency episodes	At terminal course	Common and repeated
Age at diagnosis	± 60 yr	± 50 yr
Integument	No cyanosis or clubbing	Cyanosis; rarely, clubbing
Pulmonary exam	Hyperresonance, end-expiratory wheezing, lower intercostal space retractions, accessory muscle usage	No hyperresonance, often rhonchi with coarse and wet breath sounds, no lower intercostal retractions, less accessory muscle usage

Table 15-3. Diagnostic test findings in COPD

Finding	Type A: emphysema (pink puffer)	Type B: chronic bronchitis (blue bloater)
Total lung capacity	Increased	Normal or slightly increased or decreased
Vital capacity	Decreased	Decreased
Residual volume	Greatly increased	Moderately increased
Elastic recoil	Markedly decreased	Normal
Inspiratory airway resistance	Normal to slightly increased	Markedly increased
Compliance (static)	Increased	Near normal
Compliance (dynamic)	Normal to slightly decreased	Markedly decreased
Diffusing capacity	Decreased	Normal to slightly decreased
Hematocrit	35–45%	40–55% (lower value may indicate superimposed infection with anemia)
PCO_2	35–40 mm Hg	50–65 mm Hg
PO_2	65–75 mm Hg	45–60 mm Hg
Cardiac output	Often decreased	Usually normal
Chest x-ray	Hyperlucent, hyperinflated lung with flat diaphragms; small heart, decreased vascular markings, and bullae may be evident	Large heart; increased bronchovascular shadows in lower field; evidence of old inflammatory disease

Table 15-4. Complications of COPD

Complication	Type A: emphysema (pink puffer)	Type B: chronic bronchitis (blue bloater)
Pulmonary hypertension at rest	None to mild	Moderate to severe
Pulmonary hypertension with exercise	Moderate	Worsens
Cor pulmonale	Rare (terminal event)	Common
Infectious exacerbations	Less frequent	More frequent

the normal lung there is a delicate balance between the elastase released by polymorphonuclear leukocytes (PMNs) in the lung and alpha-1 protease inhibitor (A1PI), which inhibits the elastase. Cigarette smoke disturbs this balance by increasing the concentration of PMNs and alveolar macrophages in the lung, thus increasing the reservoir of elastase, and by oxidizing the A1PI, rendering the elastin protector impotent. The net result is that cigarette smoking promotes the breakdown of elastin in the lung. This loss of elastin compromises the internal structure of the respiratory bronchioles, causing them to obstruct upon exhalation.

B. Chronic bronchitis is characterized by hypertrophy and hyperplasia of submucosal mucus-producing glands in larger airways, and small airway changes such as goblet-cell hyperplasia, inflammatory reaction, and retained bronchial secretions.

C. **Emphysema** is subdivided into two main types: **panacinar** and **centrilobular**. The panacinar form, the hereditary form, is due to A1PI deficiency, and is characterized by uniform destruction of the acinus. These patients develop emphysema at a much younger age (30–40), and many do not have a history of smoking. Alpha-1 protease inhibitor was previously known as alpha-1-antitrypsin. The centrilobular form results from smoking, and tends to leave alveoli at the margin of the acinus unaffected; it generally involves alveolar ducts and respiratory bronchioles in the center of the lobule. Clinically, emphysema is best diagnosed by spirometric tests (which correlate well with the pathologic changes that define the disease).

Pulmonary Tuberculosis
(see Colorplate D, 11)

I. **Definition.** A chronic, necrotizing, transmissible infection of the lungs caused by *Mycobacterium tuberculosis*.

II. **Clinical manifestations**

A. **History.** Most patients are asymptomatic at diagnosis. Initial constitutional symptoms: dry, nonproductive cough, night sweats, fever, anorexia, fatigue, dyspnea, hemoptysis, and pleuritic pain.

B. **Physical exam.** Will be normal in many cases. Initial sign may be rales near lung apices. As tuberculous process progresses, there may be asymmetric respiratory excursion ± tracheal deviation, dullness to percussion, ↑ tactile fremitus over involved areas, and rales.

C. **Diagnostic tests**

1. **PPD.** A positive reaction is defined as greater than or equal to 10 mm of induration at 48 hours. Up to 25 percent of newly diagnosed tuberculosis patients have a negative tubercullin skin test, particularly patients with renal failure, elderly patients, patients on steroid or immunosuppressive therapy, HIV-positive individuals, and patients with severe protein deficiency, concomitant live virus vaccination or infection, lymphoma, or sarcoidosis. Negative PPD with positive *Candida* or mumps control is highly sensitive in excluding active tuberculosis. Patients who have received **BCG vaccine** will be PPD positive.

2. **Sputum.** Acid-fast bacillus stain positive in primary tuberculosis, although it is often difficult to find the organism microscopically. Mycobacterial cultures take a minimum of four weeks to grow, and although the cultures make the definitive diagnosis, they are rarely useful in the acute setting.

3. **CBC.** Normochromic, normocytic anemia common (may be severe); WBC normal (diff may include 8–15% mononuclear cells).

4. **Urinanalysis** (U/A). Hematuria and pyuria may indicate renal involvement (**sterile pyuria** classically associated with tuberculosis). Albuminuria (secondary to amyloidosis) may be seen in prolonged infections.

5. **Chemistry:** ↓ Na (SIADH), ↓ Albumin (severe cases)

6. **CXR.** Crucial to diagnosis.

a. **Primary tuberculosis.** Patchy infiltrates in lower lung fields and hilar adenopathy.

   b. **Postprimary tuberculosis.** Patchy upper-lobe infiltrates (apical and posterior segments involved), cavitation, fibronodular infiltrates, fibrosis, and unilateral infiltrates are common.

III. **Differential diagnosis.** Tuberculosis needs to be differentiated from the following:

   A. **Acute bacterial pneumonia.** Sputum exam, response to antibiotics helpful in distinguishing from TB.

   B. **Neoplasm.** High incidence of tuberculous changes in upper lobes of older men may make the diagnosis of neoplasm difficult; sputum cytology, bronchoscopy with brushings may help distinguish.

   C. **Sarcoidosis.** Negative PPD test; lymph node biopsy through mediastinoscopy may be necessary to distinguish.

   D. **Fungal disorder (especially histoplasmosis).** Histoplasmosis and tuberculosis may coexist; skin tests for fungus and cultures help make the diagnosis.

   E. **Cavitary lung abscess.** Involves superior segments of lower lobes (most often due to aspiration); positive air-fluid level (rare in tuberculosis); no associated patchy infiltrate adjacent to cavity on CXR (common in tuberculosis).

IV. **Pathophysiology**

   A. TB infection in Western societies almost always is by **inhalation of aerosolized bacilli** ("droplet nuclei") from coughing, sneezing, or speech. Tubercle bacilli multiply slowly (maximum of 1–2 cell divisions/day) and require high O_2 concentration, which is why primary tuberculosis occurs in the lower lobes.

   B. **Disease stages**

      1. **Primary tuberculosis.** Bacterial multiplication with asymptomatic spread to regional hilar nodes; leads to lymphohematogenous spread. Seeds widely, especially to the lung apices, kidneys, vertebral column, long bones, brain, lymph nodes (organs with high oxygen concentrations). Reticuloendothelial system involved in clearance of bacilli.

      2. **Postprimary tuberculosis.** Onset 3 to 6 weeks after infection; a specific population of T lymphocytes determines pathologic response and is responsible for tuberculin reaction and cellular immunity. Quiescent tuberculosis results from immunologically contained infection.

Pulmonary Embolism

I. **Definition.** Impaction of thrombotic embolus in the pulmonary vascular bed, with subsequent obstruction of the blood supply to the lung parenchyma.

II. **Clinical manifestations**

   A. **History.** Sudden onset of dyspnea, precordial or substernal pain (may be pleuritic or nonpleuritic), sudden cough or hemoptysis, syncope, fever, diaphoresis.

   B. **Physical exam**

      1. **Pulmonary.** Tachypnea, rales, localized wheezing, pleural friction rub.

      2. **Cardiovascular.** There may be evidence of deep venous thrombosis in the lower extremities. Patients usually present with tachycardia, increased P_2 component of S_2 (acute cor pulmonale), murmur of tricuspid insufficiency, right ventricular heave, S_4 (and/or S_3), distended

neck veins, cyanosis, hypotension. There may also be positive hepato-jugular reflux, hepatomegaly, and evidence for severe right heart failure in patients with multiple chronic pulmonary embolization.

C. **Diagnostic tests**

1. **ECG.** Normal in many patients. Transient changes may include sinus tachycardia, T wave inversion in V_1 to V_4, acute cor pulmonale exhibited by "$S_1 Q_3 T_3$" pattern, P pulmonale, acute right bundle branch block, new-onset atrial fibrillation, right axis deviation, S-T segment depression in lead II, and right ventricular strain pattern.

2. **CXR.** Normal in 50 percent of patients. There may be also abrupt cutoff of vessel shadow and radiolucent area distal to the area of embolus **(Westermark's sign).** Atelectatic streaks and consolidated areas may be present, as may pleural effusion or unilateral elevation of diaphragm.

3. **ABGs.** ↓ PO_2 (on room air), ↓ PCO_2 (due to hyperventilation), and increased pH.

4. **Lung scan and arteriography.** It is impossible to diagnose pulmonary embolism on clinical grounds alone. A normal ventilation perfusion scan (V/Q scan) rules out pulmonary embolism. A V/Q scan mismatch is suggestive of pulmonary embolism, and a V/Q scan of high probability is deemed confirmatory. A V/Q scan of moderate, low, or indeterminate probability, in a patient where there is a high clinical suspicion of pulmonary embolism should receive a pulmonary arteriogram. A positive arteriogram confirms the diagnosis.

III. **Differential diagnosis.** Note that the symptoms and signs of pulmonary embolism are **nonspecific;** it is a difficult diagnosis to make.

A. **Pulmonary embolism without infarction of lung parenchyma.** Bacteremic shock, myocardial infarction, peritonitis, anxiety with hyperventilation, and cardiac tamponade.

B. **Pulmonary embolism with infarction of lung parenchyma.** Pneumonia, atelectasis, heart failure, and pericarditis.

IV. **Pathophysiology**

A. Eighty to 90 percent are due to venous thrombi originating in the lower extremities; in postsurgical patients, pelvic vein or prostatic plexus thrombi may also lead to emboli. About 10 percent of detected emboli cause infarction of lung tissue.

B. **Predisposing factors** include prolonged immobilization, peripheral vascular disease (venous), estrogen-containing oral contraceptives, right ventricular failure, pregnancy and early puerperium, postoperative state, trauma or surgery to the lower extremities or pelvis, advanced age, and history of deep venous thrombosis or pulmonary embolism, visceral carcinoma (lung, pancreatic, gastrointestinal, and genitourinary), burns, obesity, diabetes mellitus, and hematologic disease (antithrombin III deficiency, protein C deficiency, protein S deficiency, lupus anticoagulant, polycythemia vera, dysfibrinogenemia, paroxysmal nocturnal hemoglobineuria).

Pneumonia
(see Colorplate D)

I. **Definition.** An acute infection of lung parenchyma. There are several types of pneumonia: **lobar pneumonia** (infection confined to a single lobe), **segmental or lobular pneumonia** (infection confined to a segment of a lobe), **broncho-**

pneumonia (infection involves alveoli and contiguous bronchi), **interstitia pneumonia** (infection involves interstitial tissue). These distinctions are based on x-ray observations.

II. **Clinical manifestations and differential diagnosis.** The most common bacterial, viral, mycoplasma, and fungal pneumonias:

A. **Bacterial pneumonias**

1. *Streptococcus pneumoniae* (pneumococcus) (see Colorplate D, 6)

   a. **History.** The **most common cause of bacterial pneumonia,** and the most common cause of pneumonia in adults. Frequently seen in patients with COPD and alcoholism (aspiration pneumonia). **Community acquired,** usually with a history of preceding viral upper respiratory infection.

   Sudden onset with single shaking chill, which is followed by fever, pleuritic chest pain, cough, dyspnea, and purulent sputum production that is "rust" colored or blood-tinged; fever > 102°F.

   b. **Physical exam.** Patient appears seriously ill. Typical pulmonary signs of lobar pneumonia include those consistent with a consolidation: increased tactile fremitus, percussion dullness, egophony, and whispered pectoriloquy. With pleural effusions or empyema there may be percussion dullness, diminished breath sounds, or a pleural rub. The most frequent observation is simply rales.

   c. **Diagnostic tests**

   (1) **CXR.** The **most frequent cause of lobar pneumonia** is pneumococcus; the most frequent x-ray pattern among all patients with pneumococcal pneumonia is a bronchopneumonia pattern; therefore, pneumococcal pneumonia can appear as a dense contion confined to a single lobe with typical air bronchograms or a bronchopneumonia pattern.

   (2) **Microbiology.** Gram stain shows gram-positive diplococci in short chains. Gram stain is better diagnostic tool than culture, which often fails to grow organism. Positive blood cultures in 20 to 25 percent of patients allows definitive diagnosis.

2. *Klebsiella pneumoniae* (see Colorplate D, 10)

   a. **History.** Rarely causes pneumonia in previously well adult hosts. Inflicts infants and the aged; is acquired in nursing home or hospital; host is often immunocompromised.

   Sudden onset of symptoms with fever > 102°F, chills, cough, and thick, bloody ("tenacious") sputum.

   b. **Physical exam.** Characterized by upper-lobe involvement, tissue necrosis with abscess formation.

   c. **Diagnostic tests**

   (1) **CXR.** Variable; usually bronchopneumonia pattern with upper-lobe central cavitation and abscess formation.

   (2) **Microbiology.** Gram stains of sputum show large numbers of gram-negative bacilli. Positive cultures from blood, pleural fluid, or a transtracheal aspirate obtained before treatment are considered diagnostic.

3. *Staphylococcus aureus* (see Colorplate D, 2)

   a. **History.** Similarly to *Klebsiella;* inflicts infants and the elderly; is acquired in nursing home or hospital; host is often immunocompromised. Intravenous drug abusers are prone to staphylococcal tricuspid valve endocarditis with embolic pneumonia. Patients with influenza pneumonia are predisposed to staphylococcal super-infection.

Onset of symptoms similar to pneumococcal pneumonia.

b. **Physical exam.** Similar to that noted for pneumococcal pneumonia. Staphylococcus differs in its tendency to cause recurrent shaking chills, tissue necrosis with abscess formation (rare with pneumococcal pneumonia), and pneumatoceles (most common in infants and children); empyema is common. Infected skin site (portal of entry) often identifiable in IV drug abusers.

c. **Diagnostic tests**

(1) **CXR.** Variable; most common pattern is a bronchopneumonia with or without abscess formation or pleural effusion. Bronchopneumonic pattern (often bilateral) seen; cavitation and abscesses common. Lobar consolidation is infrequent.

(2) **Microbiology.** Gram stain shows gram-positive clusters like "grapes." Diagnosis is made by positive cultures from sputum or empyema fluid or transtracheal or transthoracic aspirate.

B. **Mycoplasma pneumonias** (*Mycoplasma pneumoniae*)

1. **History.** Most common cause of pneumonia in 5- to 35-year-old age group. Community acquired.

Nonspecific constitutional symptoms (malaise and sore throat) are of insidious onset with fever $> 101°F$, nonproductive hacking cough with scant mucoid sputum. Cough is dominant symptom; mild or absent cough makes the diagnosis suspect.

2. **Physical exam.** Findings may be minimal (rales, cough, but little else). Unimpressive relative to patients' complaints and x-ray findings.

3. **Diagnostic tests**

a. **CXR.** Interstitial pneumonia, usually unilateral; usually seen in lower lobes, ± small pleural effusions; radiologic findings often far more severe than clinical manifestations.

b. **Serology.** Positive complement fixation tests in 75 to 80 percent of patients.

C. **Viral pneumonias (Influenza A)**

1. **History.** Ninety percent of deaths due to influenza A occur in elderly population.

Fever up to 105°F with hacking cough; sputum often blood-tinged.

2. **Physical exam.** Pulmonary auscultatory findings may be minimal or absent; respiratory distress often far more severe than radiologic findings.

3. **Diagnostic tests**

a. **CXR.** Diffuse or generalized interstitial pattern usually seen; lobar consolidation or pleural effusion rarely seen.

b. **Microbiology.** Findings of sparse bacteria and a dominance of mononuclear cells on smears of sputum, along with a failure to recover a likely bacterial pathogen from sputum culture, support the diagnosis of viral pneumonia.

c. **Serology.** Presence of cold agglutinins are diagnostic.

D. Fungal pneumonias. Primary fungal pneumonia most commonly caused by *Histoplasma capsulatum* and *Coccidioides immitis.*

1. *Histoplasma capsulatum*

   a. **History.** Asymptomatic or mild fever, malaise, dyspnea, minimal or absent sputum with nonproductive cough; chills rare. Indistinguishable from viral upper respiratory infection.

   b. **Physical exam.** Rales, oral ulceration.

   c. **Diagnostic tests**

      (1) **CXR.** Lower lobes favored, with generalized nodular and linear infiltrates; unilateral or bilateral adenopathy may be present. Chronic cavitary form produces pulmonary lesions indistinguishable, except by culture, from cavitary tuberculosis.

2. **Microbiology.** Culture from sputum or oral ulceration is diagnostic.

3. *Coccidioides immitis*

   a. **History.** Endemic in southwestern United States, predominantly occurring in men 25 to 55 years old.

   Often asymptomatic or indistinguishable from viral upper respiratory infection, with fever, chills, moderate mucoid sputum production.

   b. **Physical exam.** Scattered rales, cervical adenopathy, skin lesions resembling erythema nodosum, pleural effusion with friction rub.

   c. **Diagnostic tests**

      (1) **CXR.** Lower lobes favored, with generalized nodular and linear infiltrates; unilateral or bilateral adenopathy may be present.

      (2) **Microbiology.** Sperules of fungus present in sputum and sputum culture positive for fungus are both diagnostic.

IV. Pathophysiology. Vastly different for each microbe. For a detailed account, consult Weinberger [26].

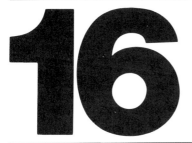

Cardiovascular Diseases

Ischemic Heart Disease: Angina Pectoris and Myocardial Infarction

> Most *serious errors made by physicians* are the result of their being unable or unwilling to consider the possibilities that they are misinformed, uninformed, or incorrect. If the patient's history and physical fail to fit neatly into some diagnostic niche, it may be that the history is incomplete, the physical incorrect, or the physician unaware of the correct niche. The patient who refuses to get better despite intensive and expensive therapy may have been treated for the wrong problem and/or, worse yet, may be toxic from the medications. Maimonides was correct: "Teach thy tongue to say I do not know and thou shall progress."
>
> **Marshall A. Wolf, M.D.**

I. **Definitions**

   A. **Angina pectoris.** Clinical syndrome characterized by pain or discomfort in chest and adjacent areas that occurs when myocardial oxygen demand exceeds supply. It is by definition **transient** and **reversible.** There are three types of angina: **stable, unstable,** and **Prinzmetal's.**

   B. **Myocardial infarction.** MI is an **irreversible** ischemic necrosis of the myocardium, resulting from an insufficient oxygen supply to that area of the heart for a prolonged period. There are two types of myocardial infarction: **transmural** and **subendocardial.**

II. **Clinical manifestations.** Diagnosis of angina is best made by history.

   A. **Angina pectoris**

   1. **History.** Each of the three types of angina presents with its own unique history.

      a. **Stable**

         (1) Usually follows a precipitating event, such as climbing stairs, sexual intercourse, a heavy meal, cold weather.

         (2) Generally same severity as previous attack; relieved by customary dose of nitroglycerin.

      b. **Unstable**

         (1) Recent onset.

         (2) Increasing severity, duration, or frequency of stable angina.

         (3) Occurs at rest or with minimal exertion.

c. Prinzmetal's

   (1) Occurs when patient is at rest.

   (2) No previous history of coronary artery disease.

d. An angina history is described in the following dimensions: **PQRST.**

   (1) Provocative-palliative factors. Aggravated by emotion, exercise, cold weather, large meals; occasionally also by recumbency (angina decubitus). Related to exertion or emotion. Cold weather, large meal also may precipitate. Common for angina to occur soon after awakening; shaving or washing may precipitate. Arm exercise may provoke more angina than leg exercise. Alleviated by rest, cessation of activity, and often by sublingual nitroglycerin. If emotionally precipitated, relieved by relaxation.

   (2) Quality. Often characterized as discomfort, not pain. May be described as pressure, tightness, heaviness, squeezing, band-like, viselike, burning, chocking, smothering, or a sensation similar to intestinal gas or dysphagia. Descriptions such as knifelike, stabbing, or cutting rarely reflect angina.

   (3) Region. Most frequently substernal. May also be in neck, lower jaw, arm, or hand areas (especially left arm, ulnar aspect), with or without chest symptoms. Precordial areas alone (e.g., left submammary, over heart) **uncommon.**

   (4) Severity. Mild to moderate severity; often patients must stop whatever they are doing. May seem less bothersome after patients exert themselves for a while (warm-up phenomenon). Occurs in crescendo-decrescendo pattern; not of sudden onset or dissipation.

   (5) Temporal characteristics. Elicit first onset and frequency. Typical attack 1–3 minutes; almost always shorter than 10 and longer than 1 minute.

   (6) Associated symptoms. Dyspnea common; nausea, dizziness, diaphoresis sometimes. Palpitation, loss of consciousness **rare** (unless angina is related to arrhythmia).

e. Past medical history. Check for hypertension, tobacco use, diabetes mellitus, hyperlipidemia, obesity.

f. Family history. Check for coronary artery disease, MI, angina, premature death in male relatives.

2. Physical exam. Often no physical signs are found during an attack of angina.

   a. Dyspnea and diaphoresis.

   b. New-onset S_4 frequently occurs because of decreased compliance of the ischemic ventricle.

   c. Arrhythmia may be present, which may or may not be the cause of the angina.

   d. Presence of a heart murmur may indicate valvular cause of angina: mitral valve prolapse, aortic stenosis, mitral stenosis, or idiopathic hypertrophic subaortic stenosis.

3. Diagnostic tests

   a. Nitroglycerin test. The unequivocal relief of chest pain or discomfort by the administration of nitroglycerin is strongly suggestive of angina pectoris, but not diagnostic.

    b. **ECG.** During episode of chest discomfort, may show transient ischemic changes such as T wave inversion or S-T segment depression or elevation.

B. Myocardial infarction. Diagnosis depends on meeting two of three criteria: (1) typical pain, (2) ECG changes, and (3) serum enzyme changes.

  1. History

    a. Chest pain or discomfort is the most common symptom. Preexisting and often worsening angina by history. The pain or discomfort is similar to angina pectoris in its quality, location, and intensity, but it is **not** transient, is not relieved by sublingual nitroglycerin, and lasts 30 minutes or longer. The pain is usually not induced by exertion, nor does it remit with rest. Approximately 15–20 percent of infarcts are painless; painless infarcts more common in diabetics and the aged.

    b. Often accompanied by nausea, vomiting (classically if MI is **inferior**), giddiness, anxiety.

    c. Key items of interest in the past medical history and family history are the same as in angina.

  2. Physical exam

    a. Patient will appear diaphoretic and pale, resulting in cold, clammy skin.

    b. Often heart rate accelerates and the blood pressure declines, sometimes to shock levels when there is extensive myocardial damage. A quadruple rhythm (summation gallop) is sometimes heard (S_4-S_1-S_2-S_3). Apical systolic murmur caused by mitral regurgitation secondary to papillary muscle dysfunction may be present.

    c. Arrhythmia may be present.

    d. Rales may appear in lung bases (pulmonary edema), indicative of congestive heart failure.

    e. Pericardial friction rub may be heard.

    f. Mild fever may be present.

  3. Diagnostic tests

    a. **ECG.** Changes appear soon after pain begins. **Sequence of evolution:** S-T segment elevation, T wave inversion, development of Q waves. Q waves usually develop over 12 to 36 hours. A subendocardial myocardial infarct (a non–Q wave infarct) is limited to the inner third to half of the myocardial wall. A transmural myocardial infarct (a Q wave infarct) encompasses the entire thickness of the ventricular wall.

    b. **Serum enzyme changes** (see Fig. 16-1). Creatinine phosphokinase (CPK) isoenzyme specific to cardiac muscle **(CPK-MB)** is released when damage occurs to the myocardium. This marker is thus a more specific indication of myocardial damage than the unfractionated CPK value. Amount of CPK-MB released correlates to size of the infarct.

III. Differential diagnosis

A. Angina. The two types of **thoracic pain** most difficult to differentiate from angina are musculoskeletal and gastrointestinal pain.

  1. Musculoskeletal. Costochondritis pain is often sharp in quality and usually persists for 1 or more hours; often worse at the end of day and

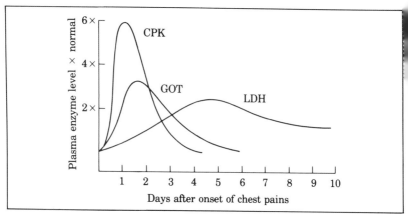

Fig. 16-1. Effect of myocardial infarction on serum enzyme levels. CPK = creatinine phosphokinase, GOT = glutonic oxaloacetic transaminase, LDH = lactate dehydrogenase.

relieved by positional changes or heat; localized (point) tenderness may be present on physical exam.

2. **Gastrointestinal.** Pain due to peptic ulcer disease, esophageal reflux, esophageal spasm, cholecyctitis, cholelithiasis, and pancreatitis. GI pain is not related to exertion, but may be related to anxiety; often related to meals; may last up to several hours; often relieved by bowel movement, antacid, and or positional change. GI pain may be relieved by nitroglycerin or calcium channel blockers (e.g., esophageal spasm) and may even be accompanied by ECG changes. Also, GI pain may precipitate anginal pain, or patient may have both GI disease and angina.

3. **Pulmonary.** Pain due to pulmonary embolism, pleurisy, pneumothorax, pneumonia with pleuritis, pulmonary hypertension.

4. **Cardiovascular.** Pain due to myocardial infarction, pericarditis, dissecting aortic aneurysm.

5. **Infectious.** Pain from herpes zoster.

6. **Psychological.** Anxiety-induced pain.

B. **Myocardial infarction.** Same differential diagnosis as angina.

See Tables 16-1 and 16-2 to differentiate among the many cardiac and noncardiac causes of chest pain.

IV. **Pathophysiology.** Angina pectoris and myocardial infarction are part of a continuum of responses resulting from myocardial oxygen demand exceeding oxygen supply.

A. **Myocardial oxygen supply** is a function of the ventricular diastolic perfusion pressure, the rate of coronary blood flow, and the oxygen-carrying capacity of the blood. Myocardial oxygen demand is a function of heart rate, ventricular wall tension, and the intrinsic contractility of the myocardium. Wall tension is proportional to left ventricular systolic blood pressure and left ventricular volume, and inversely proportional to left ventricular wall thickness. Exertion, the major cause of myocardial ischemia, increases all three determinants of myocardial oxygen demand. Due to coronary artery disease, this increase in oxygen demand cannot be met with an in-

Table 16-1. Cardiovascular causes of chest pain

Condition	Location	Quality	Duration	Aggravating or relieving factors	Associated symptoms or signs
Angina	Retrosternal region; radiates to or occasionally isolated to neck, jaw, epigastrium, shoulder or arms—left common	Pressure, burning, squeezing, heaviness, indigestion	<10 min	Aggravated by exercise, cold weather, or emotional stress, or occurs after meals; relieved by rest or nitroglycerin; atypical (Prinzmetal's) angina may be unrelated to activity and caused by coronary artery spasm	S_4, paradoxical split S_2, or murmur of papillary muscle dysfunction during pain
Rest or crescendo angina	Same as angina	Same as angina	>10 min	Same as angina, with gradually decreasing tolerance for exertion	Same as angina
Myocardial infarction	Substernal, and may radiate like angina	Heaviness, pressure, burning, constriction	Sudden onset, 30 min or longer but variable; usually goes away in hours	Unrelieved	Shortness of breath, sweating, weakness, nausea, vomiting, severe anxiety
Pericarditis	Usually begins over sternum or toward cardiac apex and may radiate to neck and down left upper extremity; often more localized than the pain of myocardial ischemia	Sharp, stabbing, knifelike	Lasts many hours to days	Aggravated by deep breathing, rotating chest, or supine position; relieved by sitting up and leaning forward	Pericardial friction rub, cardiac tamponade, pulsus paradoxus
Dissecting aortic aneurysm	Anterior chest; radiates to thoracic area of back; may be abdominal; pain may move as dissection progresses	Excruciating, tearing, knifelike	Sudden onset, lasts for hours	Unrelated to anything	Lower blood pressure in one arm, absent pulses, paralysis, murmur of aortic insufficiency, pulsus paradoxus, MI

Reproduced with permission from T. E. Andreoli et al. [2].

Table 16-2. Noncardiac causes of chest pain

Condition	Location	Quality	Duration	Aggravating or relieving factors	Associated symptoms or signs
Pulmonary embolism (chest pain often not present)	Substernal or over region of pulmonary infarction	Pleuritic (with pulmonary infarction) or anginalike	Sudden onset; minutes to < hour	May be aggravated by breathing	Dyspnea, tachypnea, tachycardia, hypotension; signs of acute right heart failure and pulmonary hypertension with large emboli; rales, pleural rub, hemoptysis with pulmonary infarction; clinically present in minority of cases
Pulmonary hypertension	Substernal	Pressure; oppressive		Aggravated by effort	Pain usually associated with dyspnea; signs of pulmonary hypertension

Pneumonia with pleurisy	Localized over area of consolidation	Pleuritic, well localized		Painful breathing	Dyspnea, cough, fever, dull to percussion, bronchial breath sounds, rales, occasional pleural rub
Spontaneous pneumothorax	Unilateral	Sharp, well localized	Sudden onset, lasts many hours	Painful breathing	Dyspnea, hyperresonance and decreased breath and voice sounds over involved lung
Musculoskeletal disorders	Variable	Aching	Short or long duration	Aggravated by movement; history of muscle exertion	Tender to pressure or movement
Herpes zoster	Dermatomal in distribution		Prolonged	None	Rash appears in area of discomfort
Gastrointestinal disorders (e.g., esophageal reflux, peptic ulcer, cholecystitis)	Lower substernal area, epigastric, right or left upper quadrant	Burning, coliclike, aching		Precipitated by recumbency or meals	Nausea, regurgitation, food intolerance, melena, hematemesis, jaundice
Anxiety states	Often localized to a point	Sharp burning, commonly location of pain moves from place to place	Varies; usually very brief	Situational anger— very brief	Sighing respirations, often chest wall tenderness

Reproduced with permission from T. E. Andreoli et al. [2].

crease in oxygen supply, an imbalance occurs, and myocardial ischemia results.

B. In addition to coronary artery disease, other conditions may result in an imbalance between myocardial oxygen supply and demand and result in ischemia. Decreased myocardial oxygen supply can result from decreased aortic perfusion pressure, due to hypotension or aortic **regurgitation,** or a decrease in the blood's oxygen-carrying capacity, due to **anemia or hypoxemia.** An increase in myocardial oxygen demand that can result in ischemia is **aortic stenosis.**

C. In general, **stable** and **unstable** angina are caused by a fixed coronary artery obstruction secondary to atherosclerosis, where **Prinzmetal**'s angina is caused by coronary artery spasm, with or without superimposed coronary artery disease. **Myocardial infarction** is most often the result of coronary artery disease (85 percent of cases). It may also result from coronary artery spasm, due to cocaine use, congenital abnormalities of coronary circulation, periarteritis and other coronary artery inflammatory diseases, or coronary embolism.

Congestive Heart Failure

I. Definition. A clinical syndrome that results from the inability of the heart to achieve cardiac output capable of supplying sufficient oxygen to the metabolizing tissues. Congestive heart failure (CHF) may be further divided into **right ventricular failure, left ventricular failure,** and **biventricular failure.**

II. Clinical manifestations, listed in order of decreasing specificity for each type of heart failure:

A. Right ventricular failure

1. Jugular venous distention.
2. Hepatomegaly.
3. Increased prothrombin time.
4. Peripheral edema.
5. Increased serum glutamic oxaloacetic transaminase (SGOT) or aspartate aminotransferase (AST).
6. Increased bilirubin.
7. Pleural effusion.
8. Decreased albumin.
9. Abdominal discomfort.
10. Anorexia.
11. Proteinuria.

B. Left ventricular failure

1. Chest x-ray with redistribution of perfusion or interstitial edema.
2. Third heart sound (S_3).
3. Cardiomegaly.
4. Pulmonary rales.
5. Paroxysmal nocturnal dyspnea (PND), orthopnea.
6. Dyspnea on exertion.

III. Differential diagnosis

A. Right ventricular failure

   1. Pulmonary embolus.

   2. Tricuspid stenosis.

   3. Tricuspid regurgitation.

   4. Right atrial tumor.

   5. Cardiac tamponade.

   6. Constrictive pericarditis.

   7. Pulmonic insufficiency.

   8. Right ventricular infarction.

   9. Intrinsic lung disease.

   10. Epstein's anomaly.

   11. High cardiac output states: anemia systemic fistulae, beriberi, Paget's disease, carcinoid, thyrotoxicosis.

B. Left or biventricular failure

   1. Aortic stenosis.

   2. Aortic insufficiency.

   3. Mitral stenosis.

   4. Mitral regurgitation.

   5. Most cardiomyopathies.

   6. Restrictive cardiomyopathy.

   7. Myocardial infarction.

   8. Myxoma.

   9. Hypertensive heart disease.

   10. Myocarditis.

   11. Supraventricular arrhythmias.

   12. Left ventricular aneurysm.

   13. Cardiac shunts.

   14. High cardiac output states.

IV. Pathophysiology. The etiologies of CHF can be divided into six general categories that have distinct pathophysiologic mechanisms. For each general category, its pathophysiology, most common etiologies, and clinical manifestations are listed. Note that cardiomyopathies, valvular heart disease, systemic hypertension, and pericardial disease are the subjects of further discussion in this chapter.

A. Cardiomyopathies

   1. **Pathophysiology.** ↓ Myocardial contractile function (most cardiomyopathies), or ↓ diastolic filling secondary to ↓ ventricular compliance (e.g., infiltrative processes); results in left or biventricular failure.

   2. **Most common etiologies.** Hypertrophic cardiomyopathy, dilated cardiomyopathy, restrictive cardiomyopathy.

3. **Clinical manifestations.** Dilated versus hypertrophic cardiomyopathies on physical exam. Evidence of systemic disease (e.g., sarcoid, hemochromatosis, connective tissue disease, amyloidosis).

4. **Diagnostic tests.** Echocardiography, radionuclide ventriculography (RVG), cardiac catheterization, myocardial biopsy.

B. **Valvular heart disease**

1. **Pathophysiology.** ↑ Cardiac work load (secondary to ↑ volume or pressure work) results in left or biventricular failure.

2. **Most common etiologies.** Aortic stenosis, aortic insufficiency, mitral regurgitation, mitral stenosis.

3. **Clinical manifestations.**

   a. Presence of significant murmur(s) on physical exam.

   b. Specific cardiovascular exam findings.

   c. Echocardiography and cardiac catheterization.

C. **Systemic hypertension (HTN)**

1. **Pathophysiology.** ↑ Cardiac work load (secondary to ↑ afterload) results in left or biventricular failure.

2. **Most common etiologies.** Essential HTN.

3. **Clinical manifestations.** ↑ Blood pressure and systemic signs of HTN disease (e.g., fundoscopic, renal changes).

D. **Pericardial disease**

1. **Pathophysiology.** ↓ Diastolic ventricular filling (causes a fixed restriction in cardiac output); results in right ventricular failure.

2. **Most common etiologies.** Viral, traumatic, radiation-induced, tuberculosis- or uremia-associated constrictive disease.

3. **Clinical manifestations.** Constrictive pericarditis: signs of right heart failure (RHF)—edema, ascites ↑ venous pressure, hepatomegaly; signs of small quiet heart.

4. **Diagnostic tests**

   a. Echocardiography, cardiac catheterization, characteristic pressure tracings.

   b. CXR may show triangle-shaped heart and calcium in pericardium.

E. **Pulmonary arterial hypertension**

1. **Pathophysiology.** ↑ Cardiac work load secondary to ↑ pulmonary (right-sided) resistance; results in right ventricular failure.

2. **Most common etiologies.** Primary pulmonary hypertension, pulmonary embolism (acute or chronic), left heart disease (↑ pulmonary venous pressure), parenchymal lung disease (e.g., COPD).

3. **Clinical manifestations.** Signs of right ventricular (RV) overload and ↑ pulmonary pressures, parasternal lift, prominent jugular venous pressure (JVP) *a* wave and *v* wave if tricuspid regurgitation (TR), ↑ intensity P_2; murmurs of pulmonic insufficiency (PI) or TR, peripheral signs of RHF (hepatomegaly, edema, pulsatile liver if TR present).

4. **Diagnostic tests.** Echocardiography, RVG; right-sided and pulmonary artery catheterization.

F. High output states

    1. Pathophysiology. ↑ Workload (secondary to ↑ metabolic demands).

    2. Most common etiologies. Thyrotoxicosis, anemia, arteriovenous (AV) fistula.

    3. Clinical manifestations. Search for systemic disease, such as:

        a. Thyrotoxicosis: hyperactive heart, wide pulse pressure, atrial fibrillation.

        b. Anemia: rapid pulse, hyperactive heart, signs of peripheral vasodilatation.

        c. AV fistula: history of prior surgery, presence of continuous bruit in abnormal location.

V. Exacerbations of CHF. Patients with well-controlled chronic CHF can experience sudden exacerbations due to some slight change in the baseline compensated state of the patient. This generally occurs secondary to:

A. ↓ **Myocardial function**

    1. Poor medication compliance: ↓ digoxin.

    2. Alcohol.

    3. New-onset arrhythmia.

    4. Myocardial ischemia, myocardial infarction, or both.

B. ↑ **Cardiac work load**

    1. ↑ Salt intake.

    2. Poor medication compliance: ↓ Lasix results in fluid overload.

    3. ↑ Activity.

    4. Infection, fever.

    5. Pulmonary embolism.

    6. Anemia.

    7. Pregnancy.

    8. Thyrotoxicosis.

    9. Acute or chronic renal failure.

Cardiomyopathies

I. Definition. Disease in which the clinical presentation is due to dysfunction of the myocardium, as a result of a process that primarily affects the myocardial tissue. Classically, myocardial changes due to systemic or pulmonary hypertension, ischemic heart disease, and valvular disease are **excluded** from this group of myocardial disorders. There are three types of cardiomyopathy: **dilated cardiomyopathy, hypertrophic cardiomyopathy,** and **restrictive cardiomyopathy.**

    A. Dilated cardiomyopathy is characterized by ventricular dilatation with decreased systolic contractile function.

    B. Hypertrophic cardiomyopathy is characterized by thickened hypercontractile ventricles.

    C. Restrictive cardiomyopathy is characterized by an abnormally stiff myocardium with impaired ventricular relaxation and filling but preserved contractile function.

II. Clinical manifestations. Table 16-3 compares the clinical manifestations of the three types of cardiomyopathy.

III. Differential diagnosis

  A. Dilated cardiomyopathy: congestive or hypodynamic

    1. Idiopathic

    2. Inflammatory

      a. Infectious: postviral myocarditis (Coxsackie B or echovirus).

      b. Noninfectious: collagen vascular disease (systemic lupus erythematosis [SLE], rheumatoid arthritis, polyarteritis), peripartum, sarcoidosis.

    3. Toxin-induced. Alcohol, chemotherapeutic agents (doxorubicin and Adriamycin), drugs (cocaine, heroin, organic solvents—"glue sniffer's heart").

    4. Metabolic. Hypothyroidism and chronic hypocalcemia or hypophosphatemia.

  B. Hypertrophic cardiomyopathy. Familial (autosomal dominant trait).

  C. Restrictive cardiomyopathy

    1. Myocardial fibrosis, scarring, or infiltration.

      a. Infiltrative disorders: amyloidosis, sarcoidosis.

      b. Noninfiltrative: idiopathic, scleroderma.

      c. Storage diseases: glycogen storage disease, hemochromatosis.

    2. Endomyocardial fibrosis, scarring, or infiltration

      a. Endomyocardial fibrosis.

      b. Hypereosinophilic syndrome.

      c. Metastatic tumors.

      d. Radiation therapy.

    3. Restrictive cardiomyopathy **shares almost identical symptoms, physical signs, and hemodynamic profiles with constrictive pericarditis.** It is imperative to distinguish between these two entities, because constrictive pericarditis is curable whereas restrictive cardiomyopathy is not. Diagnosis is made by a computed tomography (CT) scan or magnetic resonance imaging (MRI) of the mediastinum. Constrictive pericarditis has a thickened pericardium, while restrictive cardiomyopathy does not.

IV. Pathophysiology

  A. Dilated (congestive) cardiomyopathy. The hallmark is biventricular dilatation with decreased contractile function.

    1. When ventricular stroke volume falls because of impaired myocyte contractility, two compensatory mechanisms activate:

      a. There is an increase in heart rate, mediated by sympathetic tone.

      b. Because of the decreased stroke volume, the ventricular diastolic volume increases and further stretches the myofibrils to increase their stroke work (Starling's principle).

Table 16-3. Clinical manifestations of cardiomyopathies

	Dilated cardiomyopathy	Hypertrophic cardiomyopathy	Restrictive cardiomyopathy
History	History of viral illness, recent pregnancy, alcoholism, collagen vascular disorder, exposure to toxins, recent mediastinal radiation, nutritional history, drug history, dyspnea on exertion, orthopnea, paroxysmal nocturnal dyspnea, peripheral edema, symptoms of pulmonary and systemic venous congestion (biventricular CHF), palpitations	Family history of sudden death due to heart disease, angina (decreased in the recumbent position), dyspnea, syncope (usually seen with exercise), palpitations	Dyspnea on exertion, orthopnea, fatigue or weakness (due to low cardiac output)
Physical exam	Pulmonary rales, hepatomegaly, peripheral edema, sinus tachycardia, pulsus alternans, diffuse PMI, S_3, S_4, MR murmur, prominent v wave with JVP and jugular venous distention	Left ventricular heave, bisferiens carotid pulse ("spike and dome" morphology), paradoxical splitting of S_2 if left ventricular obstruction is present, bifid-trifid apical impulse, systolic ejection murmur at left sternal border or apex that increases with Valsalva's maneuver and decreases with squatting, S_4	Edema, ascites, hepatomegaly, distended neck veins
Diagnostic tests	Atrial arrhythmias (AE, premature atrial contractions), ventricular arrhythmias (premature ventricular contractions), left ventricular hypertrophy with nonspecific S-T–T wave changes, right or left BBB (or both)	Left ventricular hypertrophy with strain pattern, abnormal Q waves may be seen in anterolateral and inferior leads, Wolff-Parkinson-White syndrome	Atrial and ventricular arrhythmias, nonspecific S-T–T wave changes
Chest x-ray	Cardiomegaly (may be massive), interstitial pulmonary edema	Normal, or signs of left ventricular hypertrophy	Moderate cardiomegaly, evidence of CHF (pulmonary vascular congestion and pleural effusions)
ECG	Large, poorly contractile LV	Asymmetric ventricular hypertrophy (general left ventricular hypertrophy with even greater septal hypertrophy)	Normal-size, poorly relaxing and filling LV (due to high diastolic pressures)

2. These compensations may render the patient asymptomatic during the early stages of ventricular dysfunction, but progressive myocyte degeneration and volume overload occur, and clinical symptoms of heart failure soon follow. As cardiac output falls, a decline in renal blood flow activates the renin-angiotensin system, resulting in an **increase in peripheral vascular resistance and intravascular volume.** These compensatory effects are detrimental for two reasons:

   a. The increased resistance makes it more difficult for the left ventricle to eject blood.

   b. The rise in intravascular volume burdens the dilated ventricles further.

3. As the ventricles enlarge over time, the mitral and tricuspid valves fail to coapt adequately in systole, and **valvular regurgitation** ensues. Such regurgitation has two detrimental effects:

   a. Volume and pressure loads are placed on the atria, causing them to dilate and often leading to atrial fibrillation.

   b. Regurgitation of blood into the left atrium further decreases stroke volume and thereby cardiac output into the systemic circulation.

B. **Hypertrophic cardiomyopathy.** There is marked hypertrophy of the myocardium and a disproportionately greater thickening of the interventricular septum than that of the free wall of the ventricle: asymmetric septal hypertrophy (ASH). During midsystole the apposition of the anterior mitral leaflet against the hypertrophied septum can cause a narrowing of the subaortic area and result in left ventricular outflow obstruction. Because of this, the disease has been termed idiopathic hypertrophic subaortic stenosis (IHSS) or hypertrophic obstructive cardiomyopathy (HOCM).

C. **Restrictive cardiomyopathies.** These are less common than dilated cardiomyopathy and hypertrophic cardiomyopathy. They are characterized by abnormally rigid ventricles that impair diastolic filling but retain normal size and normal systolic function. Reduced ventricular compliance, due to fibrosis or infiltration, results in abnormally high diastolic pressure, which has two consequences: elevated systemic and pulmonary venous pressures, with signs of right- and left-sided vascular congestion, and reduced ventricular cavity size with decreased stroke volume and cardiac output.

Mitral Valve Disease

I. **Definition.** Alterations in the integrity or normal functioning of the mitral valve or its associated structures that lead to alterations in normal cardiovascular physiology. The two most common pathologies of the mitral valve are **mitral stenosis** and **mitral regurgitation.**

II. **Clinical manifestations.** Table 16-4 compares some common features of mitral stenosis and mitral regurgitation. Unless otherwise stated, mitral regurgitation refers to the **chronic** lesion.

III. **Differential diagnosis and pathophysiology**

A. **Mitral stenosis** results from rheumatic heart disease (RHD). Fifty percent of those with mitral stenosis will have a history of rheumatic fever.

B. **Mitral regurgitation** can result from RHD, mitral prolapse, or ruptured chordae tendinae or papillary muscle dysfunction post-MI.

Table 16-4. Common features of mitral stenosis and mitral regurgitation

	Mitral stenosis	Mitral regurgitation
History	Dyspnea on exertion, pulmonary edema, hemoptysis, fatigue, reactive pulmonary hypertension, right heart failure	In *chronic* mitral regurgitation, fatigue, dypnea on exertion appear gradually; if *acute*, sudden onset of CHF symptoms
Heart sounds	Loud S_1; opening snap	Diminished S_1; S_3 due to volume
Murmurs	Localized near apex; onset at opening snap (middiastolic) of a low-pitched decresendo murmur; presystolic accentuation of murmur if normal sinus rhythm present	Loudest over PMI; holosystolic; blowing; radiates to axilla
Chest x-ray	Straight left heart border; large LA, RV; mitral valve calcification; Kerley's B lines; prominent upper lung field vasculature	LV and LA enlarged; minimal pulmonary congestion if chronic
ECG	Broad, notched P waves; axis normal or right axis deviation (RAD); AF common	Left atrial dilatation; tall P waves, sometimes notched; AF common

Aortic Valve Disease

I. **Definition.** Alterations in the integrity or normal functioning of the aortic valve or aortic infravalvular or supravalvular structures that lead to alterations in the normal physiology of the cardiovascular system. The two most common pathologies of the aortic valve are **aortic stenosis** and **aortic regurgitation.**

II. **Clinical manifestations**

   A. **History**

   1. **Aortic stenosis.** CHF, angina, and syncope, are the three main symptoms; presence of **any one** indicates need for surgical therapy.

   2. **Aortic regurgitation.** CHF or angina late in course; may be asymptomatic or have subtle decreases in exercise tolerance over long period of time.

   B. **Physical exam and diagnostic tests.** Findings in aortic stenosis and aortic regurgitation are compared in Table 16-5.

III. **Differential diagnosis and pathophysiology**

   A. **Aortic stenosis** results from congenital lesions, such as bicuspid aortic valve, rheumatic heart disease, and calcific aortic stenosis.

   B. **Aortic regurgitation** results from rheumatic heart disease, endocarditis, valvular congenital structural defects, dissecting aneurysms, syphilis, inflammatory diseases, and subvalvular structural disease.

Table 16-5. Physical exam and diagnostic test findings in aortic stenosis and aortic regurgitation

	Aortic stenosis	Aortic regurgitation
Heart sounds	A_2 normal or decreased in calcific AS (may be increased in congenital AS); S_4	A_2 normal or decreased; S_4
Murmurs	Diamond-shaped systolic ejection murmur at right second intercostal space parasternally or at apex	Decrescendo diastolic murmur begins after A_2 and ends before S_1; located at left sternal border in third to fourth intercostal space
Pulse wave	Carotid pulse with gradual upstroke and prolonged downstroke (pulsus tardus and parvus)	Dictrotic pulse (pulsus bisferiens), bounding pulse (water-hammer pulse), Duroziez's sign
Chest x-ray	± Left ventricular hypertrophy, prominent ascending aorta, calcified valve	Dilated LV
ECG	Left ventricular hypertrophy	Left ventricular hypertrophy, left axis deviation (LAD)

Systemic Hypertension

I. **Definitions.** The definition of HTN is arbitrary but is at present based on studies defining the relationship between systolic and diastolic pressures and cardiovascular morbidity and mortality rates.

   A. Using the **blood pressure (BP) levels** obtained from these studies, hypertensive patients may be diagnosed as:

      1. Women at any age: BP > 160/95.

      2. Men older than 45: BP > 140/95.

      3. Men younger than 45: BP > 130/90.

      It is worth pointing out that a clear impact on cardiovascular mortality by blood pressure control has been demonstrated principally in patients with initial diastolic pressures > 105 mm Hg.

   B. **Malignant** HTN is defined as elevated pressures (usually in the > 200/140 range) with evidence of papilledema.

   C. Remember that 97–98 percent of HTN is **essential** (idiopathic).

II. **Clinical manifestations.** Findings associated with hypertension vary; the degree of symptomatology and physical exam evidence of HTN is roughly correlated with the degree of blood pressure elevation.

   A. **History**

      1. Essential hypertension is asymptomatic until complications develop.

2. With **increasing pressures,** cardiovascular dysfunction may become apparent as orthopnea, dyspnea, anginal symptoms, and even frank pulmonary edema. Ocular fatigue, decreased visual acuity, visual blurring, and occipital headaches may all be present.

3. With **high pressures,** severe headaches may develop, with associated visual impairment, drowsiness, and even encephalopathic changes. Transient paresthesias and cerebrovascular accidents tend to occur with higher pressures.

B. Physical exam. Classical findings are described for the cardiovascular, visual (retinal), and neurologic systems.

1. **Cardiovascular** findings are due to left ventricular hypertrophy, which results from increased afterload. Possible findings include a left ventricular heave, sustained apex beat, and fourth heart sound (S_4). As the hypertrophy worsens, murmurs of aortic insufficiency (AI), mitral regurgitation (MR), or both, as well as signs of left ventricular failure (e.g., S_3, pulsus alternans) may occur.

2. **Retinal** changes follow a progression based on the severity and duration of the elevation in blood pressure.

    a. **Earlier retinal changes** consist of vascular changes: constriction of retinal arterioles and arteriovenous nicking.

    b. With **higher blood pressures,** in addition to vascular changes, there are flame-shaped hemorrhages and exudates.

    c. **Papilledema,** the most severe retinal change, defines malignant hypertension.

3. **Neurologic** changes include transient weakness or numbness, paresthesias, and an increasing incidence of cerebrovascular accidents: cerebral thrombotic or hemorrhagic events.

4. **Hypertensive encephalopathy** occurs with very high blood pressures and is characterized by transient, focal central nervous system deficits, severe headache, visual disturbances, and even convulsions, stupor, and coma.

C. Diagnostic tests

1. **Urinalysis** may reveal proteinuria; hematuria can occur, usually with higher pressures.

2. **Chemistries** may show evidence of renal disease, with increased BUN and creatinine values.

3. **ECG** may show increased voltage consistent with left ventricular hypertrophy, as well as "strain" patterns of T wave flattening or inversion, especially in lateral leads (V4-V6).

4. **CXR** may show cardiomegaly, with left ventricular prominence. Dilatation or tortuosity of the ascending aorta may be a prominent feature as well.

III. Differential diagnosis. Table 16-6 lists the causes of secondary hypertension and their major clinical manifestations.

IV. Pathophysiology. The cause of essential HTN is unknown, and complications are due to tissue changes that result from prolonged exposure to a hypertensive vascular system. Table 16-7 lists the multisystem complications of hypertension.

Table 16-6. Secondary causes of hypertension

Cause	Symptoms/signs	Associations	Confirmation
Renovascular	Flank bruit, diffuse atherosclerosis	↓ K⁺, ↑ creatinine	Arteriogram, ↑ renal vein, renin level
Renal disease	Edema	Acute/chronic renal disease	↑ Creatinine, ↑ BUN
Pheochromocytoma	Paroxysmal sweating, palpitations, flushing, headache, weight loss, episodic hypertension, tachycardia, orthostatic hypotension	↑ Urine VMA, metanephrines, catecholamines	CT scan, arteriography
Mineralocorticoid excess	Weakness, muscle cramps	Hypokalemia, alkalosis, ↓ renin	↑ Aldosterone level, CT scan
Aortic coarctation	↑ BP in arm, ↓ BP in legs	Rib notching on CXR	Arteriography

VMA = vanillyl mandelic acid.
Reproduced with permission from T. E. Andreoli et al. [2].

Table 16-7. Hypertensive complications

Target organ	Hypertensive	Atherosclerotic
Brain/eye	Intracerebral hemorrhage; lacunar infarcts; encephalopathy; fundal hemorrhages, exudates, papilledema	Thrombotic stroke, TIA
Heart	Congestive failure, ventricular hypertrophy	MI, angina
Kidney	Nephrosclerosis	Renal artery stenosis
Vessels	Aortic dissection	Diffuse atheromata

Reproduced with permission from T. E. Andreoli et al. [2].

Pericardial Disease

I. **Definition.** Cardiovascular dysfunction due to acute or chronic changes involving the pericardium, either from a primary disease process or as a manifestation of systemic illness. There are two types of pericarditis: **acute** and **chronic.**

II. **Clinical manifestations.** Table 16-8 lists pertinent findings on history, physical exam, and diagnostic tests that differentiate acute and chronic pericarditis.

III. **Differential diagnosis**

   A. **Acute pericarditis**

   1. Idiopathic (possibly postviral).

   2. Infectious: viral (Coxsackie B), bacterial, tuberculous, fungal, amebic, protozoan).

   3. Collagen-vascular disease (SLE, rheumatoid arthritis, scleroderma).

   4. Postmediastinal radiation.

   5. Uremia.

   6. Post-MI.

   7. Postpericardiotomy.

   8. Rheumatic fever.

   9. Trauma

   B. **Chronic (constrictive) pericarditis**

   1. Idiopathic.

   2. Occasionally, history of acute pericarditis.

IV. **Pathophysiology.** The clinical manifestations of acute pericarditis are due to inflammation of the pericardium, while the clinical manifestations of chronic pericarditis are due to constriction of the pericardium around the myocardium. Since the right ventricle experiences lower pressures than the left ventricle, it is primarily affected by the constricted pericardium, and so the symptoms seen in chronic pericarditis are right-sided symptoms. The right ventricle cannot fill to its normal capacity due to the constriction, and as a result there is venous congestion, reduction of preload, and reduction of output.

Table 16-8. Differentiating features of acute and chronic pericarditis

	Acute pericarditis	Chronic (constrictive) pericarditis
History	Antecedent upper respiratory infection; dyspnea; sharp, substernal chest pain, often with left supraclavicular radiation; ↑ pain in supine position; ↓ pain when sitting, leaning forward; malaise, constitutional symptoms, myalgias	Exertional dyspnea
Physical exam	Fever, pericardial friction rub ± pericardial effusion, muffled heart sounds, cyanosis, pulsus paradoxus	Jugular venous distension (Kussmaul's sign), edema of the legs, hepatomegaly, ascites, pulsus paradoxus, pleural effusions, cyanosis, prominent JVP *a* wave and rapid *y* wave descent, pericardial knock in early diastole
Lab tests	Mild to moderate leukocytosis, ↑ ESR	↓ Serum albumin, lymphopenia
ECG	S-T segment elevation with decreased QRS voltage and T wave flattening; supraventricular arrhythmias (e.g., PACs, PAT, AF or flutter)	Low voltage in QRS complex, notched P wave, AF, flattened or inverted T waves in leads I and II
Chest x-ray	± Enlarged cardiac silhouette	Small heart, ± calcium in pericardium, irregular or triangle-shaped heart, dilated SVC
ECG	Effusion ± pericardial thickening	Pericardial thickening, small ventricular chamber size, enlarged atrial chamber size

PACs = paroxysmal atrial contraction, PAT = paroxysmal atrial tachycardia.

Peripheral Vascular Disease

I. **Definition.** Acute or chronic changes in the arterial or venous vasculature that lead to compromise of blood circulation in a given extremity. There are two types of arterial peripheral vascular disease, **acute** and **chronic,** as well as two types of venous peripheral vascular disease, acute and chronic.

II. **Clinical manifestations**

A. **Arterial disease.** The common clinical manifestations of acute and chronic arterial vascular disease are as follows. To diagnose acute arterial disease look for the **five P's: pain, paresthesias, polar, pallor,** and **pulselessness.**

1. **History**

a. **Acute arterial disease.** Sudden onset, pain, paresthesias, numbness. **Risk factors** for mural thrombi include AF, arrhythmias post recent MI, chronic CHF, cardiomyopathy, history of endocarditis.

b. **Chronic arterial disease.** Intermittent claudication; results in muscle ischemia and focal necrosis, causing chronic pain at rest, ± paresthesias. **Risk factors** for arterial compromise include diabetes mellitus, cigarette smoking, hypertension, obesity, hyperlipidemia.

2. **Physical exam**

   a. **Acute arterial disease.** Pale extremity, pulselessness, ↓ temperature distal to occlusion.

   b. **Chronic arterial disease.** ↓ Or absent peripheral pulse(s), ↓ temperature distal to occlusion, bruit(s) over involved area.

      (1) **Feet.** Pallor on elevation; delayed capillary blush on lowering to dependent position; rubor on dependency.

      (2) **Trophic skin changes.** ↓ Hair or nail growth, or both.

      (3) **Ulcers.** Inferior to malleoli; toes most common site.

3. **Diagnostic tests.** Arterial angiography for both acute and chronic arterial disease.

B. **Venous disease.** The common clinical manifestations of acute and chronic venous disease are compared in Table 16-9.

III. **Differential diagnosis.** Symptomatically related syndromes include:

A. **Raynaud's disease.** Symptom complex of pain and pallor in fingers, toes, or both, following exposure to cold or emotional upset.

B. **Raynaud's phenomenon.** Symptom complex of Raynaud's disease, found in association with systemic disease (e.g., collagen vascular diseases).

C. **Leriche's syndrome.** Impotence and bilateral buttock and thigh pain due to aortoiliac atherosclerotic disease.

D. **Thromboangiitis obliterans.** Vascular disease characterized by occlusion of small to medium arteries below the elbow and knee, which may lead to necrosis of the digits of hands and feet. Most commonly seen in young Jewish males who are heavy smokers. Thrombophlebitis often coexists.

Table 16-9. Clinical manifestations of acute and chronic venous disease.

	Acute venous disease	Chronic venous disease
History	Thrombophlebitis may be asymptomatic; pain: aching, tenderness over muscles; conditions leading to venous stasis: post-MI, postoperative period, hemiplegia, hypercoagulable states (e.g., polycythemia vera)	Aching pain after standing or sitting, pregnancy, ascites, abdominal tumor, excessive weight or height
Physical exam	Superficial venous distension, swelling, edema, cyanosis, measurable difference in calf circumference	Thickened, discolored (brown) overlying skin, secondary varicosities, pruritis, ulcers anterior and superior to lateral malleoli
Diagnostic tests	Noninvasive: impedance plethysmography, real-time (duplex) ultrasonography, invasive: contrast venography	Noninvasive (same as for acute venous disease) for documentation purposes only

IV. Pathophysiology

A. Acute arterial disease is the result of inadequate distal oxygenation secondary to occlusion by embolus (90 percent originates from mural thrombus in heart). **Chronic arterial disease** is the result of inadequate distal oxygenation secondary to arterial lumen stenosis caused by atherosclerotic plaques.

1. **Common sites** for acute arterial disease include narrowed areas and bifurcations: femoral artery (profunda femoris junction), aortoiliac junction. Common sites for chronic arterial disease include superficial femoral and popliteal in vast majority of patients, as well as the aortoiliac junction.

B. Acute venous disease results from impaired venous return secondary to **thrombophlebitis** mostly, but also external venous compression and trauma. **Chronic venous disease** results from impaired venous return secondary to thrombotic disruption of venous vessels and valves.

1. **Common sites** for both acute and chronic venous disease include deep and superficial veins of lower extremities.

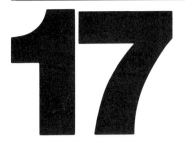

Gastrointestinal Diseases

Peptic Ulcer Disease

I. **Definition.** An ulcer found in the esophagus, stomach, or duodenum, caused directly or indirectly by gastric secretions.

II. **Clinical manifestations** (See Table 17-1.)

A. **History.** Epigastric pain, typically described as burning, aching, or gnawing.

1. **Duodenal ulcers** (DU) are typically felt when the stomach is empty, such as early in the morning or before meals, and frequently pain or discomfort awakens patients a few hours after they have gone to sleep. Usually relieved by eating.

2. **Gastric ulcers** may present similarly to duodenal ulcers, or may lack any specific pattern of pain. In some cases, pain is exacerbated or caused by eating.

B. **Physical exam.** Epigastric tenderness.

C. **Diagnostic tests**

1. Sometimes positive stool guaiac.

2. **Upper gastrointestinal (GI) series** may show ulcer craters or gastritis, with increased folds, esophagitis.

III. **Differential diagnosis.** Peptic ulcer disease (PUD) must be distinguished from gastritis, pancreatitis, diverticulitis, appendicitis, inflammatory bowel disease, and gastric carcinoma. Diagnosis is made on basis of Hx, endoscopy, x-rays, secretory study, biopsy, cytology.

IV. **Pathophysiology**

A. Pathogenesis unclear; leading theories involve both **gastric hypersecretion** and **mucosal breakdown.** Duodenal ulcer disease may be quite different from gastric ulcer disease.

B. Duodenal ulcer patients, as a group, secrete twice the acid that healthy patients do, but there is a large overlap between the two groups.

C. Mucosal junctions (esophagus-stomach, pylorum-duodenum, fundus-antrum) are the most commonly affected sites.

D. Pain may be result of nerve irritation by acid, or of increased tone in duodenum and antrum.

E. **Zollinger-Ellison syndrome.** Gastric hypersecretion associated with gastrin-secreting islet tumors of the pancreas.

F. **Complications.** Hemorrhage, perforation, penetration into adjacent organs, pyloric obstruction, gastric malignancy, chronic pain.

Table 17-1. Gastric versus duodenal ulcers

	Gastric ulcer	Duodenal ulcer
Usual site	Lesser curvature	Duodenal bulb
Male-female ratio	1:1	4:1
Pain	After meals	Relieved by meals
Pathology	May be malignant	Rarely malignant
Gastric acid	Low or normal	Hypersecretion
Vomiting	Common	Uncommon

Cholecystitis

I. **Definition.** Inflammation of the gallbladder, usually secondary to obstruction of cystic duct by a calculus.

II. **Clinical manifestations**

A. Gallstones present in 15 percent of Americans age 55–65. Predominance in Native Americans, patients with regional enteritis, diabetes mellitus. Male-female ratio 1:2.

B. **History.** Onset of classic attack often follows meal of fried or fatty foods. Steady, sometimes severe pain in epigastrium may be accompanied by nausea, vomiting, jaundice, fever. Pain may radiate to infrascapular area and subside spontaneously after 12–18 hours.

C. **Physical exam.** Right upper quadrant abdominal tenderness is frequently found, as is **Murphy's sign** (inspiratory arrest on palpation of right upper quadrant).

D. **Diagnostic tests**

1. ↑ WBC, ↑ serum bilirubin (1–4 mg/dl).

2. **Radiologic studies**

a. Plain film **x-ray** is sometimes useful, though only 10–15 percent of gallstones are radiopaque.

b. **Ultrasound** has replaced oral and IV **cholecystography** as the primary diagnostic test in cholecystitis. Enlargement of the gallbladder, dilatation of the biliary tree, and thickening of the gallbladder wall all indicate the presence of stones.

c. **HIDA** scans are the best test to use in acute cholecystitis, and are positive when the radiolabeled dye enters the common duct but not the gallbladder.

d. **Transhepatic cholangiography** or **fiberoptic endoscopy** may be used for direct visualization of the biliary tree if the preceding tests are inconclusive.

III. **Differential diagnosis.** Pancreatitis, perforated peptic ulcer, appendicitis, carcinoma, and hepatitis must be ruled out.

IV. **Pathophysiology**

A. **Cholesterol stones** are composed of cholesterol, phospholipids, conjugated bile salts. Bile salts in water form micelles, which solubilize cholesterol and phospholipids, so stone formation depends on relative proportion of all three constituents. In the United States, they account for 75 percent of stones.

B. Stages of cholesterol gallstone formation

1. **Chemical stage.** Secretion of bile supersaturated with cholesterol occurs during fasting.

2. **Crystallization stage.** Precipitation and crystallization in gallbladder.

3. **Growth stage.** Coalescence of microscopic stones into macroscopic stones.

C. Pigment stones (<10 percent cholesterol) account for 20 percent of cases in U.S. and contain mostly calcium bilirubinate and unconjugated bilirubin.

D. Choledocholithiasis (common bile duct stone) develops in over 15 percent of cholelithiasis patients. **Charcot's triad** (pain, fever, jaundice) is characteristic of an acutely obstructed duct.

Gastrointestinal Bleed

I. Definition. Acute or chronic blood loss from any point in the GI tract.

II. Clinical manifestations

A. History. Key points to elicit are site of bleeding, amount of bleeding, and duration. Ask about alcohol use, drugs (e.g., aspirin), ulcer disease, family or personal history of cancer.

B. Physical exam. Check for symptoms of shock (tachycardia, hypotension, clammy skin), tenderness or other findings on abdominal exam, blood on rectal exam. Also look for stigmata of cirrhosis and signs of other bleeding problems (e.g., other bruises). Symptoms (Sx) of shock indicate loss of 20–30 percent of total blood volume if present when patient upright; 50 percent loss if present while patient recumbent.

C. Diagnostic tests

1. The approximate extent of blood loss can be gauged by checking **blood pressure, BUN, and hemoglobin.** Systolic BP <100, hemoglobin <11 g/dl, and BUN >40 mg/dl suggest a loss of more than 1 liter of blood. Low hematocrit suggests that bleeding began at least 12 hours before; hemodilution may take 24 hours or more.

2. **Endoscopy** is usually superior to x-ray studies for finding the site of bleeding. In some cases, **angiography** may be required to find the source.

III. Differential diagnosis. Many clinical manifestations can help determine site, severity of bleed:

A. Red blood per rectum. Either lower GI lesion or massive upper GI lesion with fast transit time.

B. Hematemesis; blood in gastric aspirate. Bleeding proximal to ligament of Treitz; "coffee grounds" in aspirate suggest bleeding has stopped.

C. Guaiac-positive stools. Loss of >10 ml blood per day. Continuous occult bleeding suggests malignancy; intermittent bleeding suggests benign lesions (polyps, hemorrhoids).

D. ↑ **BUN with normal creatinine.** Result of recent GI bleed and digestion of intraintestinal blood.

IV. Pathophysiology

A. Common causes of **upper GI bleeds:**

 1. Erosive gastritis or duodenitis.

 2. Duodenal or gastric ulcers.

 3. Esophageal varices.

B. Common causes of **lower GI bleeds:**

 1. Hemorrhoids.

 2. Ulcerative colitis or Crohn's disease.

 3. Colorectal carcinoma.

 4. Benign rectal polyps.

 5. Bleeding diverticuli.

 6. Angiodysplasia (AV malformation).

Acute Viral Hepatitis

 I. **Definition.** Infection and inflammation of hepatocytes, caused by one of several types of viruses; most common agents are **hepatitis A, hepatitis B, and hepatitis C.**

 II. **Clinical manifestations.** The presentation of acute viral hepatitis is similar for all three types.

　　A. Prodrome. Lasts 2–14 days. Common findings are anorexia, nausea, vomiting, malaise, flu Sx, fever, enlarged and tender liver, abnormal SGOT, SGPT, LDH.

　　B. Icteric phase. Jaundice, ↑ lymphocytes (some abnormal), intensification of Sx, dark urine are found. Increased prothrombin time (PT) may signal hepatocellular necrosis. Circulating Hb_sAg is present in hepatitis B.

　　C. Convalescent phase-complication. Gradual resolution. Dangerous complications include fulminant hepatitis (hepatic failure and encephalopathy usually with hepatitis B) and chronic active hepatitis (5–10 percent of hepatitis B) where biopsy shows "piecemeal necrosis" and Hb_sAg persists.

 III. **Differential diagnosis.** Acute viral hepatitis must be distinguished from other viral infections (cytomegalovirus [CMV], herpes simplex virus, Coxsackie virus), cholecystitis, drug reactions. Diagnosis is often made on the basis of serologic detection of specific antigens and antibodies. Fig. 17-1 shows the time course of various antigens and antibodies that can be used for diagnosing hepatitis A and B.

 IV. **Pathophysiology**

　　A. Hepatitis A. Infectious hepatitis associated with fecal-oral transmission, fecal shedding of 27 nmol particle (?RNA virus), and incubation period of 15–40 days.

　　B. Hepatitis B. Serum hepatitis associated with transmission by way of parenteral inoculation (often infected blood products), shedding of 42 nmol Dane particle (DNA virus) with Hb_sAg surface antigen (detectable in more than 80 percent of patients with acute infection), and incubation period of 50–160 days. Some cases progress to chronic hepatitis. Commonly presents in IV drug abusers and homosexual men.

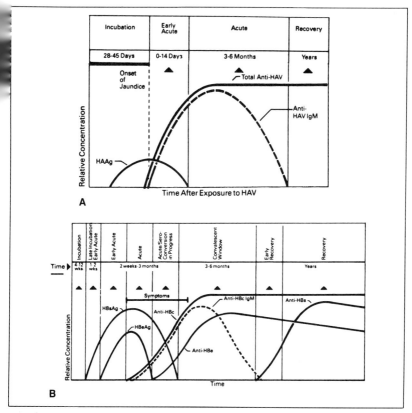

Fig. 17-1. A. Hepatitis A diagnostic profile. **B.** Hepatitis B diagnostic profile. Anti-HAV = total antibody to hepatitis A virus; confirms previous exposure to hepatitis A virus. Anti-HAV IgM = IgM antibody to hepatitis A virus; indicative of recent infection with hepatitis A virus. Anti-HBc = antibody to hepatitis B core antigen; early indicator of infection. Anti-HBc IgM = IgM antibody to hepatitis B core antigen. HBeAg = hepatitis B antigen; when present, indicates high degree of infectivity. Anti-HBe = antibody to hepatitis Be antigen; presence associated with resolution of infection. Anti-HBs = antibody to hepatitis B surface antigen; when present, typically indicates immunity and clinical recovery. (Courtesy of Abbott Laboratories, Diagnostics Division, North Chicago, Illinois. Reproduced with permission from L. G. Gomella [15].)

C. Hepatitis C. (Known previously as non-A non-B Hepatitis.) Though screened for in blood supply now, still the most common cause of posttransfusion hepatitis. Incubation period of 15–180 days; causes clinical picture similar to that of hepatitis B.

Acute Appendicitis

I. Definition. Inflammation of the appendix, often secondary to mucosal ulcerations or lumenal obstruction.

II. Clinical manifestations

A. History. Most common in patients age 10–30. Classic picture begins with periumbilical epigastric discomfort, then fever, anorexia, vomiting, nausea constipation. Within several hours, pain shifts to right lower quadrant (RLQ), sometimes localized at McBurney's point.

B. Physical exam. Abdominal tenderness, especially near **McBurney's point.** Rebound tenderness, guarding sometimes present. **Psoas** and **obturator** signs. Check for tenderness on rectal and vaginal exam. Note that patients with retrocecal appendices may present with less guarding and tenderness.

C. Diagnostic tests. Increased polys (PMNs) with left shift. Abdominal plain film is sometimes used to look for appendicoliths; ultrasound may be useful to rule out other causes of symptoms, especially in female patients.

III. Differential diagnosis.
Appendicitis must be differentiated from gastroenteritis and mesenteric adenitis. Other less common but possible diagnoses to exclude are pelvic inflammatory disease, diverticulitis, Crohn's disease, and rupture of ovarian follicle (mittleschmerz). Diagnosis is made on basis of history and physical exam.

IV. Pathophysiology

A. Incidence is much lower in undeveloped countries, suggesting that dietary factors may be involved.

B. Appendiceal obstruction often due to fecolith, but also may be caused by kinking, lymphoid swelling, foreign body, or neoplasm. Bacterial infection and lumenal necrosis often follow obstruction.

C. Complications. Perforation (followed by peritonitis); appendiceal abscess formation.

Chronic Inflammatory Bowel Disease (Crohn's Disease and Ulcerative Colitis)

I. Definition.
Crohn's disease (regional enteritis) is a chronic inflammatory disease of the GI tract (most often terminal ileum and right colon) distinguished by transmural intestinal involvement with skipped areas. **Ulcerative colitis** is a chronic inflammatory disease (usually involving the left colon more often than the right) distinguished by destruction of intestinal crypts, continuous involvement, pseudopolyposis, rectal bleeding, and occasional progression to colon cancer.

II. Clinical manifestations and differential diagnosis.
Though Crohn's disease and ulcerative colitis are closely related, their presentations, pathology, and complications are different.

A. Onset

1. Crohn's disease: gradual.

2. Ulcerative colitis: gradual or abrupt.

B. Signs and symptoms

1. Crohn's disease: intermittent crampy abdominal pain, low-grade fever, diarrhea, very little bleeding

2. Ulcerative colitis: bloody diarrhea, anorexia, urgency, fever, anemia.

C. Pathology

1. Crohn's disease: thickened intestine, ulcerated "cobblestone" mucosa, transmural lymphoid hyperplasia, fistulas, noncaseating granulomas.

2. Ulcerative colitis: "crypt abscess" formation, infiltration of lamina propria by inflammatory cells, pseudopolyps.

D. Radiologic findings

1. Crohn's disease: ileal narrowing, fuzzy mucosal pattern on barium enema.

2. Ulcerative colitis: straight and narrow colon, loss of haustra, ulcer craters, small polypoid-filling defects.

E. Complications

1. Crohn's disease: stricture obstructions, abscess formation, perforation, perirectal fistulas, gallstones, kidney stones.

2. Ulcerative colitis: colonic perforation, toxic megacolon, colonic carcinoma late in course.

III. Pathophysiology. The cause of inflammatory bowel disease is still unknown, though evidence suggests an autoimmune etiology. Despite much searching, no viral or bacterial agent has been found.

Pancreatitis

I. Definition. Acute or chronic inflammation of the pancreas.

II. Clinical manifestations

A. Acute pancreatitis

1. **History.** Severe abdominal pain continuing for hours or days; nausea, vomiting.

2. **Physical exam.** Fever, ↓ BP. Abdominal rigidity and rebound tenderness may be present. Ecchymoses on flanks **(Grey Turner's sign)** or around umbilicus **(Cullen's sign)** suggest hemorrhage or extensive inflammation.

3. **Diagnostic tests.** ↑ WBC and elevated serum amylase (sometimes marked). **Ranson's criteria** can be used to predict prognosis (see Table 17-2).

B. Chronic pancreatitis

1. **History.** Presentation may involve weight loss, glucose intolerance, or recurrent abdominal pain.

2. **Physical exam.** Signs and symptoms are generally similar to those of acute pancreatitis.

3. **Diagnostic tests.** Serum amylase levels may not be elevated if disease is advanced. X-ray may show pancreatic calcification. Before nitrogen wasting or steatorrhea become obvious, 90 percent of pancreatic tissue will have been destroyed.

III. Differential diagnosis

A. Acute pancreatitis must be distinguished from other causes of abdominal inflammation: cholelithiasis, common duct stones, intestinal obstruction or perforation, ectopic pregnancy, pelvic inflammatory disease, peptic ulcer disease.

Table 17-2. Ranson's criteria for acute pancreatitis*

On admission
Age >55
WBC >16,000
Serum LDH >350 IU/L
Blood glucose >200 mg/dl
SGOT >250 IU/L

After 48 hours
Hct decrease >10%
BUN increase >5 mg/dl
Serum CA <8 mg/dl
Arterial PO_2 <60 mmHg
Base deficit >4 mEq/L
Estimated fluid sequestration >61

---

*Used to predict mortality in patients with pacreatitis. Mortality rate rises with number of positive criteria.
Reproduced with permission from J. H. Ranson et al., Prognostic signs and the role of operative management in acute pancreatitis. *Surg Gynecol Obstet* 139:69, 1974.

- **B. Chronic pancreatitis,** which may be relatively painless, must be distinguished from malabsorption syndromes, diverticuli, pancreatic carcinoma.

- **C. Serum amylase level** is the single most valuable laboratory test for Dx.

IV. **Pathophysiology**

- **A. Acute pancreatitis** is often secondary to biliary tract disease, alcoholism, or abdominal surgery.

  Some attacks may be precipitated by impaction of gallstones in the ampulla of Vater, causing release of pancreatic enzymes and tissue necrosis. Edema, hemorrhage, and necrosis are mediated partially by release of trypsin, elastase, phospholipase A, and plasma kinins (↑ vascular permeability), leading to compressive ischemia. Pathologic changes include fat necrosis and formation of pseudocysts and abscesses.

- **B. Chronic pancreatitis** is often secondary to alcoholism. Tissue damage may be due to a variety of factors: protein malnutrition, abnormal bile formation (↑ free bile acids), direct ethanol toxicity, ↑ pancreatic secretion leading to duct obstruction.

Cirrhosis

I. **Definition.** Cirrhosis leads to a shrunken, scarred, and fibrotic liver, causing portal hypertension and hepatic insufficiency. It is most often caused by chronic alcohol ingestion, and is a leading cause of mortality and morbidity in the United States.

II. **Clinical manifestations**

- **A. History.** Seen usually late in life, in patients with a history of chronic drinking. Can present with encephalopathy, upper GI bleed from esophageal varices, or symptomatic ascites.

B. Physical exam. Spider angiomas, palmar erythma, gynecomastia, testicular atrophy, Dupuytren's contractures, and clubbing of the fingers are all frequently seen. Liver may be either firm and shrunken, or enlarged with fatty infiltration. Splenomegaly and ascites are common as well.

C. Diagnostic tests

1. **Liver function tests.** Patients with early-stage cirrhosis have elevated transaminases (AST, ALT), but later in the disease these values can return to normal because few functioning liver cells are left.

2. **BUN** <4 mg/dl is seen in cirrhosis and indicates decreased protein intake as well as inability to synthesize urea.

3. **Liver biopsy** is used to confirm the diagnosis and may help in elucidating the etiology of the cirrhosis.

III. Differential diagnosis. Causes of cirrhosis in addition to chronic alcohol intake include: severe chronic hepatitis, right-sided CHF, nutritional deprivation, hemochromatosis, Wilson's disease, and sclerosing cholangitis. In middle-aged women, primary biliary cirrhosis must be considered.

IV. Pathophysiology

A. There are two main types of cirrhosis:

1. **Micronodular,** or **Laennec's** cirrhosis, seen in alcoholics.

2. **Macronodular,** or **postnecrotic** cirrhosis, seen after chronic active hepatitis.

B. Complications of cirrhosis include variceal hemorrhage, renal failure **(hepatorenal syndrome),** encephalopathy, and malabsorption.

C. Survival rates from cirrhosis are low, with fewer than 10 percent of patients alive 5 years after the diagnosis is made.

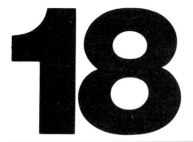

Genitourinary Diseases

Acute Renal Failure

I. **Definition.** Acute suppression of kidney filtration resulting in rapidly increasing azotemia, with or without oliguria (<500 ml daily).

II. **Clinical manifestations.** The presentation of acute renal failure (ARF) can be divided into two phases.

   A. **Oliguric phase.** Associated findings are ↓ ↓ urine output (<20 ml/hr) with rising BUN and/or serum creatinine levels; anorexia, nausea, vomiting; urine sediment consisting of protein, red cells, epithelial cells, brown granular casts; specific gravity 1.010–1.016; ↓ serum Na^+ (120–130 mEq/L); hyperkalemia; Hct 25–30 percent.

   B. **Diuretic phase.** Begins approximately 2 weeks postonset. Gradual ↑ in urine formation to 6–8 L/day, indicating nephron recovery. Continuous for 7–10 days.

III. **Differential diagnosis and pathophysiology**

   A. Table 18-1 compares lab values for prerenal versus intrinsic renal azotemia.

   B. **Etiologies**

   1. **Prerenal.** Renal compromise results from diminished renal blood flow: volume depletion; cardiac dysfunction resulting in a diminished cardiac output; diminished intravascular volume due to redistribution of fluid into interstitial spaces, as can occur with hepatic cirrhosis, sepsis, and burns.

   2. **Postrenal.** Renal compromise results from obstruction of the urinary system: benign prostatic hypertrophy, prostate cancer, calculi at the level of the prostatic urethra, pelvic or retroperitoneal tumors, and congenital anomalies. Blockage of both ureters is uncommon but can be caused by a widespread retroperitoneal process, such as lymphoma.

   3. **Renal.** Renal compromise results from intrinsic renal pathology: glomerular disease, vascular disease, tubulointerstitial disease. By far the most common cause of acute intrinsic renal disease is the category of tubulointerstitial disorders, although in hospitalized patients acute tubular necrosis is the major cause of intrinsic renal failure.

   a. **Glomerular disease.** Poststreptococcal glomerulonephritis, glomerulonephritis associated with endocarditis and abscesses, membranoproliferative glomerulonephritis, rapidly progressive glomerulonephritis (SLE, Wegener's granulomatosis, Goodpasture's syndrome, and Henoch-Schönlein purpura).

Table 18-1. Differential diagnosis of prerenal azotemia versus intrinsic renal azotemia

Determination	Prerenal	Renal
Urine osmolality	>500 mOsm/L	<350 mOsm/L
Urine: plasma creatinine	> 20	< 10
Urine: plasma urea	> 40	< 20
Urine Na$^+$	< 20 mEq/L	> 40 mEq/L

    b. Vascular disease. Renal artery thrombosis or embolism, renal vein thrombosis, scleroderma, malignant hypertension, thrombotic thrombocytopenic purpura (TTP), disseminated intravascular coagulation (DIC) with cortical necrosis.

    c. Tubulointerstitial disease. Separated into acute interstitial nephritis and acute tubular necrosis (ATN).

        (1) Acute interstitial nephritis. Caused by infiltrative disease (sarcoidosis or lymphoma), systemic infection (syphilis and toxoplasmosis), and drugs (penicillin, diuretics, nonsteroidal anti-inflammatory drugs [NSAIDs]).

        (2) Acute tubular necrosis. Caused by ischemia (shock, trauma, hypoxia, or sepsis) nephrotoxins (radiocontrast agents and aminoglycosides), myoglobinuria, and myeloma proteins (Bence Jones).

C. Damage occurs through direct **nephrotoxicity** (usually involving necrosis of tubular epithelium) and **ischemia** (often secondary to constriction of afferent arterioles).

D. Although oliguria is common, the volume of urine bears no relation to the degree of functional impairment.

Chronic Renal Failure

I. Definition. Chronic insufficiency of renal excretory and regulatory functions leading to **uremia.** Chronic renal failure (CRF) results from a progressive decrease in glomerular filtration and the loss of tubular function.

II. Clinical manifestations. The functional effects of CRF are divided into the following progressively worsening categories: diminished renal reserve, renal insufficiency, and uremia. With **diminished renal reserve,** there is a measurable loss of renal function, but homeostasis is preserved at the expense of hormonal adaptations such as secondary hyperparathyroidism and intrarenal changes in glomerulotubular balance. At the stage of **renal insufficiency,** there is slight retention of nitrogenous compounds (azotemia), reflected in elevated plasma urea and creatinine. With further renal dysfunction, fluid and electrolyte balance is disturbed, azotemia increases, and systemic manifestations of **uremia** occur.

    A. History

        1. Patients with a **diminished renal reserve** are asymptomatic, and renal dysfunction can only be detected by careful testing.

2. Patients with **renal insufficiency,** despite the elevated BUN and creatinine, suffer only from nocturia, due to the failure of the kidney to concentrate urine during the night.

3. Patients with **uremia** suffer from weakness, fatigue, and mental status changes, as well as anorexia, nausea, vomiting, early satiety, stomatitis, and an unpleasant taste in the mouth. Patients also suffer from intractable pruritis.

B. **Physical exam and pathophysiology.** Following are the physical manifestations of the multisystem effects of the **uremic state:**

1. **Cardiovascular:** hypertension (due to volume overload), dilated cardiomyopathy (due to volume overload), pericarditis.

2. **Pulmonary:** pulmonary edema and large pulmonary effusions (due to volume overload, increased capillary permeability), and Kussmaul's respirations (due to acidemia).

3. **Neurologic:** both peripheral and central nervous system derangements are seen. Progressive sensory polyneuropathy and distal motor dysfunction is usually present. Uremia unchecked will eventually result in asterixis and coma (metabolic encephalopathy).

4. **Hematopoietic:** normochromic normocytic anemia results in pallor (due to progressively decreasing erythropoietin levels), thrombasthenia (decreased platelet aggregation and adhesiveness) presents as purpura.

5. **Gastrointestinal:** increased incidence of duodenitis and angiodysplasia of stomach and proximal intestine result in ulceration and bleeding.

6. **Metabolic disturbances:** hypertriglyceridemia (hepatic dysfunction); increased insulin resistance and glucose intolerance.

7. **Skin:** yellow-brown discoloration and urea from sweat may crystallize on skin as uremic frost.

8. **Musculoskeletal:** bone pain and multiple fractures (due to renal osteodystrophy resulting from secondary hyperparathyroidism).

C. **Diagnostic tests.** Lab findings include azotemia, acidosis ($[HCO_3^-] = 15-20$ mEq/L), hyperphosphatemia, hyperkalemia, and normochromic normocytic anemia. Urine osmolarity $\sim$ 300–320 mOsm/L.

III. **Differential diagnosis.** The cause of CRF must be elucidated, because some etiologies are reversible. Etiologies of CRF include advanced and prolonged hypertension, diabetes mellitus, glomerulonephritis, tubulointerstitial disease, polycystic kidney disease, and obstructive uropathy. All result in parenchymal scarring and progressive glomerular failure.

Glomerulopathies

I. **Definition.** A group of diverse conditions including, but not limited to, glomerulonephritis, in which the disease predominantly affects glomerular function.

Based on their clinical presentation, the glomerulopathies have been divided into five subtypes:

A. **Acute glomerulonephritis (GN).** Acute onset and early resolution.

B. **Rapidly progressive glomerulonephritis (RPGN).** Acute onset and rapid progression.

C. **Idiopathic renal hematuric syndrome.** Persistent, asymptomatic, minimal urinary abnormalities.

D. **Nephrotic syndrome.** Acute onset and gradual resolution.

E. **Chronic glomerulonephritis.** Insidious onset and gradual progression.

II. **Clinical manifestations and differential diagnosis** vary, depending on the subtype. Acute glomerulonephritis and nephrotic syndrome are discussed in detail later in this chapter as they are by far the most common glomerulopathies.

III. **Pathophysiology.** Glomerular damage produces changes in glomerular capillary permeability, resulting in various degrees of proteinuria, hematuria, leukocyturia, and urinary casts.

Microthrombosis occurs, commonly accompanied by epithelial "crescents" formed from leaked fibrinogen and precipitated fibrin, and if damage is severe, hemodynamic changes may produce oliguria. Commonly tubular function is deranged by inflammatory changes in the interstitium. Measurable changes consist of reduction in the urinary concentrating capacity, acid excretion, and varying disturbances in nephron solute exchange. Because there is some inherent capacity for glomerular hypertrophy, such defects in tubular function usually occur before the **glomerular filtration rate** (GFR) is much reduced. As glomerular derangement progresses, however, the total filtration surface is significantly reduced, the GFR falls, and azotemia occurs.

Acute glomerulonephritis

I. **Definition.** Group of diseases characterized pathologically by diffuse inflammatory changes in the glomeruli and clinically by the acute onset of **hematuria, RBC casts, and proteinuria.**

II. **Clinical manifestations** of acute glomerulonephritis vary according to the disease entity that causes it. The most common cause of acute glomerulonephritis is **poststreptococcal glomerulonephritis** (PSGN).

A. **History.** History of streptococcal pharyngitis 3–4 weeks prior to onset of smoky or frankly bloody urine, oliguria, headaches, and visual disturbances (secondary to hypertension).

B. **Physical exam**

1. Hypertension.

2. Gross or microscopic hematuria.

3. Periorbital edema.

C. **Diagnostic tests**

1. **Urinalysis:** proteinuria of 1–3 gm/day, hematuria, active urinary sediment including WBC, granular, and RBC casts.

2. Positive throat culture for B-hemolytic streptococci.

3. Low C3.

4. Elevated antibodies to streptococcal antigens (antistreptolysin O or antihyaluronidase).

III. **Differential diagnosis**

A. **Postinfectious glomerulonephritis.** PSGN, subacute bacterial endocarditis, infected ventriculoatrial shunts, varicella, hepatitis B, syphilis, and malaria.

B. **Mesangiocapillary glomerulonephritis.**

C. **Lupus nephritis.**

D. **IgA nephropathy (Berger's Disease).**

IV. **Pathophysiology.** The glomerular damage seen in acute glomerulonephritis is due to immune complex deposition and the activation of the complement system that results from this deposition. An endogenous or exogenous antigen stimulates production of a specific antibody, which combines with the antigen in one of two ways: within the kidney, after the antigen has been planted; or in the circulation, to form a circulating immune complex that subsequently becomes deposited. The former mechanism is the more common process. Deposition of the immune complex in the glomerular wall in subepithelial sites activates the complement system. From the complement cascade, chemotactic factor C567 is formed, which causes polymorphonuclear leukocyte localization in the area of the immune complex deposition and the release of lysozyme. Lysozyme injures the foot processes of the podocytes, resulting in "holes" in the glomerular filter. These holes are the means by which red blood cells and protein escape into the tubular portion of the nephron.

Nephrotic syndrome

I. **Definition.** Nephrotic syndrome (NS) is characterized by proteinuria, hypoalbuminemia, lipemia, and generalized edema.

II. **Clinical manifestations**

A. **History and physical exam.** Patients usually report symptoms associated with new-onset focal edema, "foamy" urine (urine with bubbles on its surface), anorexia, and malaise.

Focal edema is usually the trigger that brings the patient with NS to a physician. Patients seek help for such varied complaints as difficulty breathing (pleural effusion or laryngeal edema), substernal chest pain (pericardial effusion), scrotal swelling, swollen knees (hydroarthrosis), swollen abdomen (ascites), and, in children, abdominal pain from edema of the mesentery.

B. **Diagnostic tests**

1. **Urinalysis: Proteinuria >3 gm/day;** urine sodium low and urine potassium high (due to increased aldosterone secretion as the body attempts to increase intravascular volume); lipiduria.

2. **Serum chemistries:** hypoalbuminemia (<2.5 gm/dl); BUN and creatinine are elevated in proportion to the degree of renal impairment; increased cholesterol and triglyceride levels.

III. **Differential diagnosis.** Diagnosis of NS made by clinical features and proteinuria (see Fig. 18-1), but determination of the etiology of the nephrotic syndrome depends on renal histology determined by renal biopsy.

A. **Primary renal diseases** account for 90 percent of cases of nephrotic syndrome in children and 75 percent in adults.

	Children	Adults
Minimal change disease (MCD)	65%	15%
Focal glomerulosclerosis (FGS)	10%	15%
Membranous glomerulonephritis (MGN)	5%	35%
Membranoproliferative glomerulonephritis (MPGN)	10%	10%
Total	90%	75%

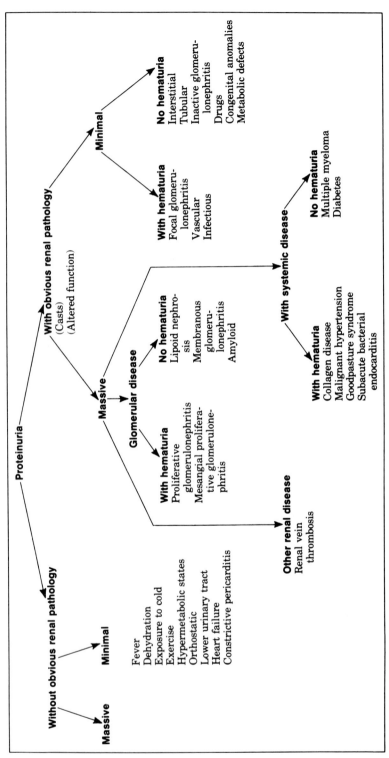

Fig. 18-1. Proteinuria with and without obvious renal pathology. (Reprinted with permission from Children's Hospital, Boston, *Manual of Pediatric Therapeutics*, 5th ed., Boston: Little, Brown, 1994.)

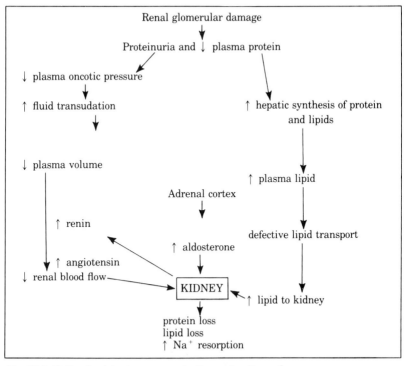

Fig. 18-2. Pathophysiologic sequence in the nephrotic syndrome.

B. **Secondary disease** accounts for 10 percent of NS in children and 25 percent of NS in adults. Secondary causes include:

1. **Metabolic:** diabetes mellitus, amyloidosis.

2. **Immunogenic:** systemic lupus erythematosis, Henoch-Schönlein purpura, polyarteritis nodosa, Sjögren's syndrome, sarcoidosis.

3. **Neoplasms:** leukemias, lymphomas, multiple myeloma.

4. **Nephrotoxins:** mercury, gold, penicillamine.

5. **Infections:** PSGN, shunt nephritis, endocarditis, syphilis, hepatitis B, varicella, malaria, schistosomiasis.

6. **Hereditary:** Alport's syndrome, Fabry's disease.

7. **Miscellaneous:** toxemia of pregnancy, malignant hypertension.

IV. **Pathophysiology.** The sequence of events leading to the nephrotic syndrome is illustrated in Fig. 18-2.

Urinary Tract Infection
(see Colorplate D, 9)

I. **Definition.** Acute or chronic infection of any portion of the urinary tract.

II. **Clinical manifestations and differential diagnosis**

A. UTI must be distinguished from other causes of dysuria, polyuria, urgency, and lower abdominal pain. These disorders include genital infections, external bladder compression, prostatitis.

B. Differentiating features of lower and upper UTI

    1. History and physical exam

        a. Lower UTI (cystitis): Dysuria; dark, foul-smelling urine.

        b. Upper UTI (pyelonephritis): headaches, chills, fever, vomiting, back pain, costovertebral angle (CVA) tenderness.

    2. Diagnostic tests

        a. Lower UTI (cystitis): bacteriuria, pyuria, normal C-reactive protein.

        b. Upper UTI (pyelonephritis): bacteriuria, proteinuria, pyuria, leukocytosis (with left shift). Chronic UTI may result in anemia, uremia, acidosis, hypertension, elevated C-reactive protein.

III. Pathophysiology

    A. Usually due to ascending urinary tract infection by fecal-perineal flora. Since female urethra is shorter, UTI generally more common in women than men (except for cases of congenital anomalies and prostatism). Instrumentation of urethra increases risk.

    B. Most common organism is *Escherichia coli.* Others include *Klebsiella, Proteus,* enterococci.

Gonorrhea and Syphilis
(see Colorplate D, 7)

I. Definition. Gonorrhea and syphilis are two common sexually transmitted diseases (STDs).

II. Clinical manifestations and differential diagnosis. The clinical features of gonorrhea and syphilis are compared in Table 18-2. Note that syphilis manifests itself in one of three stages (primary, secondary, and tertiary).

III. Pathophysiology

    A. Gonorrhea. More than 3,000,000 untreated cases in U.S.; caused by **Neisseria gonorrhoeae,** a gram-negative, kidney-shaped diplococcus usually found intracellularly (especially in polymorphonuclear leukocytes) on Gram stain.

    B. Syphilis. More than 400,000 untreated cases in U.S.; caused by **Treponema pallidum,** a spirochete. *T. pallidum* often invades the central nervous system and aorta, leading to the symptoms of meningovascular neurosyphilis, tabes dorsalis, dissecting aortic aneurysm, aortic insufficiency, and aortic scarring.

Table 18-2. Clinical manifestations of gonorrhea and syphilis

Disease	Time from exposure to onset	Clinical manifestations	Diagnostic tests
Gonorrhea	2–8 days	Dysuria, frequency, discharge; often asymptomatic; men often present with urethritis, women with PID	Discharge smears show gram-negative diplococci; selective medium and high CO_2 necessary to culture organisms
Primary syphilis	10–90 days (average 21)	Painless chancre, often in genital area; nontender adenopathy in draining modes	Fluid from lesions contains *Treponema pallidum*; must use dark fields or immunofluorescence.
Secondary syphilis	6 wk–6 mo	Mucosal lesions; generalized rash consisting of lesions (condylomata latum); generalized nontender adenopathy; fever, hepatitis, arthritis, iritis, meningitis	VDRL and FTA-ABS serologic tests almost always positive
Tertiary syphilis	2–10 yr	Charcot's arthropathy; infiltrative tumors (gummas) in liver, skin, bone; aortic aneurysms with aortic insufficiency; meningovascular involvement; neurologic: degenerative changes, tabes dorsalis, paresthesias, dementia, etc.; Argyll Robertson pupil and Romberg's sign	Often positive CSF serology

VDRL = Venereal Disease Research Laboratories; FTA-ABS = fluorescent treponemal antibody-absorption.

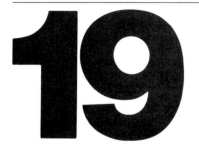

**Musculoskeletal
Diseases**

In this chapter we will discuss some important examples among the four major types of rheumatologic disease:

1. **Monoarticular arthritis:** gout, pseudogout, septic arthritis.
2. **Polyarticular arthritis:** rheumatoid arthritis (RA), osteoarthritis.
3. **Connective tissue disorders:** systemic lupus erythematosus (SLE), scleroderma.
4. **Vasculitides:** temporal arteritis.

Gout

I. **Definition.** A usually monoarticular arthritis caused by deposition of uric acid crystals in joints.

II. **Clinical manifestations**

  A. **History and physical exam.** Predominantly affects middle-aged and elderly men and postmenopausal women. Linked with excessive alcohol consumption and salicylate ingestion. Clinical manifestations of gout can be divided into three phases.

   1. An **acute attack** consists of a very painful monoarthritis, usually in the first metatarsophalangeal joint (i.e., the big toe). Recurrences may affect other joints, but usually spare the hips and shoulders.

   2. In the **interval phase** patients are asymptomatic, but as the disease progresses this period gets shorter and shorter.

   3. About 10–20 years after original onset, patients enter the **chronic phase,** in which tophaceous deposits are found in various periarticular areas, as well as commonly on the extensor surface of the forearm and pinna of the ear. Later complications include uric acid nephrolithiasis and tubulointerstitial nephritis.

  B. **Lab findings.** Gout is characterized by excess circulating uric acid and deposition of uric acid crystals in the joint fluid. A patient with a uric acid level > 10 mg/dl has a 90 percent chance of suffering from gout. Measurement of 24-hr urine uric acid after a 5-day purine-restricted diet can be used to separate uric acid overproducers from undersecretors.

III. **Differential diagnosis.** Definitive diagnosis, made by the presence of uric acid crystals in joint fluid, is important because anti-inflammatory agents used to treat gout can mask signs of joint sepsis. **Pseudogout,** the result of deposition of calcium pyrophosphate, is indistinguishable clinically from gout, except for its predilection for larger joints, such as the knee.

IV. **Pathophysiology.** Causes of increased uric acid include genetic defects in purine metabolism, increased cellular turnover (psoriasis, myeloproliferative diseases), and decreased excretion of uric acid (as in patients with interstitial nephritis, or those taking various drugs, like certain diuretics).

Pseudogout

I. **Definition.** A usually monoarticular arthritis caused by calcium pyrophosphate deposition in joints.

II. **Clinical manifestations**

   A. **History and physical exam.** Seen most frequently in the elderly and in those with hyperparathyroidism, hyperthyroidism, and hemochromatosis. Painful attacks can last up to 2 weeks and are accompanied by fever. Pseudogout usually attacks larger joints, like the knee, and not uncommonly affects more than one joint at a time.

   B. **Diagnostic tests**

   1. **X-ray** shows linear, punctuate calcifications in the knee, hip, intervertebral disks, and other joints.

   2. Definitive diagnosis is made by identifying calcium pyrophosphate crystals in synovial fluid.

III. **Differential diagnosis.** See "Gout," sec. III.

Septic Arthritis

I. **Definition.** Inflammation of one or more joints due to infection in the joint space.

II. **Clinical manifestations**

   A. **History.** Patients with preexisting arthritis are especially prone to septic joints, as are those with diabetes, a history of joint injury, immunosuppression, and chronic alcohol and IV drug abuse. Onset is rapid, and patients can range from showing no signs of systemic illness to appearing quite sick.

   B. **Physical exam.** Involved joints are warm, red, swollen, and tender, with intense pain, especially on motion.

   C. **Diagnostic tests.** Definitive diagnosis is made by Gram stain and culture of synovial fluid.

III. **Differential diagnosis.** Septic arthritis can be differentiated from other causes of monoarthritis by the signs of infection both locally (redness, warmth, swelling, intense pain on movement) and systemically (fever, enlarged nodes).

IV. **Pathophysiology**

   A. In young sexually active patients, most common cause is *Neisseria gonorrhea*. In other populations, *Staphylococcus aureus* is the most frequently encountered pathogen. Gram-negative organisms are seen especially in patients with underlying diabetes, cancer, or other serious diseases.

   B. Mechanism of infection is primarily through the hematogenous spread of microorganism.

Rheumatoid Arthritis

I. **Definition.** A chronic systemic disease characterized by inflammation of synovial membranes with resultant cartilage and joint destruction.

II. Clinical manifestations

A. History. Onset is usually insidious and may begin with small joints. Prodrome symptoms include fever, malaise, weight loss, morning stiffness, and lymphadenopathy. Joint symptoms are usually symmetric, and include pain, swelling, stiffness, and muscular weakness. In the fingers, proximal interphalangeal (PIP) and metacarpophalangeal (MCP) joints are usually involved, distal interphalangeal (DIP) usually spared.

B. Physical exam. Swelling, warmth, and tenderness of involved joints. As disease progresses, joint deformities develop, including ulnar deviation, hyperextension of PIP joint with flexion of DIP joint **(swan-neck deformity)**, and PIP flexion with DIP hyperextension **(boutonnière deformity)**.

C. Diagnostic tests

1. 85 percent have positive rheumatoid factor, usually IgM reactive against IgG. Usually increased erythrocyte sedimentation rate (ESR), with moderate anemia and sometimes positive antinuclear antibody (ANA).

2. X-ray shows periarticular osteoporosis, juxta-articular erosions, commonly subluxation of upper cervical spine.

III. Differential diagnosis.
The differential diagnosis of progressive polyarthritis includes, in addition to RA, degenerative joint disease, the seronegative spondyloarthropathies (rarer conditions like ankylosing spondylitis and Reiter's syndrome), connective tissue diseases, hypothyroidism, gout, and pseudogout.

IV. Pathophysiology

A. Etiology is unknown, most probably autoimmune; 3:1 female to male predominance. Risk factors include family history, histocompatibility locus antigen (HLA) DW4.

B. Typical **pathology** involves inflammation of the synovial membrane followed by hypertrophy and proliferation of the cells lining the synovial membrane (called pannus tissue), which erode into the soft tissue of the joint. Microscopic findings include the rheumatoid nodule, a focus of central necrosis surrounded by a palisade of connective tissue cells and granulation tissue.

C. Complications of RA can include amyloid deposits, **Felty's syndrome** (splenomegaly and neutropenia accompanying the arthropathy), **Sjögren's syndrome** (lymphocytic infiltration of the lacrimal and salivary glands), and other severe systemic vasculitides.

Osteoarthritis (Degenerative Joint Disease)

I. Definition.
A chronic, progressive, noninflammatory osteoarthropathy primarily involving the articular cartilage.

II. Clinical manifestations

A. History. Onset insidious, with stiffness, pain, crepitus. Symptoms precipitated by activity and relieved by rest. Minimal systemic involvement. Usually affects DIP and PIP joints in hand, as well as thumb, hip, knee, cervical and lumbar spine. May follow joint trauma.

B. Physical exam. Diminished range of motion, crepitation, and pain seen in interphalangeal and large weight-bearing joints. Look especially at hand for bony deformities: **Heberden's nodes** (DIP) and **Bouchard's nodes** (PIP).

C. Diagnostic tests

1. Serum tests, including rheumatoid factor, ESR, are usually normal.

2. X-ray shows narrowed joint space, increased subchondral bone density, osteophytes.

III. Differential diagnosis. Can be differentiated from RA by pattern of joint involvement, lack of systemic manifestations, normal lab tests, and characteristic x-ray findings.

IV. Pathophysiology

A. Persistent wear, trauma, aging, and obesity all contribute to this disease.

B. Classic pathology involves erosion of articular cartilage, osteophyte (bone spur) formation, and synovial hypertrophy with minimal inflammation.

Systemic Lupus Erythematosus

I. Definition. An inflammatory autoimmune disease characterized by multiple organ involvement, joint symptoms, rash, and positive antinuclear antibody (ANA) test.

II. Clinical manifestations

A. History and physical exam. SLE can affect nearly every organ system.

1. **Systemic:** fatigue, malaise, weight loss, fever, lymphadenopathy.

2. **Skin:** malar (butterfly) rash, discoid rash, photosensitivity, oral ulcers.

3. **Arthritis:** usually symmetric, involving hands, wrists, and knees.

4. **Renal:** ranges from mild proteinuria to renal failure. Nephrotic syndrome and rapidly progressive glomerulonephritis are common.

5. **Neurologic:** seizures, neuropathies, migraines, and behavioral and cognitive disturbances are all seen.

6. **Cardiac:** pericarditis, Libman-Sacks endocarditis (valvular lesions).

7. **Pulmonary:** pleuritis, pneumonitis, small bilateral exudates.

8. **Gastrointestinal:** nausea, vomiting, anorexia, abdominal pain, hepatosplenomegaly.

B. Lab findings. Normochromic normocytic anemia, leukopenia, thrombocytopenia, increased ESR, false-positive serologic test for syphilis, increased serum globulin, positive Coombs' test, lowered complement, +LE cells, +ANA (autoantibodies to nucleic acids and ribonucleoprotein).

III. Differential diagnosis. SLE must be differentiated from discoid lupus (discoid rash with no other systemic disease), RA, and drug-induced lupus syndrome (seen with hydralazine, phenytoin, and procainamide).

IV. Pathophysiology

A. The vast majority of patients are young to middle-aged women. Prevalence is approximately 1:2000 people, with 8:1 female to male ratio. High twin concordance, with increased risk to people with HLA DR2 and DR3.

B. Etiology is unclear, but there is some evidence for defective suppressor T cells allowing overactive B cells to produce antibodies. Viral infection may contribute to disease induction in susceptible hosts.

Scleroderma

I. **Definition.** A chronic debilitating disease, affecting connective tissue in multiple organ systems. Also known as **progressive systemic sclerosis** (PSS).

A. **CREST** variant of scleroderma: Patients with **c**alcinosis, **R**aynaud's, **e**sophageal involvement, **s**clerodactyly, and **t**elangiectasias; thought to have a more benign course.

B. There are two forms of **localized scleroderma** without systemic effects:

1. **Morphea,** with localized skin lesions of scleroderma that heal completely.

2. **Linear,** which appears as isolated lines of sclerotic skin on the extremities in children.

II. **Clinical manifestations**

A. **History and physical exam.** Like SLE, scleroderma affects nearly every organ system.

1. **Skin:** First, changes are usually symmetric; painless swelling of hands, with tightened, thickened skin. Later trunk, face (**"purse-string mouth"**), and more proximal extremities become involved. Also seen are telangiectasic skin rashes, subcutaneous calcinosis.

2. **Raynaud's phenomenon** is seen in 90 percent of patients with scleroderma. It is a cold-related vasospasm of vessels in distal extremities that leads to cyanosis and blanching, possibly to infarction in severe cases.

3. **Joints:** Joint stiffness and polyarthritis are common.

4. **GI:** Decreased peristalsis in lower esophagus leads to reflux, esophagitis, and Barret's metaplasia, increasing the risk of malignancy. Duodenal hypermotility leads to bacterial overgrowth and malabsorption. Wide-mouth colonic diverticula are also seen.

5. **Pulmonary.** Fibrosis leads to restrictive lung disease. Pulmonary vascular involvement can lead to pulmonary hypertension and cor pulmonale.

6. **Cardiac:** Myocardial fibrosis can lead to congestive heart failure and arrhythmias. Pericarditis can lead, rarely, to tamponade.

7. **Renal:** Can lead to progressive renal insufficiency, proteinuria, and malignant hypertension.

B. **Diagnostic tests**

1. Increased ESR, decreased complement, increased ANA. Antibodies with nucleolar staining pattern are almost exclusively seen in scleroderma.

2. **X-ray** can show resorption of tufts of the distal phalanges, radius, ulna, ribs, and mandible.

III. **Pathophysiology.** Autoimmune disease with unknown etiology.

Temporal Arteritis (Giant Cell Arteritis)

I. **Definition.** A large-vessel vasculitis that affects branches of the carotid artery.

II. Clinical manifestations

   A. History. Affects patients more than 50 years old almost exclusively. Presents with headache, jaw claudication, altered vision, fatigue, myalgias, fever, and weight loss.

   B. Physical exam. Vision changes, including sudden loss of vision in one eye, prominent and tender temporal arteries.

   C. Diagnostic test. Elevated ESR. Definitive diagnosis is made with temporal artery biopsy, but many false-negatives occur due to segmental involvement of vessel.

III. Differential diagnosis.
As many of the presenting signs and symptoms of temporal arteritis—such as headache, fever, and myalgias—are very nonspecific, the differential is usually huge. Temporal arteritis should especially be considered in any elderly patient with typical symptoms and an elevated ESR. It is an important diagnosis to make, as high-dose steroids given promptly can save a patient's vision.

IV. Pathophysiology

   A. Many feel that temporal arteritis and **polymyalgia rheumatica** (a syndrome of symmetric proximal muscle pain and stiffness) are ends of the same disease spectrum, as many patients with one syndrome also display signs of the other.

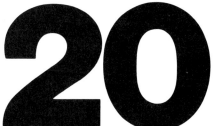

Neurologic Diseases

Seizure Disorder (Epilepsy)

I. **Definition.** A group of disorders characterized by paroxysmal transitory changes in mental status and motor activity. There are two general types of seizures: **focal,** which are limited to one part of the brain, and **generalized,** which are more global in scope.

II. **Clinical manifestations.** Different types of seizures exhibit different clinical findings.

   A. **Focal seizures**

      1. **Motor:** Premonitory aura precedes focal convulsion, and consciousness is often retained. In **Jacksonian** epilepsy, there is a characteristic "march" of motor events through the body as the seizure slowly spreads through different areas of the cortex.

      2. **Sensory:** flashing lights, tingling numbness are reported, without motor events. EEG often shows discharge in the parietal and occipital lobes.

      3. **Temporal lobe:** characterized by automatisms, emotional distress, hallucinations, autonomic dysfunctions, complex behavioral changes, such as hyperreligiosity.

   B. **Generalized seizures**

      1. **Grand mal** (tonic-clonic). Usually a sequence of tonic-clonic contractions, loss of bowel and bladder control, flaccid coma, postictal confusion. No aura or focality.

      2. **Petit mal** (absence). Brief blank spells, myoclonic jerks, akinetic seizures. Most common in children. Three-per-second spike-and-wave morphology on EEG.

III. **Pathophysiology**

   A. Initial events in seizure cycle are unclear. A group of neurons begin firing synchronously, often recruiting neighboring groups. Seizures may be precipitated by drugs, hypoxia, hypoglycemia, sensory stimulation, trauma, or intracranial masses.

   B. Focal seizures tend to be caused by local conditions, such as tumors and trauma, while generalized seizures are usually idiopathic, toxic, or metabolic.

Coma

I. **Definition.** A state of unconsciousness from which the patient cannot be aroused.

II. Clinical manifestations

A. Physical exam of patient should include vital signs, pain responses, careful inspection (note **Battle's** sign, the discoloration of skin behind the ear associated with skull fractures), pupillary and respiratory patterns, passive motion and limb-drop-maneuvers to search for hemiparesis, decerebrate or decorticate rigidity, nuchal rigidity, "doll's head" maneuver, ice-water caloric response.

B. Diagnostic tests should include: CBC, U/A, ABG, ECG, electrolytes, blood alcohol and toxicology levels, liver and kidney function tests, glucose level, PT and PTT, and, if indicated, EEG, lumbar puncture (LP), and CT scan.

III. Differential diagnosis and pathophysiology. Principal question is etiology of coma.

A. Intracranial etiologies include trauma, vascular disease, tumors, central nervous system infections, seizure disorders, increased intracranial pressure.

B. Extracranial etiologies include shock (including post-MI), metabolic disorders (hypoglycemia, hepatic disturbances, acidosis, electrolyte disturbances), drug effects, systemic trauma (hyper- and hypothermia, electric shock, anaphylaxis).

C. A useful mnemonic to remember is **AEIOU TIPS:**

Alcoholism
Encephalopathy
Insulin excess or deficiency
Opiates and other drugs
Uremia and metabolic disorders
Trauma
Infection
Psychiatric disorders
Syncope

Cerebrovascular Disorders (Stroke and Transient Ischemic Attack)

I. Definition. Acute derangement in neurologic function due to inadequate cerebral circulation. A **transient ischemic attack** (TIA) is any acute neurologic impairment that clears within 24 hours.

II. Clinical manifestations

Premonitory signs may include headache, dizziness, confusion. Actual symptoms depend on structures affected by loss of circulation. Classic TIA sign is **amaurosis fugax,** described as "a shade coming down over one eye." Strokes may also be associated with vomiting, convulsions, fever, nuchal rigidity, changed mental status.

III. Differential diagnosis. Common signs and symptoms associated with occlusion of particular arteries include:

A. Middle cerebral artery (MCA). Contralateral hemiparesis (arm and face more than leg), numbness, homonymous hemianopsia, aphasias, apraxia.

B. Anterior cerebral artery (ACA). Contralateral hemiplegia (maximal in leg), grasp and suck reflexes, incontinence.

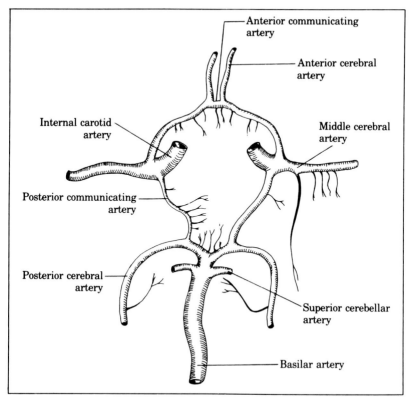

Fig. 20-1. The origins of the central arteries of the brain from the Circle of Willis.

    C. Posterior cerebral artery (PCA). Contralateral hemisensory loss, hemianopsia, visual and memory defects.

    D. Internal carotid artery. Variable; may be silent or similar to MCA stroke with profound changes in mental status. Upper extremity Sx are common.

    E. Vertebrobasilar artery. May overlap with PCA stroke; ipsilateral cranial nerve problems; contralateral or bilateral motor, sensory, cerebellar signs; staggering gait, ataxia, dysphagia, confusion.

See Fig. 20-1 for a diagram of the Circle of Willis.

IV. Pathophysiology. Strokes are caused by one of three basic disease processes.

    A. Thrombosis. Atheromatous thrombosis often involves large arteries, especially the carotid, vertebral, and basilar. **Hypertensive** thrombosis often affects small arteries within the brain itself.

    B. Embolism. Emboli can consist of calcific atherosclerotic plaques, fat, air, and the like. Although emboli often occur in "showers," they may affect individual cortical arteries, causing isolated defects that appear and resolve suddenly.

    C. Hemorrhage. Often occurs secondary to trauma, rupture of congenital aneurysms, arteriovenous malformations, tumors, intracranial hypertensive ruptures.

Meningitis

I. **Definition.** Inflammation of the meninges of the brain or spinal cord, most often due to pneumococcus, *Neisseria meningitidis, Haemophilus influenzae,* mumps, Coxsackie virus, or echovirus.

II. **Clinical manifestations**

   A. **History.** Seen most commonly in children, the elderly, and others with lowered immunity. Presents with headache, fever, chills, lethargy, vomiting, confusion, convulsions.

   B. **Physical exam.** Nuchal rigidity, **Kernig's sign** (passive resistance to knee extension from flexed thigh position), **Brudzinski's sign** (neck flexion resulting in involuntary knee flexion in supine patient). Meningococcal meningitis is often associated with petechial mucous membrane and skin rashes.

   C. **Diagnostic tests.** Increased peripheral WBC count. Cerebrospinal fluid (CSF) findings vary by etiology (see Table 20-1 for details).

III. **Differential diagnosis.** CSF findings can help differentiate etiological agents. See Table 20-1.

IV. **Pathophysiology**

   A. Entry may be through surgical or traumatic wound, or through inhaled droplets. Gram-positive meningitis may follow an infection of the lungs, middle ear, or sinuses.

   B. Infection in subarachnoid space → inflammatory reaction in pia, arachnoid, and CSF → accumulation of pus or toxin → damage to nerve roots, choroid plexuses, microvasculature, and interference with CSF flow leading to hydrocephalus.

Table 20-1. Differential diagnosis on basis of CSF fluid (see Colorplate D)

Disease type	CSF cell count	Predominant cell type in CSF	Glucose (mg/100 ml)	Protein (mg/100 ml)
Normal	<5	Mononuclear	Two-thirds serum level or ~75	<40
Bacterial meningitis	10–100,000	PMN	5–50	100–1,000
Viral				
Early phase	50–500	PMN	40–75	50–100
Late phase	20–200	Mononuclear	Normal	<100
Tuberculosis	20–1,000	Mononuclear	20–80	50–1,000
Fungal (usually) cryptococcus	25–500	Mononuclear	20–40	25–500

PMN = polymorphonuclear leukocyte.

Parkinson's Disease

I. **Definition.** A progressive neurologic disease affecting primarily the extrapyramidal tracts and characterized by tremor, bradykinesia, rigidity, and festinating gait.

II. **Clinical manifestations.** Begins insidiously with a coarse "pill rolling" resting tremor or "cogwheel rigidity." Gradually other symptoms develop: characteristic masklike facies, festinating gait, bradykinesia, dementia. Symptoms usually respond to antiparkinsonian treatment, but return if drug is withheld. Long-term control is very difficult to obtain.

III. **Differential diagnosis.** Made on basis of clinical picture and response to treatment. Parkinson's tremor must be differentiated from essential tremor (familial; faster [9–11/sec.]; no associated rigidity) and hysterical tremor (increases during stress; decreases during distraction). Always check for phenothiazine usage.

IV. **Pathophysiology**

  A. Etiologies include idiopathic as well as postencephalitic and drug-related causes (phenothiazine, reserpine, manganese, cobalt poisoning).

  B. Final pathway of disease involves decreased levels of dopamine in the basal ganglia due to degeneration of neuronal tracts in the substantia nigra.

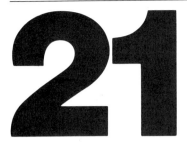

Endocrine Diseases

Diabetes Mellitus

I. **Definition.** A group of chronic systemic diseases caused by insufficient insulin action, due either to a decreased level of insulin production (type I) or to peripheral resistance to its effects (type II).

   A. **Type I** is also known as **insulin dependent** (IDDM), brittle, ketosis-prone, or juvenile-onset diabetes.

   B. **Type II** is also known as **noninsulin dependent** (NIDDM), maturity-onset, late-onset, or adult-onset diabetes. Type II diabetes seen in youths is sometimes called maturity-onset diabetes of youth (MODY).

II. **Clinical manifestations**

   A. **History and physical exam.** Classic of triad of symptoms: **polyphagia, polyuria, and polydypsia.** Additional factors:

   1. **Type I:** age less than 30 years at onset, inattentiveness in school, excessive craving for sweets, increased irritability are all early signs. Onset usually severe and progressive, with anergic lassitude, weight loss. Other symptoms include blurred vision, leg cramps, vomiting. May present in diabetic ketoacidosis (DKA); see **III.C.1**).

   2. **Type II:** common historical clues are: obesity, prior reactive hypoglycemia, history of recurrent soft tissue or mycotic infections, women with vaginitis, and women whose children's birth weight is > 9 lbs. Onset is slow; often presents on screening blood or urine test, without symptoms.

   B. **Lab findings.** Diagnosis of DM can be made in an adult if one of three criteria are met:

   1. Random plasma glucose >200 mg/dl and typical signs and symptoms of diabetes.

   2. Fasting plasma glucose >140 mg/dl on 2 consecutive days.

   3. Plasma glucose >200 mg/dl at 2 hours and at any other time up to 2 hours after ingestion of 75 gm of glucose (called a **glucose tolerance test**).

   Urine glucose can be used as a screening test, and hemoglobin A_1C levels can be used to measure degree of long-standing hyperglycemia.

III. **Pathophysiology.** Usual pathophysiology varies by type.

   A. **IDDM:** decreased or absent insulin production from pancreatic cells, thus decreased serum insulin levels. Autoimmune etiology likely linked to viral infection (e.g., Coxsackie virus). Linked to HLA-DR3 and DR4 antigens.

231

B. NIDDM: decreased or defective insulin receptors on target cells, thus usually increased or normal serum insulin levels. Linked to obesity, family history; also seen in pregnancy (gestational diabetes).

C. Complications. The many long- and short-term complications of DM are the real clinical hallmarks of the disease. You should ask every diabetic about each one.

1. **Diabetic ketoacidosis.** Seen in type I diabetics, when lack of insulin causes a chain of events leading to metabolism of triglycerides and resulting in ketoacids accumulating in the blood. Patients present with 12–24 hours of weakness, polyuria, polydipsia, **Kussmaul's respirations** (rapid, deep breathing), blurred vision, fruity-smelling breath, and abdominal pain and vomiting. They are very dehydrated, and can be in a stupor or coma. Common precipitants include infection, pregnancy, failure to keep to insulin regime, and MI.

2. **Hyperosmolar state.** Seen mainly in elderly patients with type II diabetes and extremely high blood sugars (sometimes more than 2,000 mg/dl). Ketones are absent, and acidosis is mild or not present. Can be triggered by a serious infection, such as pneumonia; GI hemorrhage; some drugs, like thiazide diuretics and steroids; and stress due to surgery. Presents with long prodrome of polyuria and polydipsia, progressing to mental status changes ranging from confusion to stupor to coma. Can present with stroke, seizures, or with other neurologic signs.

3. **Renal failure.** A major problem in both types of diabetes, presenting about 15 years after onset of diabetes. Autopsied kidneys of diabetics show Kimmelstiel-Wilson lesion (nodular glomerulosclerosis) and diffuse hyaline thickening of glomerular basement membrane. Tight blood sugar control and low protein diet may slow renal deterioration.

4. **Neuropathy.** Many presentations, including: bilateral symmetrical sensory deficits, usually seen in a stocking and glove distribution; mononeuropathy caused by infarction of nerves; and impotence and gastroparesis due to involvement of autonomic system.

5. **Retinopathy.** More than half of all diabetics develop proliferative and/or nonproliferative retinopathy within 20 years of onset of their disease. Retinal edema and exudates as well as neovascularization can be seen on ophthalmologic exam. Periodic eye screening should be done for all diabetics, as laser coagulation can slow progress of some retinopathy.

6. **Cardiovascular complications.** Diabetes is linked with increased atherogenesis through a variety of factors, and increases the risk of heart disease by a factor of two in men and three in women. Also, due to neuropathy of the cardiac nerves, many diabetics do not exhibit the characteristic symptoms of MI and thus can have silent but potentially dangerous infarctions.

Thyrotoxicosis
(Hyperthyroidism)

I. **Definition.** Clinical syndrome resulting from excess thyroid hormone.

II. **Clinical manifestations**

A. **History and physical exam.** Findings are outlined by organ system in Table 21-1.

B. **Lab findings.** Elevated T4, low thyroid stimulating hormone (TSH).

Table 21-1. Signs and symptoms of thyrotoxicosis

System	History	Physical exam
Constitutional	Fatigue, hyperactivity, insomnia, heat intolerance, ↑ appetite, weight loss	Hyperkinetism, tremulousness
Vital signs	N/A	Tachycardia, tachypnea, pyrexia, wide pulse pressure
Integument	Sweating, ↑ hair growth, pruritis, occasional urticaria	Warm, moist, fine hair; pretibial myxedema*; onycholysis; hyperpigmentation
Eyes*	Visual disturbance	Lid lag, stare, proptosis,* inflammation, ophthalmoplegia (upward gaze affected first), chemosis, periorbital edema
Neck	Neck mass	Goiter, lymphadenopathy
Cardiovascular	Palpitations, dyspnea	Hyperdynamic precordium, arrhythmias (new onset of atrial fibrillation or tachycardia)
Gastrointestinal	Increasing frequency of bowel movements, diarrhea	Active bowel sounds, splenomegaly*
Genitourinary	Nocturia, oligomenorrhea	N/A
Neuromuscular	Muscle weakness, tremor	Proximal muscle weakness, tremor, brisk deep tendon reflexes
Psychological	Emotional lability, nervousness	N/A

*Specifically characteristic of Graves's disease.

III. Differential diagnosis and pathophysiology. There are several common etiologies of hyperthyroidism.

    A. Graves's disease. TSH-like immunoglobulins stimulate a rise in thyroid hormone.

    B. Toxic multinodular goiter. Multiple autonomous areas of thyroid tissue lead to increased thyroid hormone production.

    C. Toxic adenoma. Overproduction of thyroid hormone by a single "hot" nodule.

    D. Other less common causes include: thyroiditis-related disorders, TSH-like substance production by tumors, trophoblastic tumors, thyroid carcinoma, and iatrogenic etiologies such as excess exogenous thyroid hormone.

Hypothyroidism

  I. Definition. A multiorgan syndrome resulting from inadequate levels of thyroid hormone.

II. Clinical manifestations

A. History. Patients complain of feeling cold, lethargic, depressed, with altered sense of taste and smell; myalgias, arthralgias. Also constipation, weight gain with no increased appetite, and in women heavy bleeding between periods may be noted. Friends or family may note bizarre sense of humor or psychosis. Can present with seizures.

B. Physical exam

1. Cool, coarse, rough, dry skin, with brittle hair and alopecia.

2. Periorbital edema and nonpitting puffiness (myxedema) throughout body.

3. Bradycardia and delayed relaxation phase of deep tendon reflexes.

C. Diagnostic tests. Anemia of multifactorial etiology is present in about one-fourth of patients. Low serum sodium, elevated protein in CSF, low-grade proteinuria, and moderately elevated serum cholesterol and creatine kinase are commonly seen as well. ECG shows low voltage throughout.

III. Differential diagnosis and pathophysiology

A. Hashimoto's thyroiditis is the most common cause of hypothyroidism in the U.S., and is an autoimmune attack on primarily thyroglobulin and thyroid peroxidase. Most commonly affects women 20 to 60 years old and presents with nontender, diffusely enlarged thyroid gland.

B. Iatrogenic hypothyroidism is seen in patients treated with I-131 for thyrotoxicosis, those treated with high-dose external radiation, and psychiatric patients taking lithium.

C. Iodine itself can inhibit the glandular release of thyroid hormone, and thus high doses of iodine can cause hypothyroidism (called the Wolff-Chaikoff effect). Can be seen in patients who have received a high dye load for radiologic procedures.

IV. Complications.
The most serious complication of hypothyroidism is **myxedema coma,** usually brought on by a mild illness or exposure to cold temperature. The risk of myxedema coma is not related to levels of circulating thyroid hormone or to replacement status.

Hypercortisolism
(Cushing's syndrome)

I. Definition.
Metabolic disease caused by glucocorticoid excess.

II. Clinical manifestations

A. History. Weakness, oligomenorrhea, easy bruising, mental changes.

B. Physical exam. Hypertension, purpura, abdominal striae, muscle atrophy; characteristic habitus: central obesity with buffalo hump.

C. Lab findings

1. Increased morning plasma cortisol or urinary 17-OHCS.

2. Osteopenia on x-ray.

III. Differential diagnosis.
There are four major causes of hypercortisolism:

A. Iatrogenic excess of any of several glucocorticoids.

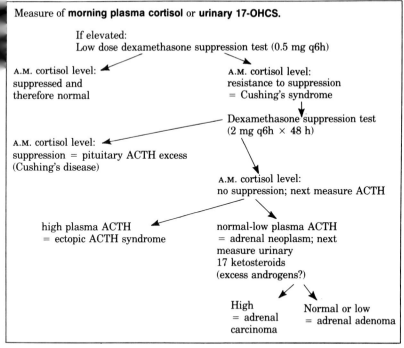

Fig. 21-1. Algorithm of lab work-up for hypercortisolism. ACTH = adrenocortico-tropic hormone.

    B. Hypothalamic-pituitary hyperfunction **(Cushing's disease).**

    C. Ectopic adrenocorticotropic (ACTH) syndrome (causing **bilateral adrenal hyperplasia**).

    D. Unilateral autonomous adrenal hypersecretion (**adrenal adenoma or carcinoma**).

    Fig. 21-1 shows lab work-up to differentiate these.

  IV. Pathophysiology. Varies according to symptom (approximate frequency of symptom shown in parentheses).

    A. Impaired glucose tolerance test (94%). Gluconeogenic effect of cortisol.

    B. Central (truncal) obesity (88%). Increased lipid mobilization, redistribution of adipose stores.

    C. Hypertension (82%). From accompanying mineralocorticoid activity, seen especially in ectopic ACTH syndrome, K^+ wasting.

    D. Oligomenorrhea (72%). Along with decreased fertility and virilism (hirsutism), caused by androgen excess.

    E. Osteoporosis (58%). Antagonism of $1,25(OH)_2$ vitamin D and inhibition of bone cell activation.

    F. Purpura and striae (42%) and **muscle atrophy and weakness** (36%). Caused by catabolic effects of steroids.

Hypocortisolism
(Addison's disease)

I. **Definition.** Syndrome consisting of many nonspecific symptoms caused by adrenal cortical insufficiency.

II. **Clinical manifestations**

    A. **History.** Fatigue, weakness, weight loss, anorexia, irritability, sleeplessness.

    B. **Physical exam.** Hypotension, hyperpigmentation of skin, loss of sexual hair in women.

    C. **Diagnostic tests.** Most common screening test is a **Cortrosyn stimulation test:** if, 30 minutes after administration of synthetic ACTH, serum cortisol remains below 20 µg/dl, adrenal insufficiency is indicated. Diagnosis needs to be confirmed with low levels of 24-hour urinary free cortisol, and diminished serum cortisol after prolonged parenteral administration of ACTH. Reduced serum sodium, increased potassium and BUN, and eosinophilia are seen in many but not all patients.

III. **Differential diagnosis.** Hypocortisolism is seen in syndromes of polyglandular failure (The **multiple endocrine neoplasia** syndromes (MEN I and II). Thus you should look for thyroiditis, DM, pernicious anemia, and hypoparathyroidism in these patients.

IV. **Pathophysiology**

    A. Causes of primary adrenal insufficiency may be autoimmune, infectious, congenital, chemical, ischemic, hemorrhagic, or infiltrative. Specific causes include HIV, TB, tumors, and such drugs as etomidate and ketoconazole.

    B. In patients with hypocortisolism, even very minor illnesses can trigger an **Addisonian crisis,** in which they present with shock, fever, nausea and vomiting, hyperthermia, hypoglycemia, hyponatremia, and hyperkalemia. This is a medical emergency that requires immediate administration of IV glucose, saline, and hydrocortisone, as well as treatment of the underlying causes.

Hypercalcemia

I. **Definition.** An elevation of ionized calcium in serum.

II. **Clinical manifestations**

    A. **History.** Many variable and nonspecific symptoms, generally related to neurologic and neuromuscular function; these include somnolence, apathy, memory loss, mental disturbances, irritability, stupor-coma (c/w acute, pronounced hypercalcemia), and proximal muscle weakness.

    B. **Physical exam.** Findings on exam are rarely helpful. Some associated findings are band keratopathy, hypertension, hypotonia, reduced deep tendon reflexes.

    C. **Diagnostic tests**

        1. **Chemistry.** Calcium levels should be evaluated after correction for amount of serum albumin present. Since albumin binds calcium, the effective (ionized) calcium level is related to albumin concentration. Thus for every 1.0-mg decrease in albumin (normal = 4 mg/dl), you

should add 0.8 mg/dl to the calcium level to get the actual calcium concentration. The reverse is true for hyperalbuminemia. For example:

If **serum calcium** = 7.5 mg/dl and **albumin** = 2.0 mg/dl (decreased by 2 mg/dl),
then the **corrected calcium** = 7.5 + 2(0.8) = 9.1 mg/dl.

Or, if **serum calcium** = 11.0 mg/dl and **albumin** = 5.0 mg/dl (increased by 1 mg/dl),
then the **corrected calcium** = 11.0 − 1(0.8) = 10.2 mg/dl.

2. **ECG** can show shortened Q-T interval, atrial arrythmias, and various AV blocks.

3. **X-ray** indicates soft tissue calcifications.

III. **Differential diagnosis.** Causes include: malignancy (most frequent cause in hospital populations), primary hyperparathyroidism (most frequent in general population), sarcoidosis, vitamin D intoxication, thyrotoxicosis, milk-alkali syndrome, adrenal insufficiency, immobilization, vitamin A intoxication, and pheochromocytoma.

IV. **Pathophysiology**

   A. Malignancies can cause hypercalcemia by several different mechanisms:

   1. **Multiple myeloma.** Osteoclastic activating factor (OAF) production.

   2. **Bone metastases** (e.g., from breast cancer). Direct bone invasion, but increased calcium probably due to local mediator production (e.g., prostaglandins).

   3. **Squamous lung cancer, renal cell cancer.** Ectopic parathyroid hormone (PTH)–like substance produced (pseudohyperparathyroidism).

   B. In **primary hyperparathyroidism,** autonomous production of PTH causes increased calcium. The interaction between the two most important regulators of calcium metabolism, **PTH** and **1,25(OH)$_2$ vitamin D,** is depicted below:

$$\uparrow \text{ renal phosphorus excretion}$$
$$\text{PTH} \rightarrow \quad \uparrow 1,25(OH)_2D \quad \text{production} \rightarrow \uparrow \text{ intestinal } Ca^{2+}$$
$$\text{mobilization}$$
$$\downarrow$$
$$\uparrow \text{ bone mobilization of } Ca^{2+} \text{ [probably synergistic with } 1,25(OH)_2D]$$

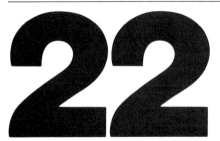

Hematologic Diseases

Bleeding Disorders

I. Definition. Disorders of any element of the hemostatic system that result in an increased tendency to bleed. Dysfunction results from **abnormal hemostatic plug formation (platelet disorder) or clot formation (defect of the coagulation cascade).**

II. Clinical manifestations

A. History and physical exam. In general, in **platelet disorders** there will be a history of bruising or bleeding during the course of another serious illness or after drug ingestion; platelet disorders are rarely hereditary, and a lifelong history of bruising and bleeding is rare. In **coagulation disorders** there will be a lifelong history of easy bruising or bleeding, with a family history of bleeding in one or both sexes.

Platelet disorders result in skin and mucous membrane petechiae, purpura, and ecchymosis, whereas coagulation disorders typically result in deep tissue bleeding (hemarthrosis, subcutaneous and intramuscular hemorrhages, intracerebral hemorrhages).

B. Diagnostic tests

1. **Bleeding time.** Platelet aggregation at the site of vascular injury results in **hemostatic plug** formation. This occurs prior to organized clotting. The bleeding time measures how long it takes a standardized skin incision to stop bleeding. The bleeding time is prolonged in all platelet abnormalities but is normal in coagulation disorders.

2. **Prothrombin time and partial thromboplastin time.** Clot formation results from the activation of the **coagulation cascade.** The cascade involves sequences of plasma protein activations in two pathways. The **intrinsic pathway** begins with activation of factor XII, while the **extrinsic pathway** begins with exposure of plasma to tissue factor, which subsequently forms a complex with factor VII. Both pathways result in the activation of factor X, which then converts prothrombin to thrombin, which in turn converts fibrinogen to fibrin. Thrombin also activates factor XIII, which converts monomer fibrin to stabilized fibrin. See Fig. 22-1 for a diagram of the pathways.

   a. **Partial thromboplastin time** (PTT) measures the ability to form a fibrin clot by the intrinsic pathway. It therefore tests for all factors except factor VII.

   b. **Prothrombin time** (PT) measures the ability to form a fibrin clot by the extrinsic pathway (see Fig. 22-1). A normal PT indicates normal levels of factor VII and those factors common to both the intrinsic and extrinsic pathways (V, X, thrombin, and fibrinogen).

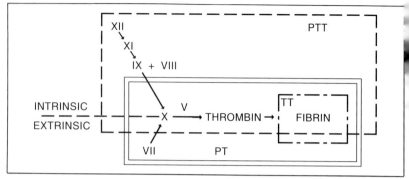

Fig. 22-1. Highly simplified scheme of the coagulation pathways. Shown are the factors involved in the intrinsic *(top)* and extrinsic *(bottom)* pathways. Also depicted by boxes are those aspects of the coagulation system tested by the three most common laboratory tests: thrombin time (TT); partial thromboplastin time (PTT); and prothrombin time (PT). (Modified from M. C. Fishman et al. [13].)

III. Differential diagnosis of common bleeding disorders

A. Platelet disorders

1. Increased destruction

a. Immune mediated

(1) Drug-induced thrombocytopenia.

(2) Idiopathic thrombocytopenia purpura (ITP).

(3) Transfusion reaction.

(4) Fetal-maternal incompatibility.

(5) Vasculitis (e.g., systemic lupus erythematosus).

(6) Lymphoreticular disorders (e.g., chronic lymphocytic leukemia).

b. Nonimmune mediated

(1) Prosthetic heart valves.

(2) Thrombotic thrombocytopenia purpura (TTP).

(3) Sepsis.

(4) Disseminated intravascular coagulation (DIC).

(5) Hemolytic-uremic syndrome.

2. Decreased production

a. Abnormal marrow

(1) Marrow infiltration (e.g., leukemia, lymphoma).

(2) Marrow suppression.

b. Inherited defect in production

(1) Wiskott-Aldrich syndrome.

(2) May-Hegglin anomaly.

c. Vitamin deficiencies

(1) B_{12}.

(2) Folic acid.

   3. Platelet sequestration and pooling (e.g., splenomegaly)

   4. Dilutional, secondary to massive transfusion.

B. Defects of coagulation cascade

   1. Inherited coagulation defects

     a. Classic hemophilia (type A).

     b. Christmas disease (type B).

     c. Von Willebrand's disease.

   2. Acquired coagulation defects

     a. DIC.

     b. Vitamin K deficiency or malabsorption.

     c. Hepatic failure.

IV. Pathophysiology and clinical manifestations of specific bleeding disorders

A. Platelet disorders

   1. ITP

     a. Pathophysiology. Peripheral platelet destruction due to antiplatelet antibody; bone marrow examination reveals normal numbers of megakaryocytes.

     b. Clinical manifestations. Platelets <50,000, petechiae, purpura; predominantly affects pediatric population.

   2. TTP

     a. Pathophysiology. Unknown etiology; microangiopathic hemolytic anemia results in arteriolar occlusion and renal and neurologic dysfunction.

     b. Clinical manifestations. Thrombocytopenic purpura, hemolytic anemia, acute renal failure, fluctuating neurologic signs (headache, seizure, acute psychosis), fever; fibrin split products usually present, suggesting DIC-like syndrome.

   3. Drug-induced thrombocytopenia

     a. Pathophysiology. Thrombocytopenia induced through marrow toxicity or platelet destruction. ETOH and thiazide diuretics suppress bone marrow production of megakaryocytes. Quinine, heparin, methyldopa, and sulfonamides induce an immunologic response that results in peripheral platelet destruction.

     b. Clinical manifestations. Severe, sudden-onset thrombocytopenia and bleeding, which usually resolves after agent discontinued.

B. Inherited coagulation defects

   1. Classic hemophilia (type A)

     a. Pathophysiology. X-linked recessive gene causes either complete inability to produce factor VIII or production of a functionally inactive factor VIII.

     b. Clinical manifestations. Episodic deep tissue bleeding (hemarthrosis, subcutaneous and intramuscular hemorrhages, intracerebral hemorrhages).

   2. Von Willebrand's disease

     a. Pathophysiology. Autosomal dominant inheritance. Disease caused by either a decrease in the amount of von Willebrand's factor (type I) or by synthesis of abnormal forms of the glycoprotein complex (types IIa and IIb). Von Willebrand's factor normally associates with factor VIII and stabilizes it; it is needed for platelet aggregation; and is needed for platelets to attach to injured vascular endothelium. All three functions are compromised in von Willebrand's disease.

    b. Clinical manifestations. Normal platelet count, severe mucous membrane bleeding (epistaxis), easy bruising, and prolonged bleeding from wounds.

C. Acquired coagulation defects

1. DIC

    a. Pathophysiology. Results from widespread activation of coagulation cascade leading to consumption of coagulation factors, prothrombin, and fibrinogen. Accompanying fibrinolysis yields high levels of fibrin split products (FSP), whose antihemostatic properties further enhance bleeding. Secondary to infection (bacterial sepsis), abnormal production or liberation of procoagulant tissue factors (tumors, fat emboli, necrotic tissue, massive acute hemolysis, obstetric catastrophe), and endothelial damage (shock, stroke, burns, acute glomerulonephritis, and Rocky Mountain spotted fever).

    b. Clinical manifestations. Increased fibrin split products; microangiopathic hemolytic anemia; embolic and thrombotic phenomena; prolonged PT and PTT.

2. Vitamin K deficiency or malabsorption

    a. Pathophysiology. Hepatocytes normal but unable to synthesize active form of factors II (prothrombin), VII, IX, X. Factor VII has the shortest half-life among the coagulation factors, and thus prolonged PT is the first evidence of vitamin K deficiency.

    b. Clinical manifestations. Prolonged PT, same clinical picture as that for hemophilia.

3. Hepatic failure

    a. Pathophysiology. Often secondary to ETOH.

    b. Clinical manifestations. Hepatocytes damaged and unable to synthesize coagulation factors II, VII, IX, X; hypoalbuminemia; portal hypertension results in decreased platelets secondary to hypersplenism; same clinical picture as hemophilia.

Anemia

I. Definition. A reduction in the oxygen-carrying capacity of the blood resulting from a decreased concentration of hemoglobin. Anemia results from either **decreased RBC production (deficiency of hematopoietic inputs or bone marrow failure) or peripheral RBC destruction or loss (hemolysis or hemorrhage).**

II. Clinical manifestations

    A. History and physical exam. For history, inquire about family and ethnic history, drug and toxic exposures, obstetric and menstrual history, external blood loss (gastrointestinal and genitourinary), dietary habits, and rapidity of onset.

In physical exam, notice general appearance, vital signs (hypotension, tachycardia), skin (pallor of the conjunctivae, lips, oral mucosa, nail beds; jaundice, petechiae, purpura), mouth (glossitis), heart (listen for flow murmurs, prosthetic valves), abdomen (splenomegaly), rectum (examine stool for occult or gross blood), lymph nodes (infiltrative lesions, infections).

B. Diagnostic tests

    1. Hematocrit and hemoglobin. Concentrations of circulating erythrocytes of Hct <36 percent or Hgb <12 gm/100 ml is considered anemic.

    2. Reticulocyte count. Indicates whether an anemia is due to destruction or loss, or to inadequate production. An anemia with a low or normal reticulocyte count is thought to be due to inadequate production of RBCs in the marrow, while an anemia with a high reticulocyte count is thought to be due to RBC destruction or loss (see Fig. 7-1 for a summary of the diagnostic approach to anemia).

III. Differential diagnosis of anemia

A. Decreased RBC production

    1. Deficiency of hematopoietic inputs

        a. Iron deficiency.

        b. Folate deficiency.

        c. B_{12} deficiency.

        d. Thalassemia.

        e. Anemia of chronic disease.

        f. Sideroblastic anemia.

    2. Bone marrow failure

        a. Drug toxicity (myelosuppressive drugs, chloramphenicol, sulfonamides).

        b. Congenital defect (Fanconi's anemia).

        c. Infections (hepatitis C).

        d. Irradiation.

        e. Neoplasm (leukemia).

        f. Toxins (benzene).

        g. Idiopathic.

B. Peripheral RBC destruction or loss

    1. Acquired hemolysis

        a. Environmental factors

            (1) Autoimmune: isohemagglutinins (transfusion reaction) or autoantibodies (warm and cold).

                (a) Idiopathic.

                (b) Drugs (penicillin, quinidine, methyldopa).

                (c) Underlying disease (SLE, non-Hodgkin's lymphoma, CLL, mycoplasma).

            (2) Nonimmune mediated

                (a) Microangiopathic (DIC, TTP, hemolytic-uremic syndrome, malignant hypertension).

(b) Hypersplenism.

(c) Prosthetic cardiac valve.

(d) Burns.

(e) Infections (malaria).

(f) Drugs (sulfonamides).

(g) Toxins (heavy metals).

b. **Membrane defects**

(1) Paroxysmal nocturnal hemoglobinuria.

(2) Spur-cell anemia.

(3) Wilson's disease.

2. **Congenital hemolysis**

a. **Defects of cell interior**

(1) Hemoglobinopathies (sickle cell anemia, thalassemia).

(2) Enzymopathies (glucose-6-phosphate dehydrogenase, or G-6-P-D).

b. **Membrane defects:** hereditary spherocytosis, elliptocytosis).

3. **Hemorrhage.** Usually acute GI or GU bleed.

IV. **Clinical manifestations and pathophysiology of specific anemias**

A. **Anemias of decreased RBC production**

1. **Iron deficiency**

a. **History and physical exam.** Pallor, fatigue, headaches, glossitis (smooth red tongue), angular cheilitis, koilonychia (spooning of the nails), pica, tachycardia.

b. **Diagnostic tests.** Hypochromic microcytic smear; target cells; anisocytosis and poikilocytosis when severe; ↓ serum ferritin; absent or low serum iron; ↑ total iron binding capacity (TIBC); reticulocytes low or normal; ↓ Hct.

c. **Pathophysiology.** Depletion of iron stores (often due to blood loss), causing defective hemoglobin production.

2. **Megaloblastic anemia**

a. **History and physical exam.** Pallor, anorexia, glossitis; B_{12} deficiency causes neurologic dysfunction (symmetric paresthesias, loss of proprioception, ataxia, psychosis: "megaloblastic madness").

b. **Diagnostic tests.** Macrocytic blood smear, hypersegmented PMNs, Howell-Jolly bodies, macroovalocytes, megablastic marrow with large erythrocyte and leukocyte precursors and abnormal megakaryocytes, low serum B_{12} or folate; Schilling test helps differentiate among the B_{12} deficiency causes of anemia; reticulocyte count low, ↓ Hct.

c. **Pathophysiology.** Faulty erythropoiesis due to ↓ nucleic acid synthesis, secondary to B_{12} or folate deficiency; B_{12} deficiency results from B_{12} intake over long period of time, deficiency of gastric intrinsic factor (pernicious anemia), bacterial overgrowth, or loss of ileal function.

3. **Thalassemias**

   a. **History and physical exam.** Pallor, fatigue, hepatosplenomegaly, facial bossing.

   b. **Diagnostic tests.** Definitive diagnosis by Hgb electrophoresis, microcytic hypochromic blood smear, target cells, ↑ reticulocytes; distinguish thalassemia smear from iron deficiency anemia smear by basophilic stippling and relatively higher Hct in thalassemia.

   c. **Pathophysiology.** Hemoglobinopathy caused by unbalanced alpha- or beta-hemoglobin-chain synthesis, results in alpha-thalassemia or beta-thalassemia. Failure of the alpha- and beta-globin chains to match up reduces the hemoglobinization of erythroblasts to concentrations inadequate for survival, and leads to intracellular accumulations of unmatched chains, which aggregate as inclusion bodies. Most erythroblasts die in the marrow, a process called ineffective erythropoiesis, and those few that make it to the peripheral circulation are unable to slip through the splenic cords, due to the inclusion bodies, and are destroyed.

4. **Marrow aplasia**

   a. **History and physical exam.** Pallor, bleeding, lassitude.

   b. **Diagnostic tests.** Normochromic normocytic anemia on blood smear, pancytopenia, "dry," fatty, hypocellular marrow found on marrow aspiration.

   c. **Pathophysiology.** Depressed hematopoiesis due to drug toxicity in 50 percent of cases (myelosuppressive drugs, chloramphenicol, sulfonamides), congenital defects (Fanconi's anemia), infections (hepatitis C), irradiation, neoplasm (myelophthisis and myelofibrosis), toxins (benzene).

B. **Anemias of RBC destruction or loss.** The four most common causes of RBC destruction are **autoimmune hemolytic anemia, mechanical hemolysis, sickle cell anemia, and G-6-P-D.** Lab findings of all hemolytic anemias include elevated indirect bilirubin, decreased serum haptoglobin, elevated reticulocyte count, and decreased Hct. Following are the clinical manifestations and pathophysiology of selected **anemias of peripheral RBC destruction.**

1. **Hereditary spherocytosis**

   a. **History and physical exam.** Pallor, splenomegaly, jaundice, gallstones, malaise.

   b. **Diagnostic tests.** Spherocytes on blood smear, ↑ osmotic fragility of RBCs, hyperbilirubinemia, elevated mean corpuscular hemoglobin concentration (MCHC).

   c. **Pathophysiology.** Autosomal dominant defect in RBC spectrin causing deficit in surface area relative to volume. The low surface-to-volume ratio creates a slightly obese, rigid structure that lacks the suppleness necessary for transversing through the tight exits of the splenic cords. Stasis in the cords subjects red cells to deficiency of glucose, low pH, O_2 free radicals discharged by the cramped macrophages, and piecemeal loss of lipid bilayer. Each transit through the splenic cords results in ↓ surface area and ↑ rigidity. Eventually the small, unbending spherocyte gets lodged in the splenic cords and is hemolyzed.

2. G-6-P-D deficiency

  a. **History and physical exam.** Pallor; hemolysis is sudden and episodic; jaundice; history of sulfonamide ingestion.

  b. **Diagnostic tests.** Abnormal G-6-P-D assay, polychromatophilia, poikilocytosis.

  c. **Pathophysiology.** Intrinsic RBC defect of G-6-P-D deficiency results in an inability of the RBC to make the reducing agent NADPH. The RBC cannot handle oxidative stresses, and hemolysis results. Sulfonamides are the most common oxidative stress to initiate hemolysis.

3. Sickle cell anemia

  a. **History and physical exam.** Pallor, fatigue, systolic ejection murmur; episodic **sickle cell crises** with fever, pain in back and joints, jaundice, vascular thrombosis, and microinfarction result in leg ulcers, functional asplenism, increased risk of aseptic necrosis of the femoral heads, and salmonella osteomyelitis; chronic hemolysis results in increased incidence of pigmented gallstones.

  b. **Diagnostic tests.** Definitive diagnosis by sickle test and Hgb electrophoresis; blood smear shows sickled cells, fragmented forms, target cells.

  c. **Pathophysiology.** Hemoglobinopathy caused by valine replacement of glutamate at the sixth position of the beta-hemoglobin chain. The altered hemoglobin, called hemoglobin S, has a strong tendency to form long crystalline aggregates when deoxygenated. These aggregates cause the RBC to assume the abnormal sickle shape. These sickled cells are then destroyed in the periphery. Intravascular sickling causes vascular sludging and thrombosis, which produces gradual but widespread tissue infarction.

4. Autoimmune hemolytic anemias

  a. **Warm-reacting antibodies**

   (1) **History and physical exam.** History of drug ingestion or underlying disease. Pallor, jaundice, hepatosplenomegaly, thrombophlebitis.

   (2) **Diagnostic tests.** Direct Coombs' test establishes the presence of bound immunoglobulin or complement on a patient's erythrocytes by demonstrating agglutination of the erythrocytes with either anti-immunoglobulin or anticomplement antibody. Blood smear shows spherocytes.

   (3) **Pathophysiology.** Most common of immune mediated hemolytic anemias. Warm-reacting antibodies have maximal effect above 31°C and are IgG antibodies. Thirty percent of autoimmune anemias are idiopathic, and 30 percent result from drug reactions. Drugs implicated include penicillin and quinidine. Penicillin attaches to the RBC membrane and serves as a hapten against which antibodies can be directed. Quinidine stimulates the production of antibodies, and drug-antibody complexes attach nonspecifically to the surface of RBCs, at which point the complement cascade is activated and hemolysis occurs. This is the most common mechanism of drug-induced hemolytic anemia. Underlying disease, such as infection (mycoplasma, Epstein-Barr virus) and lymphoproliferative disorders (CLL), have also been implicated in the formation of warm antibodies. Spherocytosis

results from the ability of the IgG to opsonize the RBC and from partial phagocytosis by the reticuloendothelial system. Progressive loss of erythrocyte membrane renders it rigid, and it assumes a spherical shape.

b. Cold-reacting antibodies

(1) History and physical exam. Pain and ulceration in chilled areas of the body, usually toes and fingers.

(2) Diagnostic tests. Diagnosis made by high titer of cold agglutinins (IgM) and low C_3.

(3) Pathophysiology. Cold-reacting antibodies have maximal effect below 31°C, are called cold agglutinins, and are IgM antibodies. Because IgM is multivalent, either hemolysis (due to complement activation) or agglutination of RBCs may dominate the clinical picture. Usually there is agglutination of RBCs resulting in vascular occlusion in the cold distal extremities. Hemolysis is highly variable, because although complement is activated, the cascade is interrupted when red cells coated with C_3 in the cool regions of the peripheral circulation return to the warm central regions where the warmed IgM rapidly dissociates and C_3 is inactivated. Cold-reacting antibodies can occur in patients with lymphoproliferative disease or infections (mycoplasma, falciparum malaria, Epstein-Barr virus), or they may be idiopathic.

Leukemias

I. **Definition.** A heterogeneous group of WBC malignancies resulting in either a rapidly progressive accumulation of immature leukocytes **(acute leukemias)** or a somewhat more indolent overgrowth by relatively mature leukocytes **(chronic leukemias).**

II. **Clinical manifestations and differential diagnosis**

A. **Acute leukemias**

1. The **clinical features** of acute lymphocytic leukemia (ALL) and acute myelogenous leukemia (AML) are compared in Table 22-1.

2. **Pathophysiology**

a. **ALL.** CNS prophylaxis crucial; CNS and testicle are "sanctuaries" for leukemic cells. Most lymphoblasts are "null" cells; T-cell ALL has worse prognosis than null-cell ALL. At least 30–50 percent of patients have chromosome abnormality in leukemic cells.

b. **AML.** DIC, leukostasis, and intracranial bleeds are common complications.

B. **Chronic leukemias**

1. The **clinical features** of chronic lymphocytic leukemia (CLL) and chronic myelogenous leukemia (CML) are compared in Table 22-2.

2. **Pathophysiology**

a. **CLL.** Malignant cell usually monoclonal B lymphocyte with defective IgG production; ↓ immune defense, so infection common; hemolytic anemia a frequent complication. Mean survival after clinical onset is 7–8 years.

Table 22-1. Clinical manifestations of acute leukemias

	Acute lymphocytic leukemia	Acute myelogenous leukemia
History	Major childhood malignancy (rare in adults), recurrent infections, weakness, bleeding, anemia, lymphadenopathy	Exposure to radiation, chemicals, viruses; recurrent infection; weakness; bleeding; anemia; lymphadenopathy. AML is uncommon.
Physical exam	Pallor, fever, ecchymoses, adenopathy, hepatosplenomegaly	Similar to ALL, but less adenopathy and hepatosplenomegaly
Diagnostic tests	↑ WBC, ↑ lymphocytes (especially immature forms), anemia, ↓ platelets, ↑ uric acid	Anemia, ↓ platelets, moderately ↑ WBC (usually myeloblasts), ↑ uric acid, abnormal LFT; 50% of patients have **Auer rods** in myeloblasts (pathognomonic); peroxidase ⊕ cytoplasmic granules often found in malignant cells

Table 22-2. Clinical manifestations of chronic leukemias

	Chronic lymphocytic leukemia	Chronic myelogenous leukemia
History	Highest prevalence of any leukemia; old age (usually >60), fatigue, weight loss, anorexia, pallor, fever, splenomegaly	2:1 male-female ratio; middle age, fatigue, weight loss, anorexia, pallor, fever, splenomegaly
Physical exam	Pallor, tachycardia, hepatosplenomegaly	Lymphadenopathy, hepatosplenomegaly
Diagnostic tests	Often extremely ↑ WBC (especially mature small lymphocytes)	↑ WBC, basophilia, mild anemia; 90% of patients have Philadelphia chromosome; usually low leukocyte alkaline phosphatase values

      b. CML. Chronic disease usually lasts 2–5 years, followed by **blast crisis,** in which mature myelocytes are replaced by immature myeloblasts, promyeloblasts, and/or lymphoblasts, with survival time of 6 months. Mean survival after diagnosis is 3–4 years.

III. Pathophysiology

    A. Cytokinetics of leukemic cells involve slow, incomplete, or defective maturation; longer-than-average cell survival time; lack of control by normal hematopoietic feedback systems.

    B. Etiology unknown; major speculations include viral agents, defective DNA repair, oncogenes.

23

Solid Tumors

The most important event in determining the success of cancer therapy is the initial management decision. *Treatment goals must be clearly defined.* If cure is the goal, then bold steps may be taken, but if palliation is the goal, then the treatment should be designed to relieve symptoms while producing as few as possible.

Samuel Hellman, M.D.

Cancer (Ca) is second only to heart disease as a leading cause of death in the United States. Fig. 23-1 shows the most common types of primary cancers in men and women, by incidence, and Fig. 23-2 shows the most common causes of death from cancer. Table 23-1 gives the most common source of metastases to several organs.

Colorectal Carcinoma

I. **Definition.** Colorectal Ca is the second most common cause (after lung cancer) of cancer deaths in the U.S. In 1990 more than 150,000 Americans developed adenocarcinoma of the large bowel, and more than 60,000 died from it. The male-female ratio is 1:1; peak incidence is in patients older than 60.

II. **Clinical manifestations**

  A. **History and physical exam.** Common presentations include change in bowel habits, abdominal pain, tenesmus, weight loss, fatigue, hemorrhoids, blood per rectum, change in stool caliber or color. Risk factors include history of ulcerative colitis, familial polyposis, Gardner's syndrome, family history of colonic cancer, and perhaps low-fiber diets and long bowel transit times.

  B. **Diagnostic tests** include tests for occult stool blood, barium enema, low hematocrit. Carcinoembryonic antigen (CEA) may be elevated, especially in patients with metastases.

III. **Pathophysiology**

  A. Fifty percent of lesions are found in the rectum, 20 percent in the sigmoid, 16 percent in the cecum; usually **adenocarcinoma.** In recent years there has been an increase in the proportion of tumors found in the right colon.

  B. **Adenomatous polyps** may be premalignant precursor; sessile polyps have higher incidence of invasive malignant foci than pedunculated polyps.

  C. Table 23-2 shows the different staging systems used with colorectal cancer, and the associated 5-year survival rates.

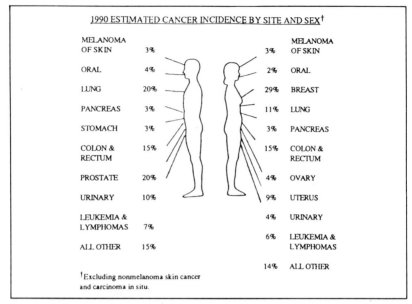

Fig. 23-1. Cancer incidence by site and sex (excluding nonmelanoma skin cancer and carcinoma in situ). (Reproduced with permission from American Cancer Society's Department of Epidemiology and Statistics, *Ca: A Cancer Journal for Clinicians* 40(1):9, 1990.)

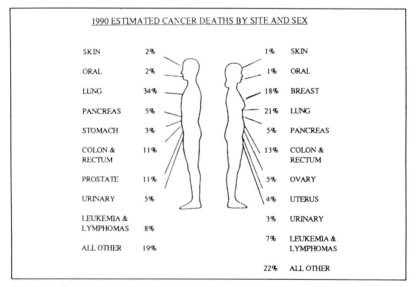

Fig. 23-2. Cancer deaths by site and sex. (Reproduced with permission from American Cancer Society's Department of Epidemiology and Statistics, *Ca: A Cancer Journal for Clinicians* 40(1):9, 1990.)

Table 23-1. The most common sources of metastases to several organs

Metastases	Common primary tumors
Bone	Breast, lung, prostate, thyroid, kidney
Brain	Lung, breast, melanoma, GU tract, colon
Liver	Colon, stomach, pancreas, breast, lymphoma
Lung	Breast, colon, kidney, testis, stomach

Table 23-2. Staging and prognosis of colorectal cancer

Classification			
Dukes	Modified Astwood-Coller	Description	5-year survival rate
A	A	Lesion limited to mucosa; nodes negative	80%
B	B_1	Extension of lesion through mucosa but still within bowel wall; nodes negative	70%
	B_2	Extension through the entire bowel wall (including serosa); nodes negative	60–65%
C	C_1	Lesion limited to bowel wall; nodes positive	35–45%
	C_2	Extension of lesion through entire bowel wall (including serosa); nodes positive	15–30%

Breast Cancer

I. **Definition.** Breast cancer is the most common malignant tumor found in nonsmoking American women; more than 150,000 cases of breast cancer are diagnosed in American women each year, and over 40,000 die each year of the disease. The American Cancer Society estimates that the average American woman has a one in nine chance of getting breast cancer in her lifetime.

II. **Clinical manifestations**

   A. **History and physical exam.** Painless breast mass, nipple discharge, erythema, dimpling of breast skin, axillary and supraclavicular adenopathy. Risk factors include family history, high-fat diet (increased steroid precursors?). Nulliparous and late first pregnancy women may be at increased risk. Unclear whether oral contraceptives are risk factors.

   B. **Diagnostic tests.** Mammography, CXR, bone scans, LFTs, CEA titer, biopsy (with estrogen receptor protein-level analysis).

III. **Differential diagnosis.** Breast carcinoma must be differentiated from benign breast masses, which include polycystic breast disease and fibrocystic changes (adenofibromas). More than 80 percent of breast masses are benign. In contrast to malignancy, benign conditions are often well delineated and mobile, without signs of retraction. While mammography is often helpful, **biopsy results are definitive.**

Table 23-3. Clinical stage vs. survival rate for breast cancer

Stage		Survival (%)	
		2 yr	5 yr
I	Tumor < 2 cm	95%	82%
II	Tumor 2–5 cm; regional nodes ⊕ or ⊖	89%	63%
III	Tumor > 5 cm, or extensions to other structures; regional nodes ⊕ or ⊖	70%	42%
IV	Distant metastases	22%	< 10%

IV. **Pathophysiology**

   A. **Histologically,** 75 percent are classified as **ductal adenocarcinomas;** other types include lobular, medullary, and colloid carcinomas.

   B. **Staging and prognosis** are shown in Table 23-3.

   C. Usual routes of **metastasis:**

   1. Regional metastasis by way of axillary and internal mammary lymph node chains.

   2. Distant metastases (lymphatic and hematogenous) to bones, lungs, liver.

Lung Cancer

I. **Definition.** Lung cancer represents 20 percent of cancers in American men, 11 percent of cancers in American women. It is the most common fatal cancer in the U.S. for both sexes. More than 160,000 cases were diagnosed in 1991, and approximately 90 percent of these patients will go on to die of their disease.

II. **Clinical manifestations**

   A. **History and physical exam**

   1. **Etiologic risk factors** include **cigarettes,** asbestos, radiation, industrial chemicals (e.g., nickel, chromate), and perhaps high endogenous concentrations of aryl hydrocarbon hydroxylase in bronchial epithelium.

   2. **Findings** depend on location and extent of tumor. Common presentations for endobronchial tumor include: weight loss, cough, wheezing, hemoptysis, dyspnea, and increased sputum production (positive cytology may be diagnostic). Chest pain or pleural effusion suggests extension to pleura and chest wall. Vena cava obstruction and tracheal-esophageal symptoms common if tumor invades mediastinum.

   3. **Paraneoplastic syndromes,** including endocrine, neurologic, connective-tissue, and cutaneous manifestations are also common, especially with small cell carcinoma.

   B. **Lab findings.** Important tests include comparison of current CXR with old films, chest CT, sputum cytology, tuberculin and fungal skin tests to rule out infectious cause of findings, and fiberoptic bronchoscopy.

Table 23-4. Clinical features of lung cancer and granulomas

Feature	Bronchogenic carcinoma	Granuloma (tuberculosis, histoplasmosis, coccidiomycosis)
Epidemiology	Smoker over age 35	Any age; geographic background important
Constitutional and respiratory symptoms	Cough, hemoptysis, wheeze, weight loss	Often absent
CXR appearance of coin lesion	Stellate border, not calcified; lesion doubles in size in 37–465 days	Calcified, with sharp margins; radiographically unchanged over 2-year period *or* grows more rapidly or slowly than carcinoma limits

III. **Differential diagnosis.** Most important differential Dx is between malignancy and benign processes (most commonly granulomas) that appear as coin lesions on CXR. Table 23-4 highlights the differences between lung cancer and granulomas.

IV. **Pathophysiology**

  A. Lung Ca is classified histologically into four types:

    1. **Squamous** or **epidermoid** (30–40 percent).

    2. **Adenocarcinoma** (30–40 percent).

    3. **Small cell,** or oat cell (20 percent).

    4. **Giant cell** (5–15 percent).

  B. **Small cell cancer** may be different from the other types, since it may arise from neuroectodermal cells. These cells contain neurosecretory granules and active aromatic amines, and may secrete a variety of bioactive polypeptides and amines. It is the most rapidly fatal of the cell types if untreated (5-year survival < 1 percent), but it is also the most responsive to chemotherapy.

  C. **Metastases** (lymphatic and hematogenous spread) occur early, most often to bones, lymphoreticular system, central nervous system, liver, and skin.

Prostate Cancer

I. **Definition.** Prostate Ca accounts for a significant number of malignancies in older men, with incidence increasing with age after about age 50. The vast majority of cases are adenocarcinoma. In 1991 more than 120,000 men were diagnosed with this disease, and more than 30,000 died of it.

II. **Clinical manifestations**

  A. **History.** Usually asymptomatic early in the course of disease. Later presents with symptoms of bladder outlet obstruction, hematuria, pyuria. Metastases to bones and lungs can cause severe pain.

B. Physical exam. Firm, nodular, irregular prostate felt on digital rectal exam.

C. Diagnostic tests

1. **Acid phosphatase** can be used as a marker for extracapsular spread, but is neither very sensitive nor specific.

2. **Prostate-specific antigen** (PSA) may be effective as a screening test, and can be used as a marker of disease progression.

3. **Ultrasound or CT** may be useful in confirming the dimensions and nature of the mass.

III. **Differential diagnosis.** With symptoms of bladder obstruction, the most common differential is between benign prostatic hypertrophy (BPH) and malignancy. BPH can also present with elevated PSA or acid phosphatase.

The differential of induration or a nodule felt on the prostate includes granulomatous prostatitis (including prostatic TB) and prostatic calculi, as well as malignancy.

IV. **Pathophysiology**

A. More than 30 percent of men over the age of 70 have microscopic prostate Ca found on autopsy.

B. American Urological Staging System

A—occult Ca found incidentally on microscopic exam
B—palpable tumor limited to prostate
C—local extracapsular spread
D—distant metastases

Pancreatic Cancer

I. **Definition.** Adenocarcinoma of the pancreas is the second most common GI tumor. It occurs more commonly in men, is seen primarily in the elderly, and is almost always fatal (overall 5-year survival rate is less than 2 percent).

II. **Clinical manifestations**

A. History. Pancreatic cancer can present in many ways, usually with vague, nonspecific symptoms. Abdominal pain (dull epigastric ache radiating to the back), malaise, weight loss, and depression are all presenting complaints. Frequently, patient can obtain relief from pain by bending forward, by assuming fetal position, or by taking aspirin.

B. Physical exam. More than half of patients are jaundiced from common bile duct obstruction. Infrequently one can see Courvoisier's sign (palpable, distended gallbladder).

C. Diagnostic tests

1. **Serum chemistry.** Fewer than 20 percent have elevated serum amylase. Elevated alkaline phosphatase, bilirubin, CEA can be seen in some patients.

2. **Radiology.** In most cases diagnosis can be made by viewing the pancreas with ultrasound, CT, or, more rarely, endoscopic retrograde cholangiopancratography (ERCP) to view ducts.

Brain Tumors

I. **Definition.** The term *brain tumor* encompasses a large number of different intracranial neoplasms. They can occur at any age but are most common in the early adult or middle years of life. Common primary childhood tumors include astrocytomas, medulloblastomas, and gliomas. Common adult tumors include meningiomas, gliomas, and astrocytomas. Metastases to the brain are commonly seen in patients with bronchogenic carcinoma, adenocarcinoma of the breast, and malignant melanoma.

II. **Clinical manifestations**

   A. **History and physical exam**

   1. General symptoms resulting from increasing intracranial pressure include headache, vomiting, change in mental status, weakness, and papilledema.

   2. Specific symptoms relate to localized effects on the brain and vary according to site of tumor. These include focal or generalized seizures, hemiplegia, mental changes, visual changes, cranial nerve signs.

   B. **Diagnostic tests.** Magnetic resonance imaging (MRI) is preferred over CT for imaging many brain tumors.

III. **Differential diagnosis.** An expanding intracranial lesion can be a neoplasm, granuloma, parasitic cyst, hemorrhage, aneurysm, or abscess.

·

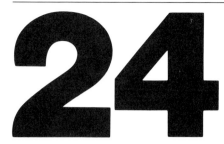

HIV and AIDS

Definitions

I.

A. Human immunodeficiency virus, type 1 (HIV-1) is a human RNA retrovirus that infects helper T cells (called T4 cells or CD4 cells) and other cells bearing the CD4 surface marker. Infection leads to lymphopenia, CD4 lymphocyte deficiency and dysfunction, impaired cell-mediated immune response, and polyclonal B-cell activation with impaired B-cell response to new antigens. This immune derangement gives rise to AIDS.

B. Acquired immune deficiency syndrome (AIDS) is a secondary immunodeficiency syndrome caused by HIV-1 and characterized by severe dysfunction of the immune system, resulting in opportunistic infections and malignancies in individuals without prior immunologic abnormality.

A patient's being HIV positive is neither necessary nor sufficient for a diagnosis of AIDS, according to Centers for Disease Control (CDC) criteria. The exact diagnosis depends on the laboratory evidence of HIV infection, as well as the presence of a number of "indicator diseases."

1. With definitive serologic laboratory evidence of HIV infection, AIDS is an acceptable diagnosis if one of the indicator diseases is diagnosed definitively or presumptively.

2. Without definitive serologic laboratory evidence of HIV infection, AIDS is an acceptable diagnosis in the absence of other causes of immunodeficiency and the definitive diagnosis of one of the indicator diseases.

3. With definitive serologic laboratory evidence against HIV infection, AIDS is still an acceptable diagnosis if there is an absence of other causes of immunodeficiency, there is the definitive diagnosis of one of the indicator diseases, and the T4 lymphocyte count is less than 400/mm.

4. The list of indicator diseases is different for each of the above categories, and the CDC changes them periodically.

C. AIDS-related complex (ARC) is a term used to describe individuals with symptoms of HIV infection but not yet diagnosed with AIDS-defining illness. Clinical picture includes recurrent oral candidiasis, lymphadenopathy, weight loss, fever, night sweats, chronic diarrhea, fatigue, lymphopenia, and skin anergy. ARC usually occurs in the middle stage of infection, but may occur earlier, later, or not at all.

II. Clinical manifestations

A. History

1. Patient belongs to a **major risk group.** Those at risk include persons who have had sexual contact with infected individuals, IV drug abusers, recipients of infected blood products, and children born to HIV-

infected mothers. The following demographics describe HIV-positive individuals in the United States as of 1991.

    a. The **adult** HIV-positive population: 66 percent are homosexual/bisexual men, 17 percent are IV drug abusers, 8 percent are homosexual male IV drug abusers, 4 percent contracted HIV through heterosexual contact, 2 percent through a transfusion, 1 percent have hemophilia or another coagulation disorder, and for 3 percent of cases the method of transmission is unknown.

        (1) New cases are showing larger percentages of heterosexual men, and women and children.

        (2) Fifty percent of heterosexually acquired HIV results from sexual contact with an IV drug abuser.

    b. The **pediatric** HIV-positive population: 79 percent have a parent with AIDS or are at an increased risk for AIDS; 13 percent of cases are transfusion associated; 6 percent have hemophilia or another coagulation disorder; for 3 percent the cause is unknown.

        (1) Forty to 50 percent of babies born to infected mothers become infected perinatally, either in utero, postpartum through exposure to HIV-tainted blood during delivery, or through breast feeding.

  2. Patient has history of having been exposed to HIV via one of the three **modes of transmission:** sexual, parenteral, perinatal.

  3. Patient is at occupational risk for contracting HIV (exposure to secretions).

  4. A detailed sexual history should always be obtained if HIV is suspected. (Ask: What is your sexual orientation? Are you a bisexual? Have you been sexually intimate with a bisexual or an IV drug abuser?)

B. Physical exam. Clinical manifestations vary according to stage of illness.

  1. Clinical manifestations seen during **acute infection:**

    a. Acute retroviral syndrome: mononucleosis-like syndrome may appear 2–6 weeks after infection in 50 percent of patients, other 50 percent asymptomatic.

        (1) Common: fever, night sweats, myalgia, anorexia, nausea, arthralgia, headache, photophobia, diarrhea, pharyngitis, lymphadenopathy, and maculopapular rash.

        (2) Uncommon: acute meningoencephalitis and peripheral neuropathy.

  2. Clinical manifestations seen during **early infection:**

    a. Asymptomatic: 1–8 years.

    b. **Dermatologic manifestations:** molluscum contagiosum, recurrent herpes zoster, persistent mucocutaneous herpes simplex, seborrheic dermatitis resistant to therapy.

  3. Clinical manifestations seen during the **middle stage** of infection:

    a. Persistent generalized lymphadenopathy (50–70 percent of all HIV-positive patients): presence of two or more extrainguinal sites of lymphadenopathy for a minimum of 3–6 months without another cause; common sites are anterior cervical and axillary.

    b. Oral lesions: thrush, hairy leukoplakia, aphthous ulcers.

c. Hematologic manifestations: idiopathic thrombocytopenic purpura (5–15 percent of HIV-positive individuals), normocytic normochromic anemia, and leukopenia.

d. ARC is manifested in this stage.

4. Clinical manifestations seen in the **late stage** of HIV infection. **AIDS-defining illnesses** manifesting themselves include:

a. Opportunistic infections: viral, bacterial, mycobacterial, fungal, protozoal.

b. AIDS-related neoplasms.

c. HIV wasting syndrome ("slim disease"): >10 percent involuntary weight loss and chronic diarrhea or chronic weakness and fever.

d. HIV encephalopathy: occurs in 50 percent of patients, progresses from impaired memory, inability to concentrate, and behavioral changes to motor dysfunction, ataxia, incontinence, and severe global impairment.

5. **Disease progression**

a. Seroconversion to HIV-positive status occurs approximately 4–12 weeks after exposure.

b. 50 percent of HIV-positive individuals progress to AIDS after a mean incubation period of 8–10 years, and 90 percent within 13 years.

c. A T4 count of less than 200/mm predicts that the patient is likely to develop AIDS within 1–2 years.

d. Once diagnosed with AIDS, 50 percent of patients die within 1 year, and 80 percent die within 2 years.

C. **Diagnostic tests**

1. Definitive diagnosis of HIV positivity: two positive ELISA and one positive Western blot.

a. Positive predictive value of ELISA depends on prevalence of HIV in the population (see Chap. 6).

b. Lab results for the three stages of HIV infection are shown in Table 24-1.

III. **Differential diagnosis of indicator diseases (opportunistic infections and neoplasms)**

A. **Viral infections**

1. **Cytomegalovirus (CMV)**

a. **Clinical manifestations:** chorioretinitis (5–10 percent of all AIDS patients), esophagitis, interstitial pneumonia, enterocolitis, bone marrow suppression, necrotizing adrenalitis.

b. **Diagnostic methods:** histopathologic evidence of infected tissue or CMV culture, characteristic findings on fundoscopic exam.

2. **Herpes simplex virus (HSV)**

a. **Clinical manifestations:** large, atypical, persistent oral, genital, or perianal mucocutaneous ulceration; esophagitis; interstitial pneumonia.

b. **Diagnostic methods:** Tzank smear, tissue biopsy, or HSV culture.

Table 24-1. Laboratory findings in HIV infection

Stage	Serologic markers	T4 lymphocytes
Acute infection	P-24 antigen positive, HIV ELISA negative	> 400 cells/mm
Early infection	P-24 antigen negative, HIV ELISA positive	> 400 cells/mm
Middle stage	HIV ELISA positive, T-cell ratio reversal (T4/T8 goes from 2:1 to less than 1:1)	100–400 cells/mm
Late stage	HIV ELISA positive or negative, depending on the amount of immune dysfunction	< 100 cells/mm

3. **Epstein-Barr virus (EBV)**

   a. **Clinical manifestations:** hairy leukoplakia, usually occurring late in the disease course.

   b. **Diagnostic method:** EBV culture.

4. **Jakob-Creutzfeldt (JC) virus**

   a. **Clinical manifestations:** progressive multifocal leukoencephalopathy (PML), which presents with altered mental status, vision loss, limb weakness, abnormalities of gait, and focal neurologic deficits.

   b. **Diagnostic methods:** brain biopsy; CT scan showing nonenhancing hypodense lesion without mass effect; MRI is most sensitive.

B. **Bacterial infections**

1. **Syphilis**

   a. **Clinical manifestations:** natural history accelerated by HIV infection, reactivation of previously treated disease, active disease with negative serology, asymptomatic neurosyphilis, and relapse after standard therapy are all commonly seen.

   b. **Diagnostic methods:** RPR, FTA-ABS, and Venereal Disease Research Laboratory (VDRL) tests; due to immunodeficiency, many HIV-positive patients who have syphilis will be seronegative.

2. **Bacterial pneumonias**

   a. **Clinical manifestations:** recurrent lobar pneumonia due to encapsulated organisms (*S. pneumoniae, H. influenzae,* group B *Streptococcus*).

   b. **Diagnostic methods:** sputum culture, bronchoalveolar lavage (BAL) if needed.

C. **Mycobacterial infections**

1. ***Mycobacterium tuberculosis***

   a. **Clinical manifestations:** miliary, extrapulmonary, disseminated disease much more prevalent than in the general population, and typical apical or cavitary lesions much more uncommon; usually presents as lower lobe infiltrates or hilar adenopathy (butterfly pattern).

   b. **Diagnostic methods:** Ziehl-Neelsen or immunofluorescent stain of sputum exhibiting acid-fast bacilli, or biopsy of tissue from an extrapulmonary site (liver, lymph node, brain); purified protein derivative (PPD) rarely positive in advanced stages of AIDS.

   2. ***M. avium intracellulare***

    a. Clinical manifestations: present in 50 percent of AIDS patients; usually seen in advanced stages of HIV disease as one of a group of concurrent infections, associated with wasting syndrome (fever, night sweats, weight loss, weakness, and chronic diarrhea); typically causes disease of the GI tract, liver, and bone marrow.

    b. Diagnostic methods: Ziehl-Neelsen or immunofluorescent stain of stool, liver, or bone marrow tissue exhibiting acid-fast bacilli.

D. Fungal infections

  1. *Candida albicans*

    a. Clinical manifestations: persistent oral thrush, esophagitis, and vaginitis.

    b. Diagnostic methods: Potassium hydroxide (KOH) prep for oral thrush and vaginitis; endoscopy with biopsy showing mucosal invasion for esophagitis.

  2. *Cryptococcus neoformans*

    a. Clinical manifestations: most common cause of fungal central nervous system disease in patients with AIDS; 15 percent of all AIDS patients will develop cryptococcal infection during course of disease. Classic presentation of cryptococcal meningitis includes mild headache and fever, malaise, no meningismus, minimal abnormalities in CSF; atypical presentation includes fulminant, disseminated disease manifested by extraneural involvement in blood, skin, lung, liver, spleen, bone, and CNS. Relapse is common with both presentations.

    b. Diagnostic methods: demonstrate organisms in CSF with India ink stain, CSF culture, or presence of cryptococcal antigen in CSF or blood.

  3. *Histoplasma capsulatum*

    a. Clinical manifestations: important pathogen in endemic areas (Ohio River Valley) presents disseminated with septicemia.

    b. Diagnostic methods: tissue biopsy or bone marrow aspiration.

  4. *Coccidioides immitis*

    a. Clinical manifestations: found in areas of American Southwest; influenzalike illness with fever and cough, 10 percent with erythema nodosum.

    b. Diagnostic methods: characteristic spherules from tissue biopsy.

  5. *Pneumocystis carinii* pneumonia

    a. Clinical manifestations: the most common opportunistic infection in patients with AIDS and the leading cause of mortality; 60 percent of HIV-positive patients will have *P. carinii* pneumonia (PCP) as the AIDS-defining illness, and 80 percent of all AIDS patients will have PCP sometime during course of illness. There is a 20–40 percent mortality rate per episode of PCP, and 65 percent of the cases will recur within 18 months of first PCP infection. Classic presentation is fever, dyspnea, and nonproductive cough, with diffuse bilateral interstitial infiltrates on chest film; atypical presentation is a mild, prolonged course, normal to minimal fever, nonproductive cough, normal chest film, and abnormal gallium scan.

    b. Diagnostic methods: demonstrate presence of organism in tissue by indirect immunofluorescent stain of induced sputum, washings from bronchoalveolar lavage and brush biopsy, or transbronchial biopsy.

E. Protozoal infections

  1. *Toxoplasmosa gondii*

    a. Clinical manifestations: present in 30 percent of individuals with AIDS; typically causes multiple CNS lesions, which range in presentation from mild headache and fever to focal neurologic deficits with profound encephalopathy, seizures, and coma. On CT scan, multiple bilateral ring-enhancing lesions found in the deep gray matter and basal ganglia. Relapse is common.

    b. Diagnostic methods: brain biopsy to demonstrate organism.

  2. *Cryptosporidium* and *Isospora belli*

    a. Clinical manifestations: chronic diarrhea.

    b. Diagnostic methods: send stool for ova/parasites, leukocytes, culture.

F. Neoplasms

  1. Kaposi's sarcoma

    a. Clinical manifestations: most common neoplasm in persons with AIDS; found in 40 percent of homosexuals with AIDS, compared with 10 percent of heterosexuals with AIDS. Nodular pigmented skin lesions with red-violet coloring; not limited to skin—can occur internally in the lungs, GI tract, brain, and lymph nodes. A single intracranial CNS lesion is most likely Kaposi's sarcoma or primary lymphoma.

    b. Diagnostic methods: biopsy of involved site.

  2. Non-Hodgkin's lymphoma

    a. Clinical manifestations: after Kaposi's, the second most common neoplasm found in AIDS patients. Unlike in general population, lymphoma in AIDS patients is often extranodal, B cell in type, and high grade, and responds less favorably to therapy. CT scan usually shows primary CNS lymphoma as a single intracranial lesion in the white matter and periventricular area, with weak enhancement and mass effect; histologic type is most often noncleaved cell (resembling Burkitt's lymphoma); lymphoma often involves intra-abdominal sites.

    b. Diagnostic methods: lymph node aspiration or biopsy of tissue from extranodal site.

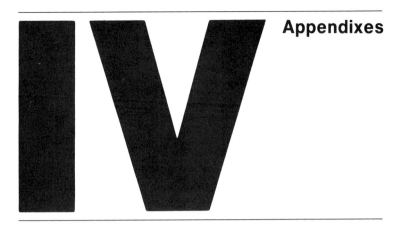

Appendixes

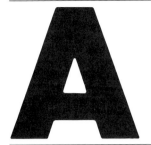

Clinical Signs

While on the wards, you will hear mentioned many clinical signs that have been named for the physicians who first described them or the phenomena they resemble. Following is a list of some of the most commonly mentioned signs. This list is meant to be used as a reference; however, we have starred (*) those signs that would be worth learning before you start on the wards.

* **Argyll Robertson pupil:** miotic pupil that responds normally to accommodation but not to light; associated with neurosyphilis.
* **Babinski reflex:** dorsiflexion of the big toe after stimulation of the lateral sole; associated with corticospinal tract lesions.
  Bagpipe sign: when patient cuts short a forced expiration while the stethoscope is on the chest, the sound of expelling air is heard to continue after his or her effort has ceased; associated with partial bronchial obstruction.
  Ballet's sign: external ophthalmoplegia, with loss of voluntary eye movements; the pupillary movements and reflex eye movements are intact; associated with Graves's disease and hysteria.
  Battle's sign: discoloration in the line of the posterior auricular artery, the ecchymosis first appearing near the top of the mastoid process; associated with basilar skull fracture.
* **Beck's triad:** distended neck veins, distant heart sounds, hypotension; associated with cardiac tamponade.
  Blumberg's sign: transient pain in the abdomen after approximated fingers pressed gently into abdominal wall are suddenly withdrawn—rebound tenderness; associated with peritoneal inflammation.
  Borsieri's sign: when fingernail is drawn along skin in early stages of scarlet fever, a white line is left that quickly turns red.
  Branham's bradycardia: bradycardia and augmentation of both systolic and diastolic arterial pressure after digital closure of an artery proximal to an arteriovenous fistula.
* **Brudzinski's sign:** flexion of the hip and knee induced by flexion of the neck; associated with meningeal irritation.
* **Chadwick's sign:** cyanosis of vaginal and cervical mucosa; associated with pregnancy.
* **Charcot's triad:** nystagmus, intention tremor, staccato speech; associated with multiple sclerosis.
* **Chvostek's sign:** facial muscle spasm induced by tapping on the facial nerve branches; associated with hypocalcemia.
* **Cheyne-Stokes respiration:** rhythmic cycles of deep and shallow respiration, often with apneic periods; associated with central nervous system respiratory center dysfunction.
  Coppernail's sign: ecchymoses on the perineum, scrotum, or labia; associated with fracture of the pelvis.
* **Courvoisier's sign:** an enlarged nontender gallbladder; associated with carcinoma of the head of the pancreas.
* **Cullen's sign:** bluish discoloration of the umbilicus; associated with acute

pancreatitis or hemoperitoneum, especially rupture of fallopian tube in ectopic pregnancy.

* **Doll's eye sign:** dissociation between the movements of the head and eyes: as the head is raised the eyes are lowered, and as the head is lowered the eyes are raised; associated with global-diffuse disorders of the cerebrum.

* **Drawer sign:** supine patient flexes his or her knee and rests foot flat on table, and examiner sits on foot to anchor it; head of tibia is pulled toward the physician to test the anterior cruciate ligament, or pushed away from the physician to test the posterior cruciate ligament; movement of more than 1 cm is indicative of a torn cruciate ligament.

Duroziez's sign: To-and-fro murmur heard on auscultation of the femoral artery; associated with severe aortic regurgitation.

Flag sign: dyspigmentation of the hair occurring as a band of light hair; seen in children who have recovered from kwashiorkor.

* **Fluid wave:** transmission across the abdomen of a wave induced by snapping the abdomen; associated with ascites.

Goldstein's sign: wide distance between the great toe and the adjoining toe; associated with cretinism and trisomy 21.

Gottron's sign: cutaneous lesions consisting of symmetrical macular violaceous erythema, with or without edema, overlying the dorsal aspect of the interphalangeal joints of the hands, olecranon processes, patellas, and medial malleoli; pathognomonic of dermatomyositis.

* **Gowers' sign:** to stand from supine position, patient rolls to the prone position, kneels, and raises himself or herself to a standing position by pushing with the hands against shins, knees, and thighs; associated with pseudohypertrophic muscular dystrophy.

* **Grey Turner's sign:** discoloration of skin of lower abdomen and flanks, caused by massive nontraumatic ecchymoses; associated with hemorrhagic acute pancreatitis.

Grossman's sign: dilatation of the heart; associated with pulmonary tuberculosis.

* **Gunn's pupillary sign (Marcus Gunn pupil):** with patient's eye fixed at a distance and a straight light shining before the intact eye, a crisp bilateral contraction of the pupil is noted. On moving the light to the affected eye, both pupils will dilate for a short period. Then on return of the light to the intact eye, both pupils contract promptly and remain contracted; associated with damage to the optic nerve.

Hamman's sign: crunching sound in the precordium; associated with acute mediastinitis, pneumomediastinum, and pneumothorax.

Harlequin sign: in the newborn infant, reddening of the lower half of the laterally recumbent body and blanching of the upper half, due to a temporary vasomotor disturbance.

Hegar's sign: softening of the fundus of the uterus; associated with the first trimester of pregnancy.

Hoffmann's sign: flexion of the thumb and other fingers, induced by snapping of the index, middle, or ring finger; associated with corticospinal tract disease.

* **Homans's sign:** pain behind the knee, induced by dorsiflexion of the foot; associated with peripheral vascular disease, especially venous thrombosis in the calf.

* **Kehr's sign:** severe pain in the left upper quadrant, radiating to the top of the shoulder; associated with splenic rupture.

* **Kernig's sign:** inability to extend leg when sitting or lying with the thigh flexed on the abdomen; associated with meningeal irritation.

Knie's sign: unequal dilatation of the pupils; associated with Graves's disease.

* **Kussmaul's respiration:** paroxysmal air hunger; associated with acidosis, especially diabetic ketoacidosis.

* **Levine sign:** clenching of the patient's fist over the sternum while describing chest discomfort; associated with angina.

Lhermitte's sign: development of sudden, transient, electriclike shocks spreading down the body when the patient flexes the head forward; associated with multiple sclerosis and cervical cord compression.

Lucas's sign: distention of the abdomen; associated with the early stages of rickets.

Ludloff's sign: sitting patient cannot flex the thigh; associated with avulsion of the lesser trocanter.

Marie's sign: tremor of the body or extremities; associated with Graves's disease.

Markle's sign: tenderness resulting from patient rising up on his or her toes, then suddenly relaxing so that the heels hit the floor and jar the whole body (jar tenderness); abdominal pain on walking is an equivalent test; associated with peritoneal irritation.

Mayne's sign: a diminution of 15 mm Hg in the diastolic pressure in the arm when it is elevated over the head, as compared with values taken when the arm is at heart level; associated with aortic regurgitation.

* **McBurney's sign:** tenderness at McBurney's point (located two-thirds of the distance from the umbilicus to the anterior-superior iliac spine); associated with appendicitis.

McMurray's sign: occurrence of a cartilage click during manipulation of the knee; associated with meniscal injury.

Müller's sign: pulsation of the uvula and redness of the tonsils and velum palati, occurring synchronously with the action of the heart; associated with aortic insufficiency.

* **Murphy's sign:** inspiratory arrest during midcycle of respiration by painful contact with fingers that are held under the liver border, where an inflamed gallbladder may descend upon them; associated with acute cholecystitis.

* **Obdurator sign:** hypogastric or adductor pain elicited by passive internal rotation of the flexed thigh, due to contact between an inflammatory process and the internal obdurator muscle; associated with obdurator nerve irritation, often as a result of appendicitis.

* **Osler's sign:** small painful erythematous swellings in the skin of the hands and feet; associated with bacterial endocarditis.

* **Psoas sign:** pain induced by hyperextension of the right thigh while lying on the left side; associated with appendicitis.

Radovici's sign: vigorous scratching or pricking of the thenar eminence causes a palomental primitive reflex, ipsilateral contraction of the muscles of the chin; associated with corticospinal tract disease, increased intracranial pressure, and latent tetany.

* **Romberg's sign:** unsteadiness or falling down when the eyes are closed and the feet are close together; associated with tabes dorsalis and labyrinthine disorders.

Romberg-Howship sign: pain down the medial aspect of the thigh to the knee due to obdurator nerve compression; associated with obdurator hernias.

* **Setting-sun sign:** downward deviation of the eyes so that each iris appears to "set" beneath the lower lid, with white sclera exposed between it and the upper lid; associated with increased intracranial pressure or irritation of the brainstem.

Siegert's sign: pinky fingers are short and curved inward; associated with trisomy 21.

Sisto's sign: constant inconsolable crying; associated with congenital syphilis in infancy.

Squire's sign: alternate contraction and dilatation of the pupil; associated with basilar meningitis.

Stellwag's sign: infrequent blinking, associated with thyrotoxicosis.

* **Tinel's sign:** tingling sensation felt from light percussion on the radial side of the palmaris longus tendon; associated with carpal tunnel syndrome.

Trendelenburg's sign: the falling of one buttock relative to the other because the muscles are not strong enough to sustain position when the femur is not engaged in the acetabulum; associated with dislocation of the hip.

Weber's sign: paralysis of the oculomotor nerve on one side and hemiplegia of the opposite side; associated with impending uncal herniation.

Westphal's sign: loss of knee jerk; associated with tabes dorsalis.

Whipple's triad: spontaneous hypoglycemia, central nervous or vasomotor system symptoms, relief of symptoms by the oral or intravenous administration of glucose; associated with insulin-producing tumors.

Williamson's sign: markedly diminished blood pressure in the leg as compared with that in the arm on the same side; associated with pneumothorax and pleural effusions.

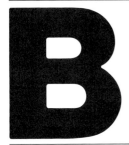

Commonly Used Drugs

Most of the patients you will see on the wards will be taking several medications. This appendix is designed to serve as a quick guide to some of the most common medications you will encounter during your ICM course. Part one lists drugs by their chemical or generic name, and part two is a similar list sorted by trade name. Part three lists drugs by class, giving common indications and their mechanisms of actions where known.

When a patient mentions a drug, look it up on the appropriate list, then turn to its drug class in part three to learn why it is probably being used and how it works. We do not mention here dosages or side effects; this is well covered in other sources (see, for instance, *Handbook of Commonly Prescribed Drugs,* 8th ed., by Digregorio and Babieri [Medical Surveillance, 1992]).

Part One: Drugs by Chemical Name

Chemical name	Trade name	Drug class
Acetazolamide	Diamox	Diuretic
Acetominophen	Datril, Tempra, Tylenol	Nonopioid analgesic
Acyclovir	Zovirax	Antiviral
Albuterol	Proventil, Ventolin	Antiasthmatic
Allopurinol	Zyloprim	Antigout
Alprazolam	Xanax	Antianxiety
Aminophylline	Aminophyllin, Somophyllin	Antiasthmatic
Amitriptyline	Elavil, Endep	Antidepressant
Amoxicillin	Amoxil, Larotid, Polymox	Antibacterial
Amoxicillin/potassium clavulanate	Augmentin	Antibacterial
Amphoterocin B	Fungizone	Antifungal
Ampicillin	Amcill, Omnipen, Principen	Antibacterial
Ampicillin/sulbactam	Unasyn	Antibacterial
Aspirin		Nonopioid analgesic
Atenolol	Tenormin	Antihypertensive
Baclofen	Lioresal	Antispastic
Beclomethasone	Beclovent, Beconase, Vancenase, Vanceril	Antiasthmatic
Bisacodyl	Dulcolax	Laxative
Bretylium	Bretylol	Antiarrhythmic
Bromocriptine	Parlodel	Antiparkinsonian
Bumetanide	Bumex	Diuretic

Chemical name	Trade name	Drug class
Captopril	Capoten	Antihypertensive
Carbamazapine	Tegretol	Anticonvulsant
Carbenicillin	Geopen, Piopen	Antibacterial
Carbidopa/levodopa	Sinemet	Antiparkinsonian
Cefaclor	Ceclor	Antibacterial
Cefazolin	Ancef, Kefzol	Antibacterial
Cefolexin	Keflex	Antibacterial
Cefotaxime	Claforan	Antibacterial
Cefoxitin	Mefoxin	Antibacterial
Ceftazadime	Fortaz	Antibacterial
Ceftriaxone	Rocephin	Antibacterial
Cefuroxime	Zinacef	Antibacterial
Chloral hydrate	Noctec	Sedative
Chloramphenicol	Chloromycetin	Antibacterial
Chlordiazepoxide	Librium	Antianxiety
Chlorpromazine	Thorazine	Antipsychotic
Chlorpropramide	Diabenese	Antidiabetic
Cholestyramine	Questran	Cholesterol lowering
Cimetidine	Tagamet	Antiulcer
Ciprofloxacin	Cipro	Antibacterial
Clindamycin	Cleocin	Antibacterial
Clonazepam	Clonopin	Anticonvulsant
Clonidine	Catapres	Antihypertensive
Clotrimazole	Lotrimin, Mazole	Antifungal
Codeine		Opioid analgesic
Colchicine		Antigout
Cortisone	Deltasone	Steroid
Cromolyn sodium	Intal, Nasalcrom, Opticrom	Antiasthmatic
Dantrolene sodium	Dantrium	Antispastic
Desipramine	Norpramin	Antidepressant
Desmopressin	DDAVP, Stimate	Hormone
Dexamethasone	Decadron	Steroid
Diazepam	Valium	Antianxiety
Dicloxacillin	Dycell, Dynapen	Antibacterial
Digoxin	Lanoxicaps, Lanoxin	Antiarrhythmic
Diltiazem	Cardizem	Antianginal
Diphenhydramine	Benadryl, Benolyn	Antihistamine
Diphenoxylate with atropine	Lomotil	Antidiarrheal
Dipyridamole	Persantin	Anticoagulant
Disulfiram	Antabuse	Antialcohol
Dobutamine	Dobutrex	Inotropic agent
Dopamine	Dopistat, Intopin	Inotropic agent
Doxepin	Atapin, Sinequan	Antidepressant
Ducosate sodium	Colace	Laxative
Enalapril	Vasotec	Antihypertensive
Erythromycin	E-Mycin, Erythrocin, Ilosone	Antibacterial
Esmolol	Brevibloc	Antiarrhythmic
Estrogen	Premarin	Hormone
Famotidine	Pepcid	Antiulcer
Fentanyl	Sublimaze	Opioid analgesic
Fluoxitene	Prozac	Antidepressant
Fluphenazine	Permitil, Prolixin	Antipsychotic
Furosemide	Lasix	Diuretic

Chemical name	Trade name	Drug class
Gemfibrozil	Lopid	Cholesterol lowering
Gentamycin	Garamycin	Antibacterial
Glyburide	Diabeta, Micronase	Antidiabetic
Griseofulvin	Fulvicin, Grifulvin, Grisactin, Gris-PEG	Antifungal
Haloperidol	Haldol	Antipsychotic
Heparin sodium		Anticoagulant
Hydralazine	Apresoline	Antihypertensive
Hydrochlorothiazide	Hydrodiuril	Diuretic
Hydrocortisone	Solu-Cortef	Steroid
Hydromorphone	Dilaudid	Opioid analgesic
Ibuprofen	Advil, Motrin	Nonopioid analgesic
Imipenem/cilastatin	Primaxin	Antibacterial
Imipramine	Tofranil	Antidepressant
Insulin		Hormone
Ipratropium bromide	Atrovent	Antiasthmatic
Isoetharine	Bronkosol	Antiasthmatic
Isoniazid	INH	Antituberculous
Isosorbide dinitrate	Isordil	Antianginal
Ketoconazole	Nizoral	Antifungal
Lactulose	Chronulac	Laxative
Levothyroxine	Synthroid	Hormone
Lidocaine	Xylocaine	Antiarrhythmic
Lisinopril	Prinivil, Zestril	Antihypertensive
Lithium carbonate	Eskalith	Antimanic
Loperamide	Imodium	Antidiarrheal
Lorazepam	Ativan	Antianxiety
Lovastatin	Mevacor	Cholesterol lowering
Medroxyprogesterone	Provera	Hormone
Meperidine	Demerol	Opioid analgesic
Metaproterenol	Alupent, Metaprel	Antiasthmatic
Methadone	Dolophine	Opioid analgesic
Methicillin	Staphcillin	Antibacterial
Methyldopa	Aldomet	Antihypertensive
Methylprednisolone	Depo-Medrol, Solu-Medrol	Steroid
Metronidazole	Flagyl	Antibacterial
Miconazole	Monistat	Antifungal
Midazolam	Versed	Sedative
Minoxidil	Rogaine	Antihypertensive
Morphine		Opioid analgesic
Nadolol	Corgard	Antihypertensive
Naproxen	Naprosyn	Nonopioid analgesic
Niacin	Nicolar	Cholesterol lowering
Nifedipine	Procardia	Antianginal
Nistatin	Micostatin, Nilstat	Antifungal
Nitroglycerin		Antianginal
Nortriptyline	Aventyl	Antidepressant
Oxacillin	Bactocill, Prostaphlin	Antibacterial
Oxazepam	Serax	Antianxiety
Oxycodone	Percocet, Percodan	Opioid analgesic
Oxytocin	Pitocin	Hormone
Pancrelipase	Cotazyme, Pancrease	Hormone
Penicillin G		Antibacterial
Pentamidine	Pentam	Antiprotozoal
Phenobarbital		Anticonvulsant

Chemical name	Trade name	Drug class
Phenytoin	Dilantin	Anticonvulsant
Piperacillin	Pipracil	Antibacterial
Prazosin	Minipress	Antihypertensive
Prednisone		Steroid
Probenecid	Benemid	Antigout
Procainamide	Procan, Pronestyl	Antiarrhythmic
Propranolol	Inderal	Antihypertensive
Propoxyphene	Darvocet, Darvon, Dolene	Opioid analgesic
Quinidine	Quinidex, Quiniglute	Antiarrhythmic
Ranitidine	Zantac	Antiulcer
Rifampin	Rifadin	Antituberculous
Secobarbital	Seconal	Sedative
Spirolonalactone	Aldactone	Diuretic
Streptokinase	Kabikinase, Streptase	Thrombolytic
Streptomycin		Antituberculous
Sucralfate	Carafate	Antiulcer
Tamoxifen	Nolvadex	Hormone
Terfenadine	Seldane	Antihistamine
Tetracycline		Antibacterial
Theophylline	Theo-Dur, Theolair	Antiasthmatic
Thiothixene	Navane	Antipsychotic
Ticarcillin	Ticar	Antibacterial
Timolol	Blocadren, Timoptic	Antihypertensive
Tobramycin	Nebcin	Antibacterial
Tolbutamide	Orinase	Antidiabetic
Triazolam	Halcion	Sedative
Trimethoprim-sulfamethoxazole	Bactrim, Septra	Antibacterial
Urokinase	Abbokinase	Thrombolytic
Valproic acid	Depakene, Depakote	Anticonvulsant
Vancomycin	Vancocin, Vancoled	Antibacterial
Vasopressin	Pitressin	Hormone
Verapamil	Calan, Isoptin	Antiarrhythmic
Vidarabine	Vera-A	Antiviral
Warfarin sodium	Coumadin	Anticoagulant
Ziduvodine	AZT, Retrovir	Antiviral

Part Two: Drugs by Trade Name

Trade name	Chemical name	Drug class
Abbokinase	Urokinase	Thrombolytic
Advil	Ibuprofen	Nonopioid analgesic
Aldactone	Spirolonalactone	Diuretic
Aldomet	Methyldopa	Antihypertensive
Alupent	Metaproterenol	Antiasthmatic
Amcill	Ampicillin	Antibacterial
Aminophyllin	Aminophylline	Antiasthmatic
Amoxil	Amoxicillin	Antibacterial
Ancef	Cefazolin	Antibacterial
Antabuse	Disulfiram	Antialcohol
Apresoline	Hydralazine	Antihypertensive

Trade name	Chemical name	Drug class
Ativan	Lorazepam	Antianxiety
Atrovent	Ipratropium bromide	Antiasthmatic
Augmentin	Amoxicillin/potassium clavulanate	Antibacterial
Aventyl	Nortriptyline	Antidepressant
AZT	Ziduvodine	Antiviral
Bactocill	Oxacillin	Antibacterial
Bactrim	Trimethoprim-sulfamethoxazole	Antibacterial
Beclovent, Beconase	Beclomethasone	Antiasthmatic
Benadryl	Diphenhydramine	Antihistamine
Benemid	Probenecid	Antigout
Blocadren	Timolol	Antihypertensive
Bretylol	Bretylium	Antiarrhythmic
Brevibloc	Esmolol	Antiarrhythmic
Bronkosol	Isoetharine	Antiasthmatic
Bumex	Bumetanide	Diuretic
Calan	Verapamil	Antiarrhythmic
Capoten	Captopril	Antihypertensive
Carafate	Sucralfate	Antiulcer
Cardizem	Diltiazem	Antianginal
Catapres	Clonidine	Antihypertensive
Ceclor	Cefaclor	Antibacterial
Chloromycetin	Chloramphenicol	Antibacterial
Chronulac	Lactulose	Laxative
Cipro	Ciprofloxacin	Antibacterial
Claforan	Cefotaxime	Antibacterial
Cleocin	Clindamycin	Antibacterial
Clonopin	Clonazepam	Anticonvulsant
Colace	Ducosate sodium	Laxative
Corgard	Nadolol	Antihypertensive
Cotazyme	Pancrelipase	Hormone
Coumadin	Warfarin sodium	Anticoagulant
Dantrium	Dantrolene sodium	Antispastic
Darvocet, Darvon	Propoxyphene	Opioid analgesic
Datril	Acetominophen	Nonopioid analgesic
DDAVP	Desmopressin	Hormone
Decadron	Dexamethasone	Steroid
Deltasone	Cortisone	Steroid
Demerol	Meperidine	Opioid analgesic
Depakene	Valproic acid	Anticonvulsant
Depakote	Valproic acid	Anticonvulsant
Depo-Medrol	Methylprednisolone	Steroid
Diabenese	Chlorpropramide	Antidiabetic
Diabeta	Glyburide	Antidiabetic
Diamox	Acetazolamide	Diuretic
Dilantin	Phenytoin	Anticonvulsant
Dilaudid	Hydromorphone	Opioid analgesic
Dobutrex	Dobutamine	Inotropic agent
Dolene	Propoxyphene	Opioid analgesic
Dolophine	Methadone	Opioid analgesic
Dopistat	Dopamine	Inotropic agent
Dulcolax	Bisacodyl	Laxative
Dycell, Dynapen	Dicloxacillin	Antibacterial
E-Mycin	Erythromycin	Antibacterial
Elavil, Endep	Amitriptyline	Antidepressant

Trade name	Chemical name	Drug class
Erythrocin	Erythromycin	Antibacterial
Eskalith	Lithium carbonate	Antimanic
Flagyl	Metronidazole	Antibacterial
Fortaz	Ceftazadime	Antibacterial
Fulvicin	Griseofulvin	Antifungal
Fungizone	Amphoterocin B	Antifungal
Garamycin	Gentamycin	Antibacterial
Geopen	Carbenicillin	Antibacterial
Grifulvin, Grisactin, Gris-PEG	Griseofulvin	Antifungal
Halcion	Triazolam	Sedative
Haldol	Haloperidol	Antipsychotic
Hydrodiuril	Hydrochlorothiazide	Diuretic
Ilosone	Erythromycin	Antibacterial
Imodium	Loperamide	Antidiarrheal
Inderal	Propranolol	Antihypertensive
INH	Isoniazid	Antituberculous
Intal	Cromolyn sodium	Antiasthmatic
Intopin	Dopamine	Inotropic agent
Isoptin	Verapamil	Antiarrhythmic
Isordil	Isosorbide dinitrate	Antianginal
Kabikinase	Streptokinase	Thrombolytic
Keflex	Cefolexin	Antibacterial
Kefzol	Cefazolin	Antibacterial
Lanoxicaps, Lanoxin	Digoxin	Antiarrhythmic, inotropic agent
Larotid	Amoxicillin	Antibacterial
Lasix	Furosemide	Diuretic
Librium	Chlordiazepoxide	Antianxiety
Lioresal	Baclofen	Antispastic
Lomotil	Diphenoxylate with atropine	Antidiarrheal
Lopid	Gemfibrozil	Cholesterol lowering
Lotrimin, Mazole	Clotrimazole	Antifungal
Mefoxin	Cefoxitin	Antibacterial
Metaprel	Metaproterenol	Antiasthmatic
Mevacor	Lovastatin	Cholesterol lowering
Micostatin	Nistatin	Antifungal
Micronase	Glyburide	Antidiabetic
Minipress	Prazosin	Antihypertensive
Monistat	Miconazole	Antifungal
Motrin	Ibuprofen	Nonopioid analgesic
Naprosyn	Naproxen	Nonopioid analgesic
Nasalcrom	Cromolyn sodium	Antiasthmatic
Navane	Thiothixene	Antipsychotic
Nebcin	Tobramycin	Antibacterial
Nicolar	Niacin	Cholesterol lowering
Nilstat	Nistatin	Antifungal
Nizoral	Ketoconazole	Antifungal
Noctec	Chloral hydrate	Sedative
Nolvadex	Tamoxifen	Hormone
Norpramin	Desipramine	Antidepressant
Omnipen	Ampicillin	Antibacterial
Opticrom	Cromolyn sodium	Antiasthmatic
Orinase	Tolbutamide	Antidiabetic
Pancrease	Pancrelipase	Hormone

Trade name	Chemical name	Drug class
Parlodel	Bromocriptine	Antiparkinsonian
Pentam	Pentamidine	Antiprotozoal
Pepcid	Famotidine	Antiulcer
Percocet, Percodan	Oxycodone	Opioid analgesic
Permitil	Fluphenazine	Antipsychotic
Persantin	Dipyridamole	Anticoagulant
Piopen	Carbenicillin	Antibacterial
Pipracil	Piperacillin	Antibacterial
Pitocin	Oxytocin	Hormone
Pitressin	Vasopressin	Hormone
Polymox	Amoxicillin	Antibacterial
Premarin	Estrogen	Hormone
Primaxin	Imipenem/cilastatin	Antibacterial
Principen	Ampicillin	Antibacterial
Prinivil	Lisinopril	Antihypertensive
Procan	Procainamide	Antiarrhythmic
Procardia	Nifedipine	Antianginal
Prolixin	Fluphenazine	Antipsychotic
Pronestyl	Procainamide	Antiarrhythmic
Prostaphlin	Oxacillin	Antibacterial
Proventil	Albuterol	Antiasthmatic
Provera	Medroxyprogesterone	Hormone
Prozac	Fluoxitene	Antidepressant
Questran	Cholestyramine	Cholesterol lowering
Quinidex, Quiniglute	Quinidine	Antiarrhythmic
Retrovir	Ziduvodine	Antiviral
Rifadin	Rifampin	Antituberculous
Rocephin	Ceftriaxone	Antibacterial
Rogaine	Minoxidil	Antihypertensive
Seconal	Secobarbital	Sedative
Seldane	Terfenadine	Antihistamine
Septra	Trimethoprim-sulfamethoxazole	Antibacterial
Serax	Oxazepam	Antianxiety
Sinemet	Carbidopa/levodopa	Antiparkinsonian
Sinequan	Doxepin	Antidepressant
Solu-Cortef	Hydrocortisone	Steroid
Solu-Medrol	Methylprednisolone	Steroid
Somophyllin	Aminophylline	Antiasthmatic
Staphcillin	Methicillin	Antibacterial
Stimate	Desmopressin	Hormone
Streptase	Streptokinase	Thrombolytic
Sublimaze	Fentanyl	Opioid analgesic
Synthroid	Levothyroxine	Hormone
Tagamet	Cimetidine	Antiulcer
Tegretol	Carbamazepine	Anticonvulsant
Tempra	Acetominophen	Nonopioid analgesic
Tenormin	Atenolol	Antihypertensive
Theo-Dur, Theolair	Theophylline	Antiasthmatic
Thorazine	Chlorpromazine	Antipsychotic
Ticar	Ticarcillin	Antibacterial
Timoptic	Timolol	Antihypertensive
Tofranil	Imipramine	Antidepressant
Tylenol	Acetaminophen	Nonopioid analgesic
Unasyn	Ampicillin/sulbactam	Antibacterial
Valium	Diazepam	Antianxiety

Trade name	Chemical name	Drug class
Vancenase, Vanceril	Beclomethasone	Antiasthmatic
Vancocin, Vancoled	Vancomycin	Antibacterial
Vasotec	Enalapril	Antihypertensive
Ventolin	Albuterol	Antiasthmatic
Vera-A	Vidarabine	Antiviral
Versed	Midazolam	Sedative
Xanax	Alprazolam	Antianxiety
Xylocaine	Lidocaine	Antiarrhythmic
Zantac	Ranitidine	Antiulcer
Zestril	Lisinopril	Antihypertensive
Zinacef	Cefuroxime	Antibacterial
Zovirax	Acyclovir	Antiviral
Zyloprim	Allopurinol	Antigout

Part Three: Drug Classes

A. Antialcohol. Indications: used to deter ethanol ingestion.

1. Acetaldehyde dehydrogenase blocker

Disulfiram (Antabuse)

Mechanism: inhibits acetaldehyde dehydrogenase, which leads to buildup of acetaldehyde after consumption of alcohol, causing nausea, vomiting, and headache.

B. Antianginal. Indications: to relieve angina pectoris (effort-induced or coronary artery spasm).

1. Calcium channel blockers

Diltiazem (Cardizem)
Nifedipine (Procardia)

Mechanism: reduces muscle contractility by blocking voltage-dependent calcium channels and thus decreasing intracellular calcium concentration.

2. Nitrates

Nitroglycerin
Isosorbide dinitrate (Isordil)

Mechanism: releases nitric oxide in smooth muscle, increasing cGMP, leading to smooth muscle relaxation.

C. Antianxiety

1. Benzodiazepines

Alprazolam (Xanax)
Chlordiazepoxide (Librium)
Diazepam (Valium)
Lorazepam (Ativan)
Oxazepam (Serax)

Mechanism: acts at a specific benzodiazepine receptor that is part of the GABA receptor–chloride ion channel complex found in many brain regions. Binding of benzodiazepines appears to facilitate inhibitory effects of GABA and glycine.

D. Antiarrhythmic. Indications: for treating abnormal cardiac rhythms (see Chap. 10).

1. Class I

Procainamide (Procan, Pronestyl)
Quinidine (Quinidex, Quiniglute)
Lidocaine (Xylocaine)

Mechanism: sodium channel blocker. Lidocaine is also frequently used as a local anesthetic.

2. Class II

Esmolol (Brevibloc)

Mechanism: beta-adrenergic receptor blocker—suppresses abnormal pacemakers.

3. Class III

Bretylium (Bretylol)

Mechanism: potassium channel blocker—prolongs the action potential and increases refractory period.

4 Class IV

Verapamil (Calan, Isoptin)

Mechanism: calcium channel blocker—most effective in arrhythmias that involve calcium-dependent cardiac tissue, such as the atrioventricular node.

5. Cardiac glycosides

Digoxin (Lanoxicaps, Lanoxin)

Mechanism: inhibits $Na^+ K^+$ ATPase of cell membrane, which increases intracellular sodium as well as calcium. Used in treating atrial fibrillation and also as a positive inotropic agent in cardiac failure.

E. Antiasthmatics. Indication: for the treatment of bronchial asthma

1. Inhaled corticosteroids

Beclomethasone (Beclovent, Beconase, Vancenase, Vanceril)

Mechanism: decreases inflammation of airways, perhaps by blocking synthesis of arachadonic acid by phospholipase A2. Also used in severe asthma are systemic corticosteroids.

2. Beta agonists

Albuterol (Proventil, Ventolin)
Isoetharine (Bronkosol)
Metaproterenol (Alupent, Metaprel)

Mechanism: increases cAMP in smooth muscle cells, inducing muscle relaxation and bronchodilation.

3. Methylxanthines

Aminophylline (Aminophyllin, Somophyllin)
Theophylline (Theo-Dur, Theolair)

Mechanism: causes bronchodilation, perhaps by inhibiting phosphodiesterase.

4. Cromolyn

Cromolyn sodium (Intal, Nasalcrom, Opticrom)

Mechanism: decreases the release of mediators such as histamines and leukotrienes from mast cells. Used more for prophylaxis than for treatment of asthma attacks.

5. Muscarinic antagonists

Ipratropium bromide (Atrovent)

Mechanism: blocks muscarinic acetylcholine receptors, preventing bronchoconstriction.

F. Antibacterial

1. Cell wall inhibitors

a. Penicillins

(1) Limited spectrum

Penicillin G

(2) Broader spectrum

Amoxicillin (Amoxil, Larotid, Polymox)
Ampicillin (Amcill, Omnipen, Principen)
Carbenicillin (Geopen, Piopen)
Piperacillin (Pipracil)
Ticarcillin (Ticar)

(3) Beta-lactamase resistant

Dicloxacillin (Dycell, Dynapen)
Methicillin (Staphcillin)
Oxacillin (Bactocill, Prostaphlin)

(4) Combinations

Amoxicillin/potassium clavulanate (Augmentin)
Ampicillin/sulbactam (Unasyn)

b. Cephalosporins

(1) First generation: against gram-positive *E. coli*

Cefalexin (Keflex)
Cefazolin (Ancef, Kefzol)

(2) Second generation: more gram negative

Cefaclor (Ceclor)
Cefoxitin (Mefoxin)
Cefuroxime (Zinacef)

(3) Third generation: crosses blood-brain barrier

Cefotaxime (Claforan)
Ceftazadime (Fortaz)
Ceftriaxone (Rocephin)

Mechanism: inhibits cell wall synthesis by preventing cross-linking of peptidoglycan chains.

2. Protein synthesis inhibitors

a. Aminoglycosides

Gentamycin (Garamycin)
Tobramycin (Nebcin)

Mechanism: binds to 30S ribosomal unit of bacteria, preventing the formation of an initiation complex. Ototoxicity and nephrotoxicity are dangerous side effects.

Chloramphenicol (Chloromycetin)

Mechanism: binds to 50S ribosomal unit of bacteria and inhibits peptidyltransferase.

Tetracycline

Mechanism: binds to 30S subunit of bacterial ribosomes, preventing the binding of aminoacyl tRNA to the ribosome.

3. Other commonly used antibacterials

Ciprofloxacin (Cipro): inhibits DNA gyrase.
Clindamycin (Cleocin): inhibits protein synthesis.
Erythromycin (E-Mycin, Erythrocin, Ilosone): binds to ribosomal sub-unit to prevent translocation.
Imipenem/cilastatin (Primaxin): inhibits cell wall synthesis.
Metronidazole (Flagyl): interferes with DNA synthesis; also antipro-tozoal.
Trimethoprim-sulfamethoxazole (Bactrim, Septra): inhibits folic acid synthesis.
Vancomycin (Vancocin, Vancoled): inhibits cell wall synthesis.

G. Anticoagulant. Indications: prevention and treatment of venous thrombo-ses, pulmonary emboli, acute arterial occlusions; prevention of emboli and occlusion in atrial fibrillation, atherosclerotic disease.

Dipyridamole (Persantin): decreases platelet aggregation.
Heparin sodium: binds to antithrombin III and blocks conversion of pre-thrombin to thrombin.
Warfarin sodium (Coumadin): inhibits vitamin K–dependent clotting fac-tors (2, 7, 9, 10).

H. Anticonvulsant. Indications: to stop the spread of aberrant electrical activ-ity in the brain.

Carbamazapine (Tegretol): for seizures refractory to other meds; blocks sodium channels.
Clonazepam (Clonopin): for petit mal, akinetic, myoclonic seizures; acts at benzodiazepine receptor.
Phenobarbital: used most commonly for children; barbiturate.
Phenytoin (Dilantin): for grand mal, myoclonic seizures; blocks sodium channels.
Valproic acid (Depakene, Depakote): for absence seizures; mechanism un-known.

I. Antidepressant

1. Tricyclics

Amitriptyline (Elavil, Endep)
Desipramine (Norpramin)
Doxepin (Atapin, Sinequan)
Imipramine (Tofranil)
Nortriptyline (Aventyl)

Mechanism: acutely inhibits reuptake of norepinephrine in the brain; however, the relationship of this mechanism to the clinical effect of the drug is not clear.

2. Serotonin reuptake inhibitors

Fluoxitene (Prozac)

Mechanism: acutely inhibits reuptake of serotonin (5-HT) in the brain; however, the relationship of this mechanism to the clinical effect of the drug is not clear.

J. Antidiabetic. Indications: for type II diabetes (non–insulin dependent).

Chlorpropramide (Diabenese)
Glyburide (Diabeta, Micronase)
Tolbutamide (Orinase)

Mechanism: these drugs, called sulfonylureas, stimulate the release of endogenous insulin from the pancreas. They may reduce glucagon release and increase the number of peripheral insulin receptors.

K. Antidiarrheal. Indications: for the symptomatic relief of nonbloody diarrhea.

Diphenoxylate with atropine (Lomotil)
Loperamide (Imodium)

Mechanism: mild narcotics that slow intestinal transit time.

L. Antifungal

1. Drugs for systemic mycoses

Amphotericin B (Fungizone): binds to ergosterol to change permeability of fungal membrane.
Ketoconazole (Nizoral): inhibits demethylation of lanosterol, decreasing ergosterol formation.

2. Drugs for superficial infections

Clotrimazole (Lotrimin, Mazole)
Griseofulvin (Fulvicin, Grifulvin, Grisactin): interferes with microtubule function.
Miconazole (Monistat)
Nistatin (Micostatin, Nilstat): binds to ergosterol.

M. Antigout

Allopurinol (Zyloprim): inhibits xanthine oxidase to reduce the conversion of purines to uric acid.
Colchicine: inhibits microtubule assembly, thus inhibiting leukocyte migration and reducing inflammation.
Probenecid (Benemid): accelerates renal excretion of uric acid by competing for reabsorption in the renal tubule.

N. Antihistamine. Indications: differ for each drug.

Diphenhydramine (Benadryl, Benolyn): for allergic reactions; sedation and treatment of extrapyramidal reactions.
Terfenadine (Seldane): for allergic rhinitis (nonsedating).

Mechanism: blockade of histamine receptors.

O. Antihypertensive

1. Angiotensin-converting enzyme inhibitors

Captopril (Capoten)
Enalapril (Vasotec)
Lisinopril (Prinivil, Zestril)

2. Beta-adrenergic receptor blockers

Atenolol (Tenormin)
Nadolol (Corgard)
Propranolol (Inderal)
Timolol (Blocadren, Timoptic)

3. Alpha-2 adrenergic agonists

Clonidine (Catapres)
Methyldopa (Aldomet)

4. Alpha-1 adrenergic blockers

Prazosin (Minipress)

5. Vasodilators

Hydralazine (Apresoline)
Minoxidil (Rogaine): also used against baldness.

P. Antimanic

Lithium carbonate (Eskalith)

Mechanism: affects generation of phosphoinositides as second messengers, but actual mechanism of action is unknown.

Q. Antiparkinsonian. Indications: ameliorates the symptoms of Parkinson's disease.

Bromocriptine (Parlodel): partial dopamine-receptor agonist.
Carbidopa/levodopa (Sinemet): levodopa is a dopamine precursor; carbidopa inhibits its activation in the periphery so that more can be activated in the brain.

R. Antiprotozoal. Indications: mainly used for *Pneumocystitis carinii*, also trypanosomiasis.

Pentamidine (Pentam)

Mechanism: unknown.

S. Antipsychotic. Indications: for relief of psychosis seen in many disorders, including schizophrenia, mania.

Chlorpromazine (Thorazine)
Fluphenazine (Permitil, Prolixin)
Haloperidol (Haldol)
Thiothixene (Navane)

Mechanism: the drugs block dopamine receptors in the CNS, but the relationship between this and the clinical effects of the medications is unclear.

T. Antispastic. Indications: used in disorders with high skeletal muscle activity, such as cerebral palsy, multiple sclerosis, stroke.

Baclofen (Lioresal): inhibits muscle firing by acting at the GABA-B receptor in the spinal cord.
Dantrolene sodium (Dantrium): reduces release of calcium from sarcoplasmic reticulum of skeletal muscle cells.

U. Antituberculous. Indication: for the treatment and secondary prevention of tuberculosis. Usually given in combination to prevent drug resistance.

Isoniazid (INH): inhibits cell wall synthesis.
Rifampin (Rifadin): inhibits DNA-dependent RNA polymerase.
Streptomycin: protein synthesis inhibitor.

V. Antiulcer. Indications: for the treatment of peptic ulcer disease.

1. H2 blockers

Cimetidine (Tagamet)
Famotidine (Pepcid)
Ranitidine (Zantac)

Mechanism: reduces acid secretion by blocking H2 (histamine) receptors in parietal cells.

2. Protective

Sucralfate (Carafate)

Mechanism: increases the tissue's resistance to acid.

W. Antiviral

Acyclovir (Zovirax): for herpes viruses (e.g., HSV, EBV, VZV); a purine analog—blocks DNA synthesis.
Vidarabine (Vera-A): for herpes simplex encephalitis; a purine analog—blocks DNA synthesis.
Ziduvodine (AZT, Retrovir): for HIV; inhibits reverse transcriptase.

X. Cholesterol lowering. Indications: for the lowering of serum cholesterol, usually to decrease the risk of atherosclerotic disease.

Cholestyramine (Questran): binds bile acids in intestine.
Gemfibrozil (Lopid): increases lipoprotein clearance.
Lovastatin (Mevacor): inhibits HMG-CoA reductase, decreasing cholesterol synthesis.
Niacin (Nicolar): reduces VLDL secretion.

Y. Diuretics. Indications: to increase renal excretion of fluid, in situations such as edema, CHF, hypertension.

1. Carbonic anhydrase inhibitors

Acetazolamide (Diamox)

2. Loop diuretics

Bumetanide (Bumex)
Furosemide (Lasix)

Mechanism: inhibits Na-K-Cl transport in loop of Henle.

3. Thiazides

Hydrochlorothiazide (Hydrodiuril)

Mechanism: inhibits NaCl transport in early distal convoluted tubule.

4. Potassium-sparing diuretics

Spirolonalactone (Aldactone)

Mechanism: inhibits aldosterone in collecting tubule.

Z. Hormones. Indications vary for each drug.

Desmopressin (DDAVP, Stimate): for diabetes insipidus, bleeding due to some hereditary coagulation defects, bed-wetting.
Estrogen (Premarin): for postmenopausal hormone replacement, contraception.
Insulin: for diabetes mellitus.
Levothyroxine (Synthroid): hypothyroid states.
Medroxyprogesterone (Provera): for secondary amenorrhea, abnormal uterine bleeding.
Oxytocin (Pitocin): for induction of labor.
Pancrelipase (Pancrease, Cotazyme): for replacement of digestive hormones (e.g., in cystic fibrosis).
Tamoxifen (Nolvadex): for adjuvant treatment of breast cancer.
Vasopressin (Pitressin): for diabetes insipidus; local treatment of GI bleeding.

Mechanism: synthetic or natural substance that acts on hormone receptors.

AA. Inotropic agents. Indications: for patients with decreased cardiac contractility; used to increase organ perfusion.

Dobutamine (Dobutrex)
Dopamine (Intopin, Dopistat)

Mechanism: stimulates beta receptors in myocardium.

BB. Laxatives. Indications: for constipation, to increase passage of stool.

Ducosate sodium (Colace)
Lactulose (Chronulac)
Bisacodyl (Dulcolax)

CC. Nonopioid analgesics. Indications: for relief of pain, swelling, fever. Some also called NSAIDs (Nonsteroidal anti-inflammatory drugs). Aspirin used as antiplatelet drug as well.

Acetominophen (Datril, Tempra, Tylenol)
Aspirin
Ibuprofen (Advil, Motrin)
Naproxen (Naprosyn)

Mechanism: inhibits cyclooxygenase, slowing the conversion of arachidonic acid to various prostaglandins and thromboxane.

DD. Opioid analgesics. Indications: mainly used to relieve pain; other uses include sedation, cough suppression, and treatment of diarrhea.

Codeine
Fentanyl (Sublimaze)
Hydromorphone (Dilaudid)
Meperidine (Demerol)
Methadone (Dolophine)
Morphine
Oxycodone (Percocet, Percodan)
Propoxyphene (Darvocet, Darvon, Dolene)

Mechanism: acts on specific opioid receptors in the CNS and periphery.

EE. Sedatives

Chloral hydrate (Noctec)
Midazolam (Versed)
Secobarbital (Seconal)
Triazolam (Halcion)

Mechanism: unclear for most drugs in this category. Benzodiazepines (Midozalam, Triazolam) act at specific receptors in the CNS to facilitate the inhibitory actions of GABA.

FF. Steroids. Indications: antiinflammatory drugs used in a wide variety of conditions, including arthritis, gout, asthma, allergic conditions, and collagen-vascular diseases.

Dexamethasone (Decadron)
Prednisone
Cortisone (Deltasone)
Hydrocortisone (Solu-Cortef)
Methylprednisolone (Depo-Medrol, Solu-Medrol)

Mechanism: acts at steroid receptors in the nucleus of cells to alter gene expression.

GG. Thrombolytics. Indications: acute arterial and venous thrombosis, acute MI.

Streptokinase (Streptase, Kabikinase)
Urokinase (Abbokinase)

Mechanism: degrades fibrin by activating plasminogen to plasmin.

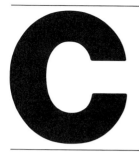

Normal Laboratory Values

These are reference values for some of the most common laboratory tests you will encounter during your first months on the wards. Many of these values will vary slightly by hospital; these are the ones used at the Barnes Hospital in St. Louis. It is best to check with your hospital lab for its range of normal before deciding a test result is abnormal.

Values for each test are for adults, given in the units most commonly used in American hospitals. Many other areas in the world use SI (Systeme International) units; a complete list of normal values in SI units, as well as multiplication factors for converting between the two systems, can be found in the Washington University *Manual of Medical Therapeutics* [28]. Normal hematologic test values can be found in Chap. 7.

Test	Reference value
Albumin	3.6–5.0 gm/dl
Alkaline phosphatase[a]	38–126 IU/L
Aminotransferases	
Alanine (ALT, SGPT)	7–53 IU/L
Aspartate (AST, SGOT)	11–47 IU/L
Ammonia (plasma)	19–43 μmol/L
Amylase	35–118 IU/L
Bilirubin	
Total	0.2–1.3 mg/dl
Direct	0–0.2 mg/dl
Blood gases (arterial, whole blood)	
pH	7.35–7.45
PO_2	80–105 mm Hg
PCO_2	35–45 mm Hg
Calcium	
Total	8.9–10.3 mg/dl
Free	4.6–5.1 mg/dl
CO_2 content (plasma)	22–31 mmol/L
Chloride	97–110 mmol/L
Cholesterol, total[b]	
Desirable	<200 mg/dl
Borderline high	200–239 mg/dl
High	>240 mg/dl
Complement	
C3	77–156 mg/dl
C4	15–39 mg/dl
Copper	70–155 μg/dl
Creatine kinase (CK)	
Male	30–220 IU/L
Female	20–170 IU/L
MB fraction	0–12 IU/L
Creatinine[c]	0.5–1.7 mg/dl

Test	Reference value
Ferritin	
Male	36–262 ng/ml
Female	10–155 ng/ml
Fibrinogen	150–360 mg/dl
Folate (serum)	1.7–12.6 ng/ml
Glucose (fasting, plasma)	65–110 mg/dl
Glycated hemoglobin	4.4–6.3%
Haptoglobin	44–303 mg/dl
HDL cholesterol[c]	27–98 mg/dl
Immunoglobulins	
IgA	91–518 mg/dl
IgM	61–355 mg/dl
IgG	805–1830 mg/dl
Iron	
Total	50–175 μg/dl
Binding capacity	250–450 μg/dl
Transferrin saturation	20–50%
Lactate (plasma)	0.3–1.3 mmol/L
Lactate dehydrogenase (LDH)	90–280 IU/L
Lipase	2.3–20 IU/L
Magnesium	1.3–2.2 mEq/L
Osmolality	270–290 mOsm/kg
Phosphate	2.5–4.5 mg/dl
Potassium (plasma)	3.3–4.9 mmol/L
Protein (total)	6.5–8.5 gm/dl
Sodium	135–145 mmol/L
Thyroid function tests	
TSH	0.45–6.20 μU/ml
T4 (total)	3.0–12.0 μg/dl
T3	80–200 ng/dl
Free thyroxine	1.0–2.3 ng/dl
Triglycerides (fasting)	<250 mg/dl
Urea Nitrogen (BUN)	8–25 mg/dl
Uric acid[b]	3.0–8.0 mg/dl
Vitamin B_{12}	200–800 pg/ml

Notes:
a. Higher values can be normal in people <20 years old.
b. See Chap. 8 for further discussion.
c. Variation occurs by age and sex. These values take into account both sexes, >5 years old.

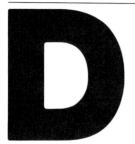

The Essential Clinical Library

As a medical student, you are faced with a bewildering choice of books that can help you as you begin work on the wards. You may have a tendency either to buy no books at all or to buy every text that looks like it might be useful. Following is a list of books we have found to be particularly useful—to own or to borrow; more information about the authors and publishers can be found in the References, which follow.

I. **Medical dictionary.** A good medical dictionary is essential for looking up new terms you come across on the wards. We recommend *Dorland's Illustrated Medical Dictionary,* which has especially good sections on physical signs and medical etymology.

II. **Major medical textbooks.** Although these are expensive, every student should own at least one to use as a reference.

    A. *Cecil's Essentials of Medicine* [2] is probably the best introductory text; it is well organized, eminently readable, and easy to digest.

    B. *Harrison's* [27] still sets the standard for comprehensive medical textbooks. You will learn to appreciate it more and more as you gain clinical experience. While the book is best used as a reference, the introductory chapters are worth reading in their entirety.

III. **Brief summaries and overviews.** These books provide good introductions and reviews. Keep them in your locker for those times when you need a 5-minute consult before presenting a patient or starting your reading on a particular topic.

    A. *Medicine* [13] is a highly readable, pathophysiology-oriented summary of the diagnosis and treatment of the most common diseases. It is well worth reading in your first few weeks on the wards.

    B. The *Merck Manual* [20] is a concise treatment of common diseases. It is less complete than *Harrison's,* but more complete than *Medicine.*

IV. **Books to carry on the wards**

    A. Washington University *Manual of Medical Therapeutics* [28] is an up-to-date summary of medical treatments pitched at the level of a medical student or intern. If you carry only one book with you, this should be it.

    B. *Problem-Oriented Medical Diagnosis* [14] is a handy guide to the work-ups of the most common medical problems, with good lists of differential diagnoses and diagnostic algorithms.

    C. *Manual of Clinical Problems in Internal Medicine* [23]. Reading the pertinent sections of this book just before you present your case on rounds will give you an idea of the current issues and controversies in diagnosis and management.

V. History and physical exam

A. *The Clinical Encounter* by Billings and Stoeckle [5] is an excellent treatment of patient interviewing techniques, especially for difficult subjects like the sexual history.

B. Bates [4], is probably the best physical diagnosis text for the novice. It has many excellent diagrams and pictures. Many students choose to borrow rather than purchase it, because it is useful for only a few months.

C. DeGowin and DeGowin, *Bedside Diagnostic Examination,* 5th ed. (New York: McGraw-Hill, 1987) is complete and authoritative, but many parts are too detailed for the second-year student.

D. *Clinical Diagnosis,* by Judge et al. [17], is less well known, but it offers a very good, complete treatment of the physical exam, with excellent illustrations.

VI. Clinical laboratory

A. Serum chemistry and hematology. Wallach's *Interpretation of Diagnostic Tests* [25] contains reasonably complete lists of most serum chemistry and hematology results. This book is perhaps too complete to be really useful for a second- or third-year student, but it can be helpful when constructing differential diagnoses of lab abnormalities.

B. ECG interpretation

    1. Dubin [10] is a simple and straightforward approach to ECGs. Try to borrow rather than buy this, as you will absorb it in a few evenings.

    2. Mudge [21] has the best collection of abnormal ECGs of any introductory text. The unknowns are particularly helpful.

C. Radiology. Squire [24] is the classic introductory text for diagnostic radiology, and every student should read it.

VII. Other texts

A. Lilly [19] is a good treatment of pathophysiology of the heart, written by medical students for medical students.

B. Weinberger [26] is an extremely well organized discussion of pulmonary diseases. A model for good writing.

C. *Cope's Early Diagnosis of the Acute Abdomen* [22] is the classic text on clinical evaluation of tender bellies.

D. *Clinical Neurology,* 2nd ed., by Greenburg, Aminoff, and Simon (Norwalk, Conn.: Appleton and Lange, 1993) contains a great treatment of cranial nerves and neural pathways.

E. *Surgical Secrets* [1] and *Medical Secrets* [29] present the basic material you will be expected to know on the wards, in question-and-answer format. Great for preparing for rounds.

References

1. Abernathy, C. M., Harken, A. H., *Surgical Secrets* (2nd ed). Philadelphia: Hanley and Belfus, 1991.
2. Andreoli, T. E., et al., *Cecil's Essentials of Medicine* (3rd ed). Philadelphia: Saunders, 1993.
3. Aronson, M. D., Delbance, T. L., *Manual of Clinical Evaluation*. Boston: Little, Brown, 1988.
4. Bates, B., *A Guide to Physical Examination and History Taking* (5th ed). Philadelphia: Lippincott, 1991.
5. Billings, J. A., Stoeckle, J. D., *The Clinical Encounter: A Guide to the Medical Interview and Case Presentation*. Chicago: Yearbook, 1989.
6. Broze, G., "The Role of Tissue Factor Pathway Inhibitor in a Revised Coagulation Cascade," *Seminars in Hematology,* 29(3): 159–69, 1992.
7. Carleton, R. A., et al., "Report of the Expert Panel on Population Strategies for Blood Cholesterol Reduction: A Statement by the National Cholesterol Education Program," *Circulation* 83(6): 2154–232, 1991.
8. Chopra, S., May, R. J., *Pathophysiology of Gastrointestinal Diseases*. Boston: Little, Brown, 1989.
9. Curran, J. W., et al., "Epidemiology of HIV Infection and AIDS in the U.S.," *Science* 239 (Feb. 2): 610–16, 1988.
10. Dubin, D., *Rapid Interpretation of EKGs: A Programmed Course* (4th ed). Tampa, Fla.: Cover Publishing, 1992.
11. Durbridge, T. C., et al., "An Evaluation of Multiphasic Screening on Admission to Hospital," *Medical Journal of Australia,* 1:703, 1976.
12. Ferri, F. F., *Practical Guide to the Care of the Medical Patient* (2nd ed). Chicago: Mosby Yearbook, 1991.
13. Fishman, M. C., et al., *Medicine* (3rd ed). Philadelphia: Lippincott, 1991.
14. Friedman, H. H., *Problem-Oriented Medical Diagnosis* (5th ed). Boston: Little, Brown, 1991.
15. Gomella, L. G., *Clinician's Pocket Reference* (7th ed). Norwalk, Conn.: Appleton and Lange, 1993.
16. Jandl, J. H., *Blood: Pathophysiology*. Boston: Blackwell Scientific, 1991.
17. Judge, R. D., Zuidema, G. D., Fitzgerald, F. T., *Clinical Diagnosis* (5th ed). Boston: Little, Brown, 1989.
18. Katzung, B. G., *Basic and Clinical Pharmacology* (5th ed). Norwalk, Conn.: Appleton and Lange, 1992.
19. Lilly, L. S., *Pathophysiology of Heart Disease*. Philadelphia: Lea and Febiger, 1993.
20. *Merck Manual of Diagnosis and Therapy* (16th ed). Rahway, N.J.: Merck Research Labs, 1992.
21. Mudge, G., *Manual of Electrocardiography* (2nd ed). Boston: Little, Brown, 1986.
22. Silen, W., *Cope's Early Diagnosis of the Acute Abdomen* (18th ed). New York: Oxford University Press, 1991.
23. Spivak, J. L., Barnes, H. V., *Manual of Clinical Problems in Internal Medicine*. Boston: Little, Brown, 1990.
24. Squire, L., Novelline, R. A., *Fundamentals of Radiology* (4th ed). Cambridge, Mass.: Harvard University Press, 1988.

25. Wallach, J., *Interpretation of Diagnostic Tests: A Synopsis of Laboratory Medicine* (5th ed). Boston: Little, Brown, 1992.
26. Weinberger, S. E., *Principles of Pulmonary Medicine* (2nd ed). Philadelphia: Saunders, 1992.
27. Wilson, J. D., et al., *Harrison's Principles of Internal Medicine* (12th ed). New York: McGraw-Hill, 1991.
28. Woodley, M., Whelen, A., *Manual of Medical Therapeutics* (27th ed). Boston: Little, Brown, 1992.
29. Zollo, A. J., *Medical Secrets*. Philadelphia: Hanley and Belfus, 1991.

Index

Index